HEALTH &
SUFFERING
in AMERICA

HEALTH & SUFFERING in AMERICA

The Context and Content of Mental Health Care

With a new introduction by the author
Robert T. Fancher

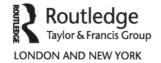

Routledge
Taylor & Francis Group

LONDON AND NEW YORK

Originally published in 1995 by W. H. Freeman and Company

Published 2003 by Transaction Publishers

Published 2017 by Routledge
4 Park Square, Milton Park, Abingdon, Oxon OX14 4RN
605 Third Avenue, New York, NY 10017

Routledge is an imprint of the Taylor & Francis Group, an informa business

Library of Congress Catalog Number: 2003040299

Library of Congress Cataloging-in-Publication Data
Fancher, Robert T.
    Health and suffering in America: the context and content of mental health care / Robert T. Fancher.
        p. cm.
    Rev. ed. of an earlier ed. published under the title: Cultures of healing.
    Includes bibliographical references and index.
    ISBN 0-7658-0544-8 (pbk. : alk. paper)
    1. Psychiatry—United States—Philosophy. 2. Cultural psychiatry.
    3. Psychotherapy—Social aspects. 4. Mental health services. 5. Healing.
    6. Suffering. I. Fancher, Robert T. Cultures of healing. II. Title: Cultures of healing. III. Title.

RC437.5.F337 2003
616.89'001—dc21   2003040299

ISBN-13: 978-0-7658-0544-7 (pbk)

FOR RON CHERNOW
AND THE MEMORY OF GAY MCRAINEY,
AND FOR MY PARENTS,
EWILDA AND JAMES FANCHER

CONTENTS

TRANSACTION INTRODUCTION

Around the time *Health and Suffering in America** first appeared, several like-minded critiques of mental health care sounded similar concerns—Phillip Cushman's magisterial *Constructing the Self, Constructing America*, Robin Dawes's devilishly clever *House of Cards*, and Paula Caplan's righteously (and rightly) indignant *They Say You're Crazy*, for instance. Despite generally fine reviews by heavyweight writers in prestigious venues, these books, taken together, have had about zero influence.

Maybe we were all wrong.

Or maybe the time just isn't quite right for our voices to make much difference.

Whatever else has happened in mental health care in recent years, this much is sure: The rise of managed health care coalesced with an insistence on "parity" for mental health problems—a legal requirement that mental health treatment be paid for just like physical health problems. As with so many well-intentioned proposals, "parity" had unintended, highly dubious effects.

To start with, justifying "parity" requires heightening, not lessening, mental health professionals' pretense to scientific surety. We would be extremely foolish to think that mental health professionals would say, "Now that we have parity, we can admit that most of what we've claimed about ourselves is false."

Furthermore, insurance parity offers a pot of gold to mental health professionals—a huge market of patients who could (or would) never have paid for care out of their own pockets. While some therapists rail against managed care—mostly those who already have successful private practices, or those who wish to practice without having to answer to those who purchase their services—more compete to get insurance money.

---

* Under its original title, *Cultures of Healing: Correcting the Image of American Mental Health Care*.

To survive financially, insurance companies have narrowed their definitions of mental illness and acceptable treatment. Who can blame them? A patient who goes to insight-oriented therapy twice a week at $125 a pop spends $12,500 in a year, while paying nothing close to that in insurance premiums. However, the expense of sending a patient to a dozen or so sessions of cognitive-behavioral therapy, and giving that patient an adjunctive prescription for medication, is more than covered by the insurance premiums he or she (or the employer, more likely) pays on the patient's behalf.

Thus, you can now get insurance coverage mostly for "Axis I" disorders—mostly things like depression and anxiety—and you mostly get a variety of short-term treatments or drugs. You get little or no coverage for "Axis II" disorders, though historically those have been most frequently diagnosed. Miraculously, in a few short years Axis II disorders have virtually disappeared from most official diagnoses. Long-term depth analysis is rarely covered, though until recently it was the treatment of choice.

To justify these changes, insurance companies and the therapists who profit from them make the strongest possible rationalizations that really, after all, the quick and cheap way is the best way. That creates a whole new "culture of healing" dedicated to "scientific" studies proving what they already believe. Rather than admitting the limited scientific basis of mental health care, and looking for broader, more inclusive ways of understanding suffering, we have seen a rise in studies that rationalize limiting the expense of care.

My purpose isn't to say that mental health care is any worse than it was a decade ago. I'm not sure that's true, and I am most certainly not going to say that some golden age of good mental health care has been corrupted! My point is different: The mental health professions' changes are not what they seem, and the assertions that justify them are mostly functions of "cultures of healing," not truth.

I offer here just one example. One of the strangest developments has been insurance companies and mental health professionals treating studies of clinical effectiveness as if they were science. In all of health care, the distinction between science—which seeks to understand and explain what is real and how it works—and clinical studies—which simply tell us whether certain procedures accomplish certain things, without pretending to show how or why—is commonplace. In the current climate of competition for mental health dollars, various cultures of healing have begun treating as science what everyone has always known is obviously not science.

As if that were not enough, only double-blind, randomized clinical trials get baptized with the name of science. That is surely singular: In every other field of inquiry, method must fit the subject of study. By the fiat pronouncement that only double-blind, randomized clinical trials are science, thousands of studies carefully crafted to fit their subject matter, some actually intended as science, get ruled out of court *a priori*—and any subject that cannot be studied in a randomized double-blind manner is banished forever from investigation.

Still, though the level of pretense in mental health care has increased, in one specific sense leaders and professional organizations in the mental health establishments now agree with us critics, if only up to a point. Everyone now that says that mental health care *has been* unscientific.

Psychiatrists generally hold that only since the dethroning of psychoanalysis, the advent of biological psychiatry, and the development of DSM-IV has psychiatry become scientific. Meanwhile, the poor psychoanalysts, so out of fashion, have now, somehow, decided that psychoanalysis was always art, not science. Psychologists generally hold that only since cognitive-behavioral psychotherapy developed has psychology been put on a sound basis. Social workers, trying to portray themselves as more than the poor relations of the doctors, have become advocates for social justice, not practitioners of scientific treatment, often adopting "postmodern" claims that science isn't all that great, anyway.

Each of these arguments implies a main point of *Health and Suffering in America*—that the mental health professions won their status and authority through false claims of scientific surety.

But such admissions have provoked precious little humility and self-examination. You might think it obvious that they should—for instance, asking whether the mental health professions should still be accorded the status and privileges they won falsely, or whether we need to change what we expect of—and allow to—those professions. But they don't.

Such lack of self-criticism follows from a commonplace of contemporary cultures of healing: *Now we* are *really* scientific! The new age has arrived! The old claims were wrong, but since our claims are correct, there is nothing to reexamine. Finally, *we* are fulfilling the promise of the mental health professions. Finally, *we* deserve what our predecessors worked so hard to achieve—in fact, we deserve even more status and authority than we've already gained.

So they say.

In truth, the last decade or so has seen an explosion of extraordinary developments in the sciences of the mind, and no one who values sound knowledge should fail to be grateful and excited. But those developments—which have taken place mostly outside the clinical mental health disciplines, anyway, in neurology, general psychology, and cognitive science—simply have not yet resulted in much understanding of psychopathology. Someday, no doubt, they will. For now, they raise more questions than they answer—and they disprove many common claims of mental health professionals.

For instance, the critique I offer here of cognitive-behavioral therapy has been strengthened by recent research, even as mental health types claim that "science"—their clinical studies—has shown "CBT," as they call it, to be sound.

The general consensus among scientific researchers now says that emotions themselves are forms of judgment, which precede high-level cognition—as should be obvious, since even animals, who lack neocortex, have emotions that shape their behavior. Emotions are not caused by or dependent on high-level cognition. Quite the contrary—we do not bother to think about or remember what lacks emotional salience, a fact well reflected in the very structure of the brain.

Moreover, most cognition takes place outside of awareness, and little of it is accessible to consciousness under any circumstances. While high-level cognition certainly plays some role, we do not know just what it is—but we know it isn't what the CBTers say.

As if that were not enough, very good scientific research has shown that trying to stop "automatic thoughts" just makes things worse.

For those who care, this is the most exciting time in the history of studies of the mind. Finally, we begin to have some "critical mass" in ideas and technologies. But note that these advances have taken place by relaxing disciplinary boundaries, reaching beyond narrowly defined "professions" to include every sort of concern, from philosophy to anthropology to engineering, in studies of the mind. As studies of the mind have exploded through rediscovering interdisciplinary ventures, the mental health professions have become more insular and less inclusive than ever. For the most part, you simply cannot teach in a clinical psychology department unless you are a clinical psychologist, a social work school unless you are a social worker, or a psychiatry program unless you are a psychiatrist. This is a significant change—a couple of decades ago, each sort of department employed a variety of professionals as professors.

When I wrote *Health and Suffering in America*, I was most concerned with the false claims of the mental health professions leading us to devalue other important, non-scientific ways of thinking about suffering. Now, I am just as alarmed that the cultures of healing preclude mental health professionals' making good use of the astounding science beginning to emerge.

In a climate of exploding discovery, the cultures of healing bind our minds to orthodoxies of method and belief that are at odds with the most provocative and interesting of current research possibilities. Even as serious science opens new vistas, raising new questions and offering ways of thinking about minds no one has conceived before, the clinical fields help reinforce, even insist, that their believers should rest content and anxiety-free within limited or patently false beliefs that they simply will not allow the new science to question.

For example, in real science, the notions of unconscious processing, unconscious emotion, and tacit knowledge—that is, beliefs we acquired so long ago that we can no longer call them to consciousness readily—have made a serious comeback. When we look at the work of Antonio Dimasio, Joseph Ledoux, Stephen Kosslyn, Daniel Wegner, and a host of others, we find that *within science* the unconscious has become critically important to understanding minds. You can easily get a mental health degree without ever knowing much about this, though, and certainly without giving any serious thought to what it might imply about the process of talk therapy.

For another example, the sorts of things that mental health professionals pronounce from their armchairs about adultery, jealousy, and various difficulties of marriage bear little resemblance to what evolutionary psychologists now understand about those phenomena. Apparently a great many problems of living that clinicians treat as psychopathology are altogether, and all too sadly, entirely normal. That does not make them good or unproblematic, but it means that curtailing them requires very different notions than "healing." By and large, clinicians seem not even to notice that their understandings of these phenomena are decrepit. Quite the contrary. At precisely the time that we realize, scientifically, that many problems of marriage have little to do with pathology, and everything to do with human nature, many prestigious psychiatrists want to bring the whole realm of family relationships within their jurisdiction. As reported by the *New York Times* (Sunday, September 1, 2002; page A01), psychiatrists calling for the creation of a "Relational Disorders" category of mental health problems, led by a former DSM editor, Michael First of Columbia University, say that troubled relationships are the reason many people seek psychiatric help—which is true. But that doesn't change the fact that now we have very sound evidence—scientific evidence—that these problems are not health deficits.

I thought of rewriting *Health and Suffering in America* to make my case even stronger, along the lines I've suggested here. My main work has moved to other concerns, though, so that going back to the topic of *Health and Suffering in America* really isn't on my own agenda.

I thought, then, of just letting the book pass on, an analysis that arrived at the wrong time. That bothered me for obvious reasons—ego, of course, and not wanting my baby to die. More significant, *Health and Suffering in America* continues to have a small following, and a few folks continue to teach from it at various colleges and universities here and abroad. And I believe more than ever that the basic argument is right and important.

I do not argue that mental health care is a bad thing. We need it—we need professionals who spend all their time trying to understand and ameliorate suffering. But mental health care isn't what it claims to be, or what we think it is, so we accord to mental health professionals an authority they do not deserve. We should never treat mental health professionals as experts on how to live, and we should always submit their recommendations to social and moral criticism. For "health," in most cases, consists of how a particular culture of healing says it would be good for us to be. That is, "mental health" is an ethical ideal, not a scientific discovery. Each assertion about what is "healthy" should be examined as a moral recommendation.

I offer this reprint edition without any illusion that suddenly it will change the world. I only hope that others will be inspired to develop the perspective more forcefully and effectively, and that in due course that will help create sounder, wiser mental health care.

Robert T. Fancher
2003

ACKNOWLEDGMENTS

All thinking and writing is fundamentally conversational, I think, and this book constitutes such a conversation. The participants include parties who will become evident in the text, teachers, friends, persons less amicably related to me, and generally those whose influence and opinion matter to me one way or another. To acknowledge all of them would certainly be impossible; some, like a college biology teacher who was a most helpful slave driver, I cannot even remember by name. Joe Cooper, Kim Plochmann, Charles Scott, John Post, Bert Weinblatt, and Bill Sykes are among the teachers whose influence has been foremost in the internal conversation that makes up this book.

Jerome Kagan read both the initial proposal for this book and the penultimate draft, and his encouragement and wise comments served a multitude of helpful purposes. Ron Chernow talked me through several perplexities, as well as reading the first chapters of the penultimate draft and advising on the expectable anxieties of a first-time book writer. In an extraordinary act of generous kindness, Carol Tavris—whom I had never met, and who had no reason but her own good will, gave a late draft of the book a thorough and perceptive reading and offered guidance at a very crucial point. Raymond Corsini read half the first draft, when it was a sprawling mass half again as large as the finished version; his comments were very helpful in bringing some discipline to the manuscript. Donald Spence and Elliot Valenstein provided careful readings and productive comments. Marvin Clawson gave the near-final draft an excellent reading.

None of these readers, of course, is responsible for the final form, especially since each will find places where, for good or ill, I followed my own counsel despite their thought-provoking commentary.

For being able to bring this project to completion, I am indebted to many friends for support. Karen Eaton, Lucy Winer, John and Lisa Steinhardt, Buffy Friedman, Lisa Tumbleson, Susan Egert, Bill Milling, Randy Fort, Christina Noriega, Adrian Fisher, Liz Marra, and Alice Nagel were crucial sources of comfort and perspective. My parents, James and Ewilda, and my brothers, Frank and James, provided camaraderie and nurtured my perseverance, though at the large geographic distances that separate us. Rereading my mother's books during this process gave me a standard of clear and engaging writing that I only hope I have approached.

My patients are also due a special acknowledgment. I maintained a full caseload in the course of writing the book, and as I have burrowed into the various cultures of healing, my work has shifted in various directions. At times I have been substantially perplexed about what therapy amounts to. My patients have graciously persisted in getting better even in the face of my clinical wanderings and perturbations and in giving their work with me credit. What I know of therapy has much to do with their responses to the diverse efforts they have endured from me through the years. That, I know, means that what I know of therapy has less to do with science than the particularities of my experiences with those who have entrusted their well-being to me. I am grateful for those experiences.

Deciding on the dedication of this book, my first "solo" volume, required much soul-searching. Many people have been crucial in my life and development, personally and professionally, and I owe them all so much. To Gay McRainey (who has died too young, of a brain tumor) and Ron Chernow, I owe the possibility of being in the position of writing any book at all. Each supported and taught me when my own hope and courage threatened to fail. Each has been pivotal in my learning such things as I know about attending watchfully to the lives and needs of persons. They have taught me that a life of value and well-being requires the wise and gracious care—in the deepest sense of grace—of those beyond one's self. I am grateful.

Like almost every person who has attained adulthood, I owe more to my parents than I can say. In my particular life, and for the purposes of this book, I must especially (and with much pleasure and appreciation) give credit that my parents taught me to seek understanding, to think for myself, to care about what is true, and to value following my conscience more highly than conforming to what others would prefer of me. With them I have also learned that profound disagreement is completely consistent with profound love and respect. The gifts they have given me and continue to give are responsible for much that is best in my person and my work; I hope to have shown myself faithful to those gifts.

When the time came to look for a new publisher for this book, Transaction was the first—and only—place I contacted. The reasons were straightforward. First, I wanted to be in the august company of their list! Second, no other press maintains a greater commitment to keeping in print important works that challenge conventional thinking in social science and cultural studies.

When Irving Horowitz wrote to me within a matter of days expressing his wish to publish the book, I was stunned and delighted. I consider this one of the most gratifying compliments I have ever received. Though no one would confuse me with a shrinking violet, my own questions whether I was kidding myself to think this book has continuing value niggled at me, and Dr. Horowitz's enthusiasm touched me deeply.

The staff at Transaction has been a delight. Special thanks to Michael Paley for handling the editorial tasks.

Robert T. Fancher
2003

FOREWORD

All societies seek to relieve suffering through rituals conducted by specially trained healers. Societies invest these healers and their methods with power and prestige as persons who have participated in special rites derived from the society's world-view. In contemporary American society, the diagnosis and management of suffering are primarily entrusted to the medical profession. With some prominent exceptions reflecting the pluralism of our society, the healing profession gains its power and status by being grounded in the scientific world-view, according to which understanding and control of phenomena in the outside world is to be gained by systematic observation and analysis. Application of the scientific world-view to physical phenomena has yielded such massive advances in control of these phenomena that in this realm it has superseded all other cosmologies. The preeminence of the scientific perspective is so unquestioned that it is really assumed to be valid for the full understanding of all phenomena, including those in the psychological and sometimes even spiritual spheres. To the degree that these contain an irreducibly subjective component, however, the scientific method can yield at best only an incomplete understanding. This is especially true of the phenomena of therapy, since these involve culturally and personally determined meanings of suffering and the methods of its alleviation.

Many students of psychotherapy, a discipline that consists almost entirely of manipulating these meanings, have been struggling with how best to incorporate this insight into their world-views. Most try to stretch the methods of scientific investigation to encompass psychotherapy by conceiving it as an applied behavioral science to which these methods, if sufficiently ingenious, are appropriate. Others dare to raise the question of whether conceptualizations other than the scientific one might provide a better grasp of this perplexing field. One is the author of this book. He immediately nails his colors to the mast by bluntly stating that the claim of mental health care to scientific status is false. Instead, schools of therapy "induct people into understanding life in certain ways that are artifacts of the cultures of healing—that is, schools of care—rather than facts about human nature." (p 4). *Cultures of Healing* is an illuminating explication and defense of this provocative thesis.

In the introductory chapters the author points out that the urgent need to do something about suffering leads healers and their followers to exaggerate the amount of their knowledge and to cling to speculations, more or less justified by facts, as if there were any certainties. Fancher provides a concise, balanced historical overview of modern psychiatry in the United States.

The body of the book consists of detailed analyses and astute critiques of four influential American cultures of therapy: psychoanalysis, behaviorism, cognitive therapy, and biological therapy. Fancher's emphasis is how heavily their concepts and methods are determined by their cultures rather than by empirical data. Particularly appealing are Fancher's recognition of the virtues of each culture as well as its limitations, and the fact that his appraisals are based on a wide and thorough acquaintance with the relevant literature.

Fancher shows that all cultures of psychotherapy embody certain tacit assumptions of their societies as to what constitutes mental health and illness on the one hand and what constitutes desirable life and undesirable stress on the other. The exposition is thoughtful, well organized, and based on familiarity with a wide range of contributions from philosophy, science and literature. It is couched in a clear, readable style, enlivened by vivid metaphor.

By placing psychotherapy squarely within the context of culture rather than science and explicating the consequences of this view, this book has taken a major step toward clarification of the persistent, murky, and wide-ranging issues that bedevil psychotherapeutic theory and practice.

Jerome D. Frank

Introduction

. . . THERE ARE CIRCUMSTANCES IN WHICH PEOPLE ARE JUST WRONG ABOUT WHAT THEY ARE DOING AND HOW THEY ARE DOING IT. IT IS NOT THAT THEY LIE . . . BUT THAT THEY CONFABULATE; THEY FILL IN THE GAPS, GUESS, SPECULATE, MISTAKE THEORIZING FOR OBSERVING. THE RELATION BETWEEN WHAT THEY SAY AND WHATEVER IT IS THAT DRIVES THEM TO SAY WHAT THEY SAY COULD HARDLY BE MORE OBSCURE . . . [THEY] ARE UNWITTING CREATORS OF FICTIONS, BUT TO SAY THEY ARE UNWITTING IS TO GRANT THAT WHAT THEY SAY IS, OR CAN BE, AN ACCOUNT OF EXACTLY HOW IT SEEMS TO THEM.

—Daniel C. Dennett
Consciousness Explained

※ ※ ※ ※ ※ ※ ※ ※ ※ ※ ※ ※ ※ ※ ※ ※ ※ ※ ※

※ THE DISTANCE BETWEEN what we know and what we wish we knew is too great to bear, and we fill it with believing. To believing we add doing, and to both we add institutions that elaborate, justify, enforce, and perpetuate these ways of ours. This book explores the believing that fills the gap in that area of life we call, in our time, psychopathology: those sorts of mental or emotional suffering that seem so severe or unrelenting that we think of them as diseases or defects or disorders of mind.

This is a very personal book, in a significant sense; it has resulted from my attempts to understand the profession I have become part of and to find a way to offer care for mental and emotional distress. I entered training as a psychotherapist at the age of thirty-one—after earning a Ph.D. in philosophy, teaching for two years, and working for three years in public policy analysis—in hopes this would be a field that granted a scientifically sound way to be of use. The arid arcana of philosophy and the propaganda passing as scholarship in policy analysis both left me hungry for something empirically true, conscientiously arrived at, and demonstrably useful. The world of psychotherapy, it turns out, is not so different as I had hoped. In mental health care, most of what passes for scientific theory would be more accurately called philosophy. The philosophy is juicier, more concerned with real problems of real people, than in the discipline of philosophy proper, but the price for this "juice" is philosophy of a much less careful and rigorous sort. Propaganda passing as science and scientific work infected with partisan concerns mark mental health care as much as they do public policy work. In public policy work, I learned never to take a "scientific study" seriously until I had discerned the ideology it was intended to serve. That now seems wise to me in mental health care, as well.

One of the greatest perplexities for a thoughtful clinician is the multitude of immense bodies of literature pursuing different views of mental distress, health, and care—and the general inconclusiveness *within* each body. Persons who ascribe to one school of thought take certain parts of a particular body of literature as illuminating, while others dismiss (or blithely refuse to consult) it—preferring a different literature, which in turn is dismissed by everyone else. What one counts as good research depends very much on what one is already prepared to believe. What one is prepared to believe has much to do with philosophical commitments and one's personal and professional biases.

If we had a good science of psychopathology, that would be a good thing. It would tell us about human nature and how pathological distress comes about and how it can be cured. That is what the mental health professions have *claimed* to provide, by virtue of which they have achieved status in society. As we shall see, their claims radically outrun the science they have done. We do not have this thing that would be good—mental health care based on a sound science.

Mental health care exerts an influence on the basis of its claim to scientific status, but that claim is false. Thus, mental health care has a place in our society that it does not deserve, and we think about it wrongly. What it actually does, I argue here, is induct people into understanding life in certain ways that are artifacts of the cultures of healing—that is, the schools of care— rather than facts about human nature. That is, it "enculturates" them. Since people in pain certainly need such help as we can offer, having cultures of healing is legitimate. We need to understand, though, how substantially the cultures of healing differ from our ordinary concept of what mental health professionals are doing. We need to think about mental health care differently than we now do. For its mission in our society is certainly important, but our current misunderstanding of what it amounts to undermines our ability to think about it wisely.

People's lives are changed by therapy, but the direction of the change has to do with what is believed in the culture they happen into. *If* schools of care were informing us of truths, we would all have to accommodate those truths and we could rely on them to be helpful. Since they are not, we do not have to accommodate them, and we rely on them with some risk. But patients, their families and colleagues, and society in general are influenced by therapy, so we have to have some way of thinking about what to believe and what not to. We should not acquiesce to or rely on the "authority" of mental health care, because that authority is based on a false claim. I have come to think that *mental health care is fundamentally part of the public conversation that constitutes life in our society, and its recommendations are essentially moral and social programs.* Thus, we have to think like social and cultural critics in evaluating the ideas and recommendations of mental health care professionals. Thus, I argue in this book that *understanding the culture of a school of care, and thinking about it as social, cultural critics, is our best bet.*

I do not argue that it should ever be thus—only that at present that is the best way to look at it. I do accept the "medical model" of psychopathology that brought the mental health care professions into existence, though I do not accept the claim that psychiatrists are the only people fit to deal with mental health problems—our divisions within the mental health care community have more to do with the history and sociology of the developing professions than with scientific or therapeutic competence. I think it would be good if we *could* classify as mental health problems only those forms of distress that result from a demonstrable failure of some essential function of the human mind. If we could say, "We know what minds are supposed to do, in the same way that we know what livers and kidneys are supposed to do," we could then delineate between forms of distress due to defects or malfunctions of mind and forms of distress due to life's hardships and injustices—or to individuals' altogether normal but problematic proclivities. At present, as Gerald Klerman—one of the most important psychiatric researchers and statesmen of our times—has said, ". . . mental illness and mental disorder are social constructs: they are among the inventions of modern society . . . They are not facts given in nature, but ideas developed by social groups and legitimized by consensual validation."[1]

The aim of science has always been to develop methods of investigation that give us truths about nature independent of any particular investigator's bias. That a bias is shared by all members of a particular society does not make it any less a bias. In mental health care, I think we should aim to identify attributes of mental functioning that are normal or abnormal, regardless of how they fit or fail to fit into a particular society. Someday we may know which kinds of enduring distress are due to failures in essential functions of human psychology—or biology—and which are matters of the clash between how we evolved and how we live. For now, for the most part, we don't. We should not pretend that our social judgments are science. That may give current mental health professions greater authority in present society—it lets them participate in the authority of science—but it impedes the effort to distinguish between what does not work under prevailing conditions and disorders of the mind.

My hope is to contribute to better thinking about the problems of patients, better evaluation of care that is offered, and better care. Making that contribution requires a great deal of brush clearing. We have far too much bias (and wish and speculation) passing as science in mental health care. We have far too little appropriate criticism, and we accord the mental health

---

[1] Gerald Klerman, "Classification and DSM-III-R," in Armand Nicholi, Jr., ed., *The New Harvard Guide to Psychiatry* (1988). Klerman also thinks other forms of illness *and* such basic scientific discoveries as electrons fit the same description. That, I think, is special pleading, an attempt to make serious scientific achievements look as shaky as the achievements of mental health research. Electrons are electrons, everywhere and always, before we knew anything about them and in societies where no physics is taught. Similarly, liver failure is liver failure, even in societies where no one knows anything about livers.

The philosophy of science has gone through a number of phases in this century, and social scientists and many psychiatrists have tended to fasten on those philosophies of science that deny science tells us how things "really are." After a vogue in the 1960s and 1970s, such views have declined among philosophers of science; the trend seems to be back toward a "realist" view of what science accomplishes. See, for instance, *The Making of Memory*, in which Steven Rose (who is as sophisticated a writer as I know on the social and political dimensions of science) provides useful comments on this issue, as well as a superb example of how real science gets done.

professions an autonomy they do not deserve. I strongly believe, with C.S. Peirce, that doubt is the surest avenue toward truth. I hope my criticisms here will unsettle the "social constructs" of the mental health professions that, in my view, need to be radically doubted so that all of us who think mental health care matters can become better at truth. More important, I hope that seeing mental health care as social and moral recommendations will let us think more appropriately as we move past the brush I hope I have cleared.

I intend this book for a general audience:[2] The issue of the image of the mental health professions is principally a social issue, just as the existence of those professions is the result of social dynamics. Each chapter includes an explication of the views of the particular culture of healing, along with my analysis of that culture. Persons who have no expertise in particular cultures, then, can engage each culture nonetheless.

I think a general audience is more likely than mental health professionals to consider my argument dispassionately—except for that (perhaps substantial) body of mental health professionals who are genuinely perplexed at what to make of their profession. To the extent that we look to established experts for reform of the image of their profession, we put ourselves in a peculiar position: To become established as an expert, one has to join a culture of healing and imbue oneself with its ways of looking at the world. One has to spend a career within its institutions, contributing to that particular perspective—addressing *its* questions, within *its* frame of reference, and advancing *its* cause. Presumably this means that the meaning and value of one's life's work becomes entwined with that perspective. We ask quite a great deal of such

---

[2] For the most part, I have chosen works to cite with a recognition that this book is for a general audience. I have tried to minimize references to professional journals and works that require proficiency in reading technical writing. Where references to professional literature are inevitable, I have tried to refer to books or to articles anthologized in books, and I have tried to consolidate references to as few anthologies as possible. The rationale is simple: Acquiring a few books is generally easier than acquiring multiple issues of professional journals. For the most part, works cited should be available and accessible to most educated readers through good public libraries or commercial booksellers. Access to an academic library should not be essential.

persons, to think they can stand back and consider carefully whether they may have accomplished something very different from what they think they have spent their lives accomplishing. We extend immense credulity if we think that their commitments to the cultures in which they have made their lives, and their investments in their images of themselves within those cultures, will not color their analysis.

My aim is to provoke a reconsideration of mental health care precisely so that its work and its place in society will be more wisely crafted. I do not believe that mental health care does what our image of it pretends it does, though I think it does important things. Those whose interests are vested in maintaining the current image of mental health care will see my book as profoundly negative: No one likes being told that one's views about the world are artifacts of culture, not facts about the world. No one likes having a positive self-image refuted, even if a more accurate image would be quite benign. No one likes having the economic status of the institutions and work on which one depends threatened by having their false advertising revealed. Persons who have achieved a measure of authority do not like to have its legitimacy eroded. I believe that more disinterested readers will recognize that the thrust of this book is to help us think clearly, and that can only be positive.

I offer this book as part of the conversation that shapes the life of our society—the conversation, in this case, that shapes how we comport ourselves toward mental and emotional distress and the professions that deal with them. No doubt a great many people, whether or not they have vested interests, will be inclined to take issue with some or all of it, and that is good. My purpose is to be part of that conversation, to reshape it, not to say how it should come out. What matters is not that I (or any other particular participant in this conversation) be right, but that the conversation move toward being true. I hope this book contributes to that goal.

In writing this book, I had to face two particularly vexing problems. One was choosing which of the hundreds of cultures of healing to expound. I decided to offer a history of how mental health care in America came to be as it is (chapter two), in order to show the social issues and some of the professional dynamics that created the mental health professions. Then I look at the most important cultures that have been taken to have attained scientific credibility—that is, the cultures by virtue of which mental health care has come to acquire its claim to authority in our society. Each of these has, in its own way, taken the issue of science seriously. That is more than can be said for a great many—perhaps most—cultures of healing.

Psychoanalysis (chapter three) and behaviorism (chapter four) have been the two most important, historically. Each claims to be, and has sold itself to the public as, scientific—while also building extensive institutions for promulgating this notion. Each fairly quickly went into decline, undermined from within as much as usurped from without, and in both we now see more diversity than agreement among their adherents. This constitutes an important object lesson. Neither of these cultures had the scientific basis it claimed, yet each in its own way convinced itself and the public that it did. Once the institutions and professions were in place, the absence of a set of scientifically valid beliefs set the stage for decline into a host of variant versions. Increasing scientific validity standardizes clinical practice; it does not fragment it. This fragmentation, though, takes place from within the basic cultural tenets established by the ideology that brought the school into existence, so that the multiple progeny of the original culture constitute its subcultures.

Cognitive therapy (chapter five) is currently the hottest of the talk therapies, and biological psychiatry and its psychopharmacological adjunct (chapter six) lead a charge back toward looking at mental health problems as biological illness. Both, like psychoanalysis and behaviorism before them, claim a scientific validity that justifies their ascendancy. In neither case, I shall show, is this claim justified. More important, each suffers deficiencies as a participant in our society's life. Both need to be rethought, not only scientifically, but culturally.

By looking at these four, I do not mean to suggest that the hundreds of others are not subject to analysis from the perspective of culture. Certainly they are—indeed, the proliferation of subcultures and microcultures supports the argument of this book, and perhaps this book will serve as a model for interrogating each of these from a cultural perspective. One must, though, respect the limits of time and book size, and my case had to be made for the strongest and most influential cultures first. That is how I chose the sample to review. By looking at these four, we will be able to see something of how cultures arise and fall, and we will be able to see the restrictions on exploration and the indulgence in beliefs exceeding the evidence that characterize the cultures of healing.

The other problem was how to present a view of the sample cultures without writing an entire book on each. Because these are cultures rather than sciences, in each we find significant subgroups who disbelieve various of its main tenets—there are, after all, Democrats who oppose welfare programs, Republicans who believe in government protection of the poor, Catholics who believe in abortion, and even vegetarians who eat chicken. In the cultures of healing, we have the additional problem of persons who claim to believe the central tenets of their school but say and do all sorts of things that neither follow from nor cohere with them. In a genuine science, such incoherence eventually reveals itself in difficulties with experimental design or theoretical deductions. In cultures, it persists for as long as members of the culture want it to. Generally, I have tried to solve this problem by presenting the most coherent view consistent with the tenets that brought the culture into existence in the first place. In some cases, this means I have presented a more coherent view than some adherents of the cultures themselves possess. In each case, a culture starts off with *something* that seems plausible, appealing, and—by its lights—capable of scientific validation. We have to understand that about each culture, then see what happens when reality sets in.

My biases concerning these cultures will be apparent, but I should make them clear up front. The behaviorist tradition and biological psychiatry do the best science, though in each case the science is so restricted that we should be extremely cautious about accepting those cultures' views. Cognitive therapy has actually been little influenced by cognitive science, so that—while I think all therapies alter cognition and altering cognition is extremely important (not least because it is the principal tool for generalizing the therapeutic encounter into the wider ranges of a patient's life)—contemporary cognitive therapy has little scientific validity. I also doubt that it addresses the kinds of cognition that need changing in most psychopathology, and I am reasonably sure its methods are inadequate for significant cognitive change. Psychoanalysis offers the richest interpretive repertoire, but its refusal to do good science has led it to a deserved state of disrepute. We actually have very little idea which parts of it are worth taking seriously. While psychodynamic psychotherapy may offer a useful vehicle of change for many patients, psychoanalysis is probably a good idea for almost no one. Its expense, intensity, and aim at deep personality change are grossly out of proportion to its intellectual credentials. My prediction is that in the long run biological and cognitive sciences will be the most important means of getting a science of psychopathology (especially as the recent move toward serious study of emotion matures), with contributions from the behaviorist tradition, social psychology, and anthropology. Psychoanalysis, like literature and other humanistic disciplines, will have value for a science of psychopathology only by suggesting hypotheses to be studied—and by providing a stance from which to critique the narrowness of views that develop along the way.

We are a great long distance from anything resembling an adequate science of human nature and its problems, but we are immersed in a world in which many people seem to need mental health care. Mental health care, like most human endeavors, is a field in which we do the best we can, by whatever ideas and activities seem to work, to solve what seem to us to be problems. Communities of like-minded people develop beliefs and practices, teach them to each other, reinforce them as the standard beliefs of the community, and lose sight of the fact that those beliefs and practices are their own make-do creations. Settled beliefs deal passably well with matters of concern, and deeper thought that would put those beliefs in question is eschewed, to protect their stability. Most of life is like this, not like science (pure or applied). The scientific image of mental health care needs to be supplanted by an image of pragmatic efforts to solve a variety of problems posed by life. The scientific image is mostly a matter of public relations—but the mental health professions have made the egregious error of believing their own press releases. I believe that by clearing away this mistaken image we can do a better job of utilizing, listening to, and reshaping mental health care.

In the first chapter, I hope to elicit in the reader the same puzzlement and disgruntlement that started me on this project and to point toward how we can rethink mental health care. The five following chapters should both deepen the reader's concern about the state of the art and help with how to think about it. In the concluding chapter, I offer my views on what should be done about mental health care, given all we shall have seen in the course of the book. In the appendix, I draw out implications on how to choose and evaluate therapy for oneself.

Though this is a very personal book, as I have explained, I have refrained from offering my own views on how therapy can or should be *done*, for that is not my purpose. While my own work, I hope, falls within the general guidelines I offer for how therapy should be reformed and practiced, I have no intention of founding yet another culture of healing. The thrust of this book is toward greater awareness in our society of what the mental health professions do and do not, can and cannot, do, and of how we might wisely think of them. I am concerned with how people in general, in our society, *think about* mental health care, not that every mental health professional should do it the way I do. Furthermore, the conclusion of this book calls for greater participation by more people in shaping mental health care, and it argues that diversity within this conversation is a good thing. It would, at best, distract from the point of the book—and probably just be logically silly—for me unilaterally to offer my own way of doing therapy as some sort of standard. That would be like arguing, "Our present form of government is wrong, we need to replace it with a form of government of type *x*, and Pat Smith should be the head of government." The form of government and who should head the government are very different issues, and confusing one with the other ensures bad thinking. Thus, I do not offer my particular candidate for how therapy should be done.

One question that is really quite beside the point of the book needs to be addressed anyway: A number of readers (all of them mainstream mental health professionals) have asked me, "How can you be a therapist, when you are so critical of extant schools?" That question, in my view, is very sad: It assumes that one cannot be devoted to an enterprise unless one buys into its myths. The thinking behind it is exactly like the thinking behind the "America: Love it or leave it" attitude toward social critics. Such thinking is exactly like that of people who say that feminists, because they radically critique current forms of family life, are opposed to the family. I have been amazed to find that some people who would never utter such nonsense about political or social criticism genuinely think one cannot take the position I take here and still be a devoted member of the mental health community.

The question, in fact, is a reflection of precisely the problem I am addressing in this book: that at the present time, mental health professionals are insufficiently aware of and thoughtful about the true status of our profession. In my view, every therapist should think very critically about one's beliefs, practices, and commitments, for a simple reason: As therapists we are supposed to be dedicated to the truth of our patients' lives. As serious intellectuals have known for a couple of dozen centuries, one cannot pursue truth without thinking critically. As Karl Popper has shown, the enterprise of science is principally a matter of assiduous efforts at refuting conjectures—scorching criticism showing extant beliefs to be wrong is absolutely the heart of scientific investigation. One main difference between good and bad science (and perhaps between the genuine sciences and most putative science in mental health care) is precisely the precision and relentlessness of the self-criticism to which good scientists subject their own findings and ideas. Furthermore, as I say many times in the course of this book, most of life lacks a solid knowledge base, and we are always having to form beliefs far in excess of anything we know. There is nothing self-contradictory in being a therapist and recognizing that therapy, like most of life, is like this. My desire is to help us think soundly, given that this is the reality of the situation. My goal is to expand the resources that get used in thinking about therapy, to clear out ill-formed views, and to enable us to think better. My position, as I spell out clearly, is that we need to invoke a wide variety of modes (not just scientific modes) of disciplining our thought in order to develop better ideas within and about mental health care. I do not say anything in this book that calls into question the likelihood that such efforts result in workable therapeutic beliefs and practices. The reader who finds himself bewildered by how a practicing therapist could write this book needs to reflect carefully on his assumptions about how thinking works and how it fits with practice—and about how thinking and practice go together in solving problems.

I think that within our society we have the resources for a reformation that will make of the mental health professions something we can rely on—if we learn to think about them as I suggest. I think, though, that our mistaken image of mental health care has led to a great many views being foisted on patients and the public without sufficient appropriate—cultural, social, and moral, as well as scientific—criticism and investigation. My argument, to put it rather grandly, is about the place of mental health care in the current state of the human condition. My position is that *mental health care is legitimate, but many of its claims to truth and authority are not.* The corrected image of mental health care I try to provide here aims to substantiate its legitimacy and to let us think more wisely as we replace those claims that are not legitimate.

Chapter One

CARE AS CULTURE

BOTH DEMOCRATIC AND SCIENTIFIC IDEALS TEND TO CAUSE MANY AMERICAN PSYCHOTHERAPISTS TO UNDERESTIMATE THE EXTENT TO WHICH PSYCHOTHERAPY IS A PROCESS OF PERSUASION. MEMBERS OF A DEMOCRACY DO NOT LIKE TO SEE THEMSELVES AS EXERCISING POWER OVER SOMEONE ELSE, AND THE SCIENTIST OBSERVES—HE DOES NOT INFLUENCE. . . . [M]OST PSYCHOTHERAPISTS IN AMERICA CLAIM TO BE BOTH DEMOCRATIC AND SCIENTIFIC, THOUGH IN MANY RESPECTS THEY ARE NEITHER.

—*Jerome D. Frank*
Persuasion and Healing

SUFFERERS WHO SEEK help assume—hope—their helpers know what they are doing: a hope so strong, it becomes faith. This faith springs from the need to believe that suffering is not ceaseless. Unless we believe that our helpers know something about helping, why believe they can help? Unless we believe our helpers can help, why consult them?

Sufferers who seek professional care for emotional pain or mental distress hope at least as strongly as anyone else that the helpers in whom they put their trust know what they are about. By one measure, their hope—faith—seems to be rewarded: Most studies in recent years seem to show that most patients of mental health care believe themselves to have benefitted from it. Informally, it seems that most people who have had serious encounters with mental health care look upon it with fondness and appreciation. For every horror story about insensitive or inept or outright destructive therapists, there seem to be at least hundreds, maybe thousands, of former patients who remember their therapists with affection and attribute to their treatment substantial benefits. Givers of care, by the same token, talk thoughtfully and with apparent wisdom about how to help patients, which patients get better, and what role the therapy played in the improvement.

Yet care for psychopathology—the technical term for mental and emotional distress that constitutes or comes from illness or abnormality—is quite a murky field. Joseph Adelson, a psychologist at the University of Michigan, offers this summary of our situation:

> Does psychotherapy work? As it happens, we have had a vast number of studies carried out on the question—over a thousand, in fact. Through a statistical *tour de force* called meta-analysis, this plethora of investigations has now been

reduced and analyzed, so that we can conclude that it does indeed work. Yet having discovered this much, over the years and painfully, we now find that we can say little more. We do not know whether any given form of therapy is more effective than any other, or which therapists do good work and which do not—that is, whether it is the training that counts, or the theory, or the personality, or the experience, or the mode of treatment, or whatever. We cannot tell with any degree of confidence which patients are likely to get better, and which are not.[3]

Understanding how to think clearly within this murky situation is the task we face in this book.

The Fluid World of Mental Health Care

The concept of psychopathology, and the attendant professions of healing, are relatively recent inventions. People have always recognized that some persons suffer distress and exhibit odd behaviors that do not yield to any ordinary ways of dealing with life's problems. In some cultures, these oddities are not regarded as problems so much as blessings or gifts. Many cultures institutionalize ways of explaining and dealing with these—whether divine visitations, demon possession, communication with the dead, spells and curses, bad blood, "markings" from the mother's experiences during pregnancy, moral or spiritual failings, laziness, or whatever. Only in the last century has the idea been widely accepted that these perplexing preternatural problems are in fact natural—that they are psychopathology, to be explicated by sciences of healing. We can find various references in the great thinkers of Western civilization to "diseases of the mind," and since the Renaissance many major thinkers who have concerned themselves with distress have looked for naturalistic explanations.

---

[3] Joseph Adelson, "The Social Sciences and the Humanities," in *Challenges to the Humanities* (1986).

Until the last several decades, though, explanations of distress as disease have been minority opinion. Even today, significant numbers of people refuse to accept the idea of psychopathology, explaining chronic or recurrent psychological distress as due to moral or spiritual failings. Significant numbers of physicians themselves seem not to recognize the notion of psychopathology, explaining patients' emotional complaints in terms of a need for more exercise and the like.

Yet the concept of psychopathology is now fully ensconced in our society's institutions and categories of explanation, if not unfailingly accepted. Because secular care for the distress we call psychopathology was vested in doctors (for reasons of historical happenstance that we shall come to understand in the course of this book), the concept of psychopathology is fundamentally a concept of disease, of deficiencies relative to normal functioning due to some illness. The *idea* of psychopathology as disease antedates any discovery of psychological diseases—indeed, the idea is what drives the minimally successful attempt to find them. The attempt to delineate diseases of the mind still lags behind the idea that there *are* such diseases. What gets counted as a mental illness, at any given point in medical history, seems to be settled as much by politics and fashion as by discovery.

The century and a half of work to discover psychopathologies and methods of cure has not resulted in any generally accepted, authoritative body of evidence defining illnesses, their causes, and their cures. Depending on who is counting, between fifty and five hundred different forms of therapy exist, each with the full panoply of professional organizations, journals, and training programs. For modern Westerners, this seems very odd. We have created *professions* of healing, requiring arduous courses of education and training, precisely because we *believe* that knowledge makes a difference. We do not license psychotherapists on the basis of their personal characteristics or intrinsic healing powers. We base our professions on the idea of *expertise*, and for us this is a profoundly knowledge-based notion. The authority that our culture vests in givers of mental health care—to define what is problematic, its nature, and its cure—and the trust that patients place in them rest on the assumption that these members of our society know something that the rest of us do not. Accordingly, we should think that what the therapist knows (or believes), and what he does on the basis of this knowledge, would determine the effectiveness of professional help. To date though, this hardly seems the case, except to those who are dead set on believing it.

Every time a new method and theory comes into existence, its practitioners proclaim a "revolutionary" advance and publish astounding research results showing success—results that generally prove not to be reproducible by more disinterested observers or even, a few years later, by the proponents of the school of care themselves. Every significant school of care can claim successes, though each claims to have some distinct superiority. Indeed, one of the most robust phenomena in psychotherapy research is the rough equivalence of success of all the schools that have been studied—Bergin and Garfield (two of the most respected authorities in the field) have said, in a comprehensive review of outcome research, that "the equal outcomes phenomenon may be the most frequent and striking theme."[4] If success comes as readily with one method as another, as it seems to, we are given pause. What do the various claims of the schools of care for psychopathology amount to? Are they truths about human nature or irrelevant verbiage—or something else? We like to believe that lawyers know true things about the law, that doctors know true things about the body, and that auto mechanics know true things about cars. We presume that the effectiveness of lawyers, doctors,

---

[4] S. L. Garfield and A. E. Bergin, *Handbook of Psychotherapy and Behavior Change*, 3d ed. (1986). The classic work on this topic can be found in M. L. Smith, G. V. Glass, and T. I. Miller, *The Benefits of Psychotherapy* (1980). Many of the essays in Marvin R. Goldfried, ed., *Converging Themes in Psychotherapy* (1982), report on and refer to the immense body of research on outcome studies.

This is a controversial topic; no school of care wants to acquiesce in the idea that it lacks special efficacy. Anyone can, if one chooses, identify a subset of studies supporting one's particular school. The fact is that any study claiming to establish the special effectiveness of a particular school must be interpreted in light of the hundreds of studies over forty years of research that show roughly equal outcomes.

We should note, as well, that *which* schools of care *get researched* is a function of political and sociological realities: what schools happen to be in the ascendancy at a given time, with a given research agency or funding board. Most schools of care do not get included in most comprehensive research programs—giving researched schools a specious air of superiority.

and auto mechanics is due substantially to their knowledge. It would seem reasonable to expect psychotherapists to know true things about the human psyche and its problems, and to expect that this knowledge is essential to effective therapy.

Recent research has complicated this issue even further: The therapist, perhaps more than the technique, seems to be what counts. When therapists use prescriptive manuals, so that all of them are doing reasonably similar things, a therapist who gets good results with one method tends to get it with others. A therapist who gets poor results with one, similarly, gets poor results across the board. Somehow it seems the person, more than what she knows, determines success. At least, whatever knowledge is involved seems not to be the sort of technical knowledge by which mental health professionals claim expertise. Such data are quite consistent with the possibility that personal characteristics or intrinsic healing powers, not professional expertise, account for results.[5]

As we shall see in detail in chapter two and beyond, there has never been a period in American (or other) mental health care in which some substantial body of reliable knowledge clearly showed which human problems ought to be considered "pathological," nor has there ever been a period in which anything approaching unanimity among practitioners has obtained. Nor has there ever been a substantial period in which it has even been agreed who should be recipients of care, what that care should look like, or where it should be administered. Yet, since

---

[5] Lester Luborsky, long one of the most respected of clinical researchers, is a pioneer in this provocative research (e.g., "Therapist Success and Its Determinants," *Archives of General Psychiatry*, vol. 42, pp. 602-611). Luborsky thinks that such therapist characteristics as the ability to form a warm, supportive relationship will turn out to be central. This seems plausible but very partial. Some highly successful therapies—like Albert Ellis's Rational-Emotive Therapy, Ormond and Spotnitz's "modern psychoanalysis," and Masterson's treatment of borderline personality disorders—do not seem obviously warm and supportive.

Morton Hunt, in his chapter on psychotherapy in *The Story of Psychology* (1993), suggests that failure to recognize and control for therapist effectiveness factors may be one reason that outcome studies have shown roughly the same success for all forms of therapy. Pierre Janet, the great French psychiatrist, essentially offered the same idea over a century ago—that an able clinician could effect improvement using whatever method he chose (quoted in Gerald Grob, *The Mad Among Us* [1994]).

the mid-nineteenth century, there have been organized professions of healing, each with its orthodoxy, each claiming to know who is ill, with what, and how to deal with it. Each claims the right to be granted licenses and other legal sanctions and protection. American mental health care has been in constant flux since its beginnings, but in spite of this, "experts" have created professions, achieved social status and government endorsement, and claimed authority.

We have substantially given the mental health professions what they have asked—for a reason. We would like to believe that they are all participants in a stable, cumulatively progressing tradition. The flux and chaos of mental health care have been obscured by the need of all of us to *believe* that we have in our culture professionals who understand and can help us master emotional and mental sufferings. We *want* authoritative professions of healing, so that we can believe suffering is not ceaseless. Our professions, with the collusion of society, have created an illusory image of what mental health care amounts to. The fluidity and diversity of American mental health care have been hidden from view by our image, and the self-images, of the professions.

The State-of-the-Art in Diagnosis

One would think that a profession devoted to mental health and mental illness for a century and a half would possess clear ideas of just what constitutes mental illness—and health. In the nineteenth and early twentieth centuries, a host of nosologies of mental illness developed, but few managed to last long. (Emil Kraepelin's descriptions of different kinds of schizophrenia is one of the notable exceptions.) In the 1940s through the 1970s, when psychoanalysis ruled, little attention was given to identifying and defining specific diseases. There was no need: Psychotics were hospitalized, and everyone else was basically treated the same way, with some form of psychoanalysis (or one of its derivative forms of therapy). By the 1970s, though, with psychoanalysis in disrepute and the desire of the psychiatric profession to put itself on a more scientific basis and increase its credibility in the medical community, definition and diagnosis of psychopathology became an active concern.

The result was the third edition of the American Psychiatric Association's *Diagnostic and Statistical Manual of Mental Disorders.* The APA committee that now oversees the manual came into existence in 1974, and in 1980 it produced its first version of the manual—referred to as DSM-III, since it is the third edition of this hoary reference tome. In 1987, a further revision appeared, called DSM-III-R.[6] In 1994, just as this book was completed, a new edition, DSM-IV, was published.[7]

The new DSMs represent an effort to construct from the chaos of contemporary diagnosis some logical and orderly structure—by committee. Hardly anyone bothers to deny that the outcome had a great deal to do with politics. Hans Eysenck says, "DSM-III has little reaction to scientific research and represents rather the power structure of contemporary feudal baronetcies."[8] Sol Garfield, less provocatively, says that DSM-III is "a compromise between different groups with different value systems."[9]

Politics or not, one dimension of the efforts behind the new DSMs seems altogether legitimate: to create uniformity of definition of diseases, so that researchers (and clinicians) can refer

---

[6] Theodore Millon and Gerald Klerman have edited a very useful volume, *Contemporary Directions in Psychopathology: Toward the DSM-IV* (1986). The opening essays, by Klerman and Millon respectively, provide an interesting glimpse into how the new DSMs came to be (as well as extensive references to the literature of the debate over it).

[7] Since DSM-IV appeared literally in the week this book was completed, there obviously does not yet exist a body of critical literature assessing it. What is clear is that politics has been at least as heavy around this edition as previous ones. Pre-publication hype about DSM-IV claims, as similar hype has claimed about earlier additions, that the new edition is more scientific. Higher standards of reliability were set for *new* categories. However, virtually none of the old diagnoses were dropped, though most do not meet the new standards, because "we didn't want to disrupt clinical practice," according to Dr. Allen Frances, the head of the DSM-IV project. This means that most of DSM-IV does not even meet its own standards! See, for instance, "Revamping Psychiatrists' Bible," *The New York Times,* 19 April 1994.

[8] Hans Eysenck, "A Critique of Contemporary Classification and Diagnosis," in Theodore Millon and Gerald Klerman, eds, *Contemporary Directions in Psychopathology: Toward the DSM-IV* (1986).

[9] S. L. Garfield, "Problems in Diagnostic Classification," in Thedore Millon and Gerald Klerman, eds., *Contemporary Directions in Psychopathology: Toward the DSM-IV* (1986).

to the same sets of observable signs and symptoms as constituting the same diseases. Before the new DSMs, the terms purporting to describe psychopathology possessed no uniform definitions, so that clinicians and researchers in one place would be looking at a different set of phenomena than clinicians and researchers in another place, and it was never clear how to compare results. As a research tool and a step toward clearer communication, the DSMs seem altogether laudable.

The DSMs do not attempt to describe causes of the disorders listed, for a very good reason. As Gerald Klerman puts it, ". . . most of the disorders we currently encounter in psychiatry have no established etiological [i.e., causal] or even pathophysiological basis."[10] Rather, the DSMs give operational definitions of the disorders—lists of the observable characteristics necessary for someone to be classified as having a disorder.

The DSM diagnostic categories have been extensively tested for reliability—that is, they have been tested to see whether the definitions are sufficiently precise and well formed that different diagnosticians, looking at the same patient, will place him in the same diagnostic category. This research has been fairly heavily criticized. For one thing, much of the testing was done among an "in-group" of physicians: persons who had worked on the document and their students, sometimes conferring with each other on how to classify patients. For another, the evaluators set themselves fairly loose standards of agreement: If two doctors placed the patient in different disease categories, this still counted as agreement, so long as both diseases were of the same sort, such as anxiety disorders. Whether or not such criticism is just, whether or not the reliability has been established, no one claims that many of the DSM definitions have been shown to be *valid*. No one claims that we know these definitions to refer to actual disease processes. One of the members of the DSM committee, Nancy Andreasen, says, "A . . . limitation, and perhaps the most cogent criticism of DSM-III, is that it may gain reliability at the

---

[10] Gerald Klerman, "Classification and DSM-III-R," in Armand Nicholi, Jr., ed., *The New Harvard Guide to Psychiatry* (1988).

expense of validity."[11] Millon tells us that "the categorical syndromes of the DSM-III are conceptual prototypes and not tangible entities."[12] Klerman makes very clear that "reliability does not guarantee validity" and emphasizes the need for further research to establish validity.[13]

The distinction between reliability and validity is vitally important. We can make up a list of definitions, and we can teach people to use them. We can then go out and find which things fit into the categories. That will not mean that the things fitting the categories share any important natural feature that gives them the characteristics detailed in our definition. So, for instance, we could say that all predominantly white flying entities are to be referred to as whargles, and we could easily then go out and identify all the whargles in the world—and whargles would include, among other things, baseballs, some airplanes, some birds, some laundry that has flown off the line and been caught by the wind, and so forth. "Whargle" would be a *reliable* category, since independent observers can agree on what things fit the definition. It would not be a *valid* category, because there is no natural property that all the members of the category share that causes each to be both predominantly white and flying.

We do not know yet which, if any, of the diagnostic categories refer to extant natural processes. Conceivably, some of them may refer to real processes, yet these processes may not be sources of the distress that bring patients for care. Thus, even when a person clearly satisfies the diagnostic criteria, we do not know whether that means she has a particular natural process going on, nor (if so) do we know whether that process is responsible for her distress. So, for instance, we may find a hundred people who fit the criteria for narcissistic personality disorder; but we know

---

[11] Nancy Andreasen, *The Broken Brain* (1984).

[12] Theodore Millon, "On the Past and Future of the DSM-III: Personal Recollections and Projections," in Theodore Millon and Gerald Klerman, eds., *Contemporary Directions in Psychopathology* (1986).

[13] Gerald Klerman, "Historical Perspectives on Contemporary Schools of Psychopathology," In Theodore Millon and Gerald Klerman, eds., *Contemporary Directions in Psychopathology* (1986).

neither whether there is some natural process they all share that accounts for these characteristics, nor whether their distress results from this concatenation of qualities we have dubbed a "personality disorder." Similarly, the vast number of people who meet the criteria for major depression may, so far as we know, suffer from any number of different processes, of different causation and prognosis. When we have a valid disease category, we can say, "The course of this disease is usually p, q, and r. If we do x, that affects the disease in the direction of y." Thus, valid categories tell us important things. For few, if any, of the categories in the DSM's can we say these things.

Yet substantial parts of the mental health community act as if the DSMs were, in fact, a list of known diseases. Carol Tavris has said, "It has succeeded in standardizing the categories of who is, and is not, mentally ill. Its categories and terminology have become the common language of most clinicians and textbooks."[14] This seems an instance of something Willa Cather observed long ago: "Give the people a new word and they think they have a new fact."[15] Official hospital and clinic diagnosis is now universally done in DSM terms, textbooks and journal articles are now written in these terms, and insurance companies make decisions about covering care on the basis of such categories. Research—including massive epidemiological surveys that get wide exposure in the popular media—gets done using these categories *prior to* the establishment of their validity. There are even treatment manuals being written for these "disorders," though many have not been shown to be genuine pathological processes. The diagnostic categories of the DSMs have become a new language for mental health care, and the ubiquity of the language hides the uncertainty of its accuracy.

That may well be the main function of the DSMs. Since diagnosis in DSM terms does not tell us what (or whether a) process

---

[14] Carol Tavris, *The Mismeasure of Woman* (1992). This book contains an excellent discussion of the new DSMs, in the context of how substantially it has been shaped by the longstanding male bias of the psychiatric profession.

[15] Quoted in William Safire, "On Language," *The New York Times Magazine*, 12 December 1993.

is going on, what causes it, and what to do about it, such diagnosis does not serve any substantial treatment function. This seems a curious phenomenon. Why has this poorly validated, politically influenced document become the standard in mental health care? Perhaps because it provides a language that lets us act as if we were saying true things, though we have little reason to know that we are. At least we are all referring to the same things with our new language, even if we do not know whether we are referring to natural processes, pathological processes, or the sources of distress at all. The ability to use a new language masks how little we know under a veneer of common terms.

Schools of Care as Cultures

We have had professions of mental health for about a century and a half. These professions claim to be expert on mental illness and its treatment. They have organized themselves, secured legal protection, and acquired authority in our society. Unfortunately—as we shall see in some detail—they do not agree on what constitutes health or illness, and they lack sound bases in science or reason. Effectiveness of treatment seems to have little to do with the various bodies of knowledge and techniques that constitute the mental health professionals' claims to expertise. At present, success seems to have something to do with *something* about the therapist himself—though at present we can only guess what that is. The claims of the mental health professions seem quite at odds with much of what seems obviously true of those professions. How are we to understand these claims—and the diverse schools of care that make them?

Our schools of care for psychopathology, as we shall see, have not been born of advancing understanding of pathological problems. Rather, they have been born of our *hope* that life might be good: that suffering is avoidable, or at worst meaningful and manageable. We do not correctly understand our efforts to isolate and ameliorate psychopathology unless we understand it as the pursuit of our ideal that a normal life is one that is reasonably happy and meaningful. What we have done in pursuit of this ideal is rather different from the way we have *explained to ourselves* what we are doing. We have invented a host of ideas and practices to try to make life better; we have claimed to understand what we are up to better than we really do. We have claimed we can understand mental health care as the application of scientific discovery, but this (as we shall see) will not bear scrutiny.

We can understand mental health care better if we explain it in terms of cultures that have been created to meet a social need and wish. Beginning in the nineteenth century, our society's need for professions that would take care of certain sorts of suffering was combined with faith in medical science, and the result was what we now call mental health care. The science to found and buttress these professions did not yet exist, though society was ready to have such professions. Those professions therefore had to invent ways of thinking about the problems they were supposed to solve and convince themselves that these were scientific truths.

The sufferings of persons afflicted with psychopathology still dwarf what the givers of care know, on any objective appraisal of what we really know about "suffering of the spirit"—the literal meaning of "psychopathology." Neither patients nor therapists customarily admit the meager measure of solid information we possess. For there is knowing, and then there is *knowing*. *Objective* knowing—whether from laboratory, ethnography, or natural history—is a small part of what givers of care and their patients know. *Subjective* knowing—a certain feeling of confident belief, a reliance beyond all reason—is a different matter. In this, care for psychopathology abounds. We tend to confuse our subjective certainty for objective knowing, and we explain this certainty as if it derived from objective knowing. Subjective certainty, shared by a group of people who mistake it for objective knowing, is characteristic of cultures: The process of enculturation imparts ideas and practices, and the social functioning of the culture reinforces and perpetuates that belief. Social scientists developed the concept of culture precisely to explain, among other things, how beliefs and practices that are not necessitated by nature or evidence become widespread among a people and appear to them to be truths of nature.

The concept of culture, which was formulated by social scientists less than a century ago, is commonplace now. The civil rights and various liberation movements, on one hand, and rising contact with the cultures of other societies (as technology, travel, and immigration have disrupted provinciality), on the other, have given all of us some familiarity with how cultures work. Hardly anyone (at least, hardly anyone who is likely to be reading this book) is unaware of the ways that our society's beliefs about race, for instance, were shaped by economic and social dynamics. None of us can fail to recognize how culturally determined notions of gender inform our thinking and action. We have all become acutely aware of substantial differences between American and Japanese notions of individuality and social participation. Sociologists and anthropologists work hard to discern the processes of socialization that enculturate persons into their society's culture—and to analyze how social institutions support and solidify cultures. For our purposes, intricate knowledge of such matters is less important than the general understanding of culture most of us, as persons who are aware of contemporary reality, possess.

A culture teaches its members how to think, act, value, and even how to feel. The ways our culture shapes us are so integral to our lives that how we think seems perfectly natural. How we feel seems to be caused by what we feel about. Our values seem right. Our ways of acting seem obviously suited to what they are supposed to accomplish. Yet, as we all know now, someone from a different culture thinks, feels, values, and acts differently—and sees her ways as natural, too. So deeply embedded in our lives are the ways of our culture that changing them is often difficult. Think of how pervasive we find sexism to be, once we begin thinking about it, and how difficult making sense of what to do about it can be. Think of how easily and "naturally" we fall into habits of sexism, and how surprised we are when we suddenly recognize sexism where we had not even noticed it before.

This is the sort of thing that takes place in the schools of thought and practice that constitute our cultures of healing. Quandaries and complaints and aspirations of patients (and quandaries and complaints and ambitions of members of the profession) cry for attention. Practices and ideas to deal with them develop, out of trial and error, speculation, wishful thinking, and sometimes discovery. Further ideas develop to rationalize the practice, and further practices develop from the implications of the ideas. The process, once started, becomes self-generating: A vast web of ideology and action builds up to explain, elaborate, safeguard, and protect what has developed. Institutions of various sorts develop—training programs, stylized methods of care, special language and manners of speech, professional organizations, defined roles for patient and therapist. Rewards, punishments, and sanctions of other kinds enculturate new members and keep old members loyal. All of this shapes how members of the culture see and think and value and feel and act. "Skillful" members are those so thoroughly enculturated that the culture's "take" on the world seems natural, right. "Brilliant" members extend the culture's beliefs and practices into further elaborations and transformations. The culture comes to define a world, which provides a context for the lives of its members and exercises an influence over those who do not join but pass through as pilgrims.

To say that schools of care constitute cultures is not necessarily to condemn them. To understand care as culture is not to dismiss it. Though we may initially be disturbed that the cultures of healing create, preserve, promulgate, and enact all sorts of beliefs and practices beyond reason and evidence, we really should not be surprised by it. When people need help they *need* it, and pain does not forestall its visitations until we understand it. *Something* must be done when people are in pain, and both patient and healer need to believe that what they are about is true. This is the wrenching burden of clinicians and the license and capital of quacks. Equally important, social institutions cannot be created and sustained without *some* ideology and some set of practices that define who is competent and who is not, who gets to hold authority, and what should be done under what conditions. If no sufficient body of scientifically valid beliefs and methods is available, *something else* must be put in place.

Having cultures of healing, however short they may be on scientific knowledge, is better than not having them, in our current state of knowledge. A culture gives its members identity, orientation, and meaning. To be enculturated gives one a sense of which problems need attention and a set of ways of attending to them. To be firmly enculturated gives one a sense of security, a way of thinking about things, a repertoire of ways of coping with various mundane and trying situations, an assurance of the acceptability of one's actions, and a consequent obviation of anxiety. One's sense of legitimacy and meaning resides with one's place in the larger culture, and insofar as one is confident of one's place, one's life has meaning.

Indeed, we can understand a great deal of the appeal of both psychoanalysis and behaviorism—and psychosurgery, for that matter—precisely in these terms. The egregious intellectual shortcomings of each of these ways of looking at psychopathology were immediately obvious when it was first introduced— yet each spread like wildfire. For while none had compelling intellectual justification, each provided a way of thinking about and dealing with the vexing problems of patients. Whether or not the patients got better, the practitioners were given a sense of what to do, why, and what to make of the results. We may guess that each fostered an illusion of knowledge that relieved the anxieties of practitioners and allowed them to perpetuate the naive hopes of patients in good conscience.

In our current state of rudimentary knowledge, patients and practitioners alike would probably be unable to tolerate the anxiety that would result from giving up all that goes beyond the scientific in the cultures of healing. When people (including givers of professional care) face intense suffering that we have no idea how to relieve, we become anxious and frightened— even (perhaps especially) when we are observing and enduring the pained entreaties of the sufferers rather than undergoing the suffering ourselves. When we have some idea of what to do, no matter how farfetched, we feel less helpless and anxious. Each culture of healing provides its practitioners with ideas that relieve our anxious recognition of our ignorance and helplessness in the face of the sufferings of patients. Perhaps this allows us to remain as attentive and responsive to patients as is currently possible, and perhaps this allows us to do such good as we actually can. To condemn our cultures of healing, simply because they go far beyond anything that is known, is too simpleminded:

That would consign the profession to the dismal, consuming fires of despair.

That clinicians make their best guess in the absence of sound knowledge is no crime; that scared and anguished people make up and believe in fairy tales to find some relief is no sin. That we create social institutions and professions to try to deal with pain before we have the necessary science does not bespeak perfidy. That we believe beyond reason (and ignore our unreason) so that we can live and act in spite of the terrors engendered by pain does not reflect dishonesty. These are simply facts of the human condition—sad facts, perhaps, to those of us who highly value sound knowledge, but facts nonetheless. Perhaps they testify to our adaptive resilience even in the face of ignorance.

We would like to believe, of course, that our schools of care for psychopathology are schools of scientific knowledge and its application. That is what most of them claim to be, and we grant them cultural authority by virtue of our participation in this myth—authority to tell us what is healthy and what is sick, what is normal and abnormal, how to get from one to the other, what truths we must accept about life. Where they reveal themselves as cultures is in the particular empirical questions they actually investigate, the methods of investigation they countenance or reject, what they make of their discoveries, what they have to say about competing schools of psychotherapy, and—most of all—what they teach that goes beyond any reasonable appraisal of evidence. We shall see that even the most self-righteously "scientific" of the psychotherapies live more off philosophy than science, wisdom than truth, conjecture than knowledge. That would not be particularly remarkable—most of life is like that—except that neither patients nor therapists (nor the teachers of therapists nor therapists engaged in collegial debate) customarily admit the true measure of what these psychotherapies propound.[16]

---

[16] I am *not* making the naive claim that science transcends culture in any simple way. Certainly even the most rigorous scientific endeavors have their cultural determinants and constitute cultures in their own right, and there is no inherent reason that a culture could not include as one of its defining characteristics a rigorous devotion to scientific soundness. But by the same token—and this is the crucial point for our present concerns—there is no inherent *congruence* between science and culture. The point I am making in this book is that we can explicate the schools of care *as cultures*, whereas we *cannot* successfully explicate them, at this point in their evolution at least, as applications of sound science.

So What?

The idea that care for psychopathology *should* be scientific is something of an historical accident, as we shall see. Schools of care need not be scientific to be effective. On reflection this seems obvious: To say that a practice must have a scientific base would be exactly like saying that before the discovery of physics, people could not build bridges, houses, or ships. Most practices and professions in most societies get on reasonably well without any special scientific basis. If we know that various forms of mental health care work, what does it matter whether they are scientific or cultural?

To say that the cultures of healing "work" is to say less than we might think. For one thing, this is a rather vague notion. What does it mean to say that a form of therapy works? Different schools of thought differ in what they see as illness and improvement. Marvin Goldfried and Wendy Padawer have said, "In many ways, outcome [i.e., effectiveness] measures represent the Achilles heel of psychotherapy research. Unlike other applied fields, where changes can be more readily discerned and agreed upon, the field of psychotherapy has done relatively little to achieve a consensus on the goals of therapeutic intervention and the methods by which such goals may be measured."[17] When we say that the schools of care that have been researched "work," there are a few things we can mean. One is that, if we give each school its own yardstick, each—patients and practitioners agree— makes patients better. Another is that when different methods are compared in the same study, using the same criteria for each, generally we find all of them working roughly equally well.

Various meta-analyses of therapy outcome studies show that, averaging across the many different kinds of scales that are used in studies, roughly two-thirds to four-fifths of patients benefit from therapy, without substantial or consistent differences between the forms of therapy tested.[18] In what is probably the most important single study to date, four different forms of care

---

[17] Marvin R. Goldfried and Wendy Padawer, "Current Status and Future Directions in Psychotherapy," in Marvin R. Goldfried, ed., *Converging Themes in Psychotherapy* (1982).

[18] Morton Hunt, *The Story of Psychology* (1993).

for depression were compared by the same measures. Cognitive therapy (based on the work of Aaron Beck and his colleagues), interpersonal therapy (derived from the work of Harry Stack Sullivan by Gerald Klerman and colleagues), an antidepressant drug known to be highly effective, and a placebo drug were compared. All the forms of care were superior to placebo, and the differences between the three were not of great substance.[19]

The consistency of this sort of result has led many eminent researchers to conclude that "nonspecific" factors must be causing the change—though the effectiveness of drugs complicates this, since drugs clearly have specific effects. At least for the non-chemical psychotherapies, though, we do not know whether it is the therapy that is working or some adventitious characteristic that may not be specific to therapy. Hans Strupp, one of the premier researchers into psychotherapy effectiveness, has said (in this instance, with Grady L. Blackwood): "Although there is both clinical and empirical evidence that in a very broad sense psychotherapy is beneficial, the more important question of whether or not the techniques of modern psychotherapy transcend in their effectiveness a baseline set by common sense, unsystematic approaches has not been answered definitively."[20]

But even if we agree that the cultures do work, and work *about as well* as one another, none of them works as well as we would like. No mental health procedure is analogous to the smallpox vaccine; no mental illness has ever been eradicated by the development of an understanding of it and a treatment for it. Persons who suffer from psychopathology rarely enjoy the kind of prognosis of someone who suffers, say, pneumonia or gonorrhea or hypothyroidism—or termites or a bad carburetor, for that matter. Mental health care is still fairly hit or miss, and there are hardly any surefire cures. We need better care for psychopathology, and

---

[19] I do not know of a presentation of this hotly debated study written for a popular audience. It is presented in a series of articles in *Archives of General Psychiatry*, including papers in October 1992, November 1989, June 1990, and August 1991.

[20] Hans Strupp and Grady L. Blackwood, Jr., "Recent Methods of Psychotherapy," in Harold I. Kaplan and Benjamin J. Sadock, eds., *Comprehensive Textbook of Psychiatry*, 4th ed. (1985).

the supposition that good science may be crucial to this is not wildly unreasonable.

"Effective," furthermore, can be a fairly crude measure. Amputating a hand would be a splendidly effective way of curing warts around the fingernail, but no one recommends it. Drunkenness effectively relieves a world of woes, but it impairs one's ability to carry on a variety of important activities and brings woes of its own. Sleeping with one's boss is a reasonably reliable way to get special treatment at work, but it may have a variety of less desirable consequences. Cultures may institute practices that effectively ameliorate the problems patients present them with, but at a great cost to other concerns of the patient or the patient's family and friends and compatriots. To say that a school of care or some particular practice is effective—even to prove it conclusively by rigorous outcome studies—is not necessarily to say much that is helpful.

In any case, different practices have different effects on patients' lives, whether or not they have different effects on the complaints that bring patients to treatment. This is a simple logical principle: A difference makes a difference; different events have different consequences. One school of thought may teach increased autonomy and self-assertion, while another may teach greater openness to dependency and love. Both may help their patients overcome depression. The patients, having been taught substantially different things, will probably live very differently from each other. Each will believe, most likely, that maintaining the way of life he has been taught is essential to remaining free from depression. Each has the authority of the therapy to justify that way of life. Furthermore, a therapy's influence on a patient has implications for people in the patient's life. The changes that the patient has come to believe are essential to his welfare simply have to be accommodated by the patient's significant others—in effect, because the therapist says so. The differences between cultures of healing do matter, then, and we can reasonably hope that science will eventually help us choose between them. For now, lack of a comprehensive science leaves us to the diverse vagaries of these many cultures.

The situation may be even worse. Therapists may actually teach people things that cost them and their associates a great deal without being any help at all—though they may appear to have caused improvement. A great many psychological problems cure themselves. Beginning in the early 1950s, a variety of studies showed that prospective patients on waiting lists improved as much as persons who actually received treatment. More recent epidemiological studies show that a great many people have suffered an episode of psychopathology that remitted spontaneously, without treatment, and did not recur. Since psychopathology can clear up spontaneously, what patients have learned from therapists probably has little or nothing to do with improvement in many cases. They have nonetheless acquired from therapy a host of beliefs and practices that affect their lives, sanctioned by the authority of the therapist, and both therapist and patient *believe* that the therapy caused the improvement. What the therapist says, though, may have more to do with fictions embedded in her culture, or with the current fashions of that culture, than with anything that helps.

When we mistake cultural norms for facts about nature, we create for ourselves a number of difficulties. When we claim that a culture's beliefs and practices are scientifically valid, these difficulties become more deeply embedded and more tenacious. Our ordinary tendency to stick with what we know gains reinforcement from the illusion of scientific validity, making our beliefs and practices more imperious than usual. Cultural norms seem all the more true and necessary when backed by the claim of scientific validity, and they become much harder to dislodge.

When social scientists developed the distinction between culture and nature, one of their major motivations was the belief that *what is cultural is optional and changeable*, in a manner more rapid and susceptible to choice, than what is natural. Presumably, mistaking culturally determined characteristics for naturally determined traits leads to serious misunderstandings over what is inevitable and what are matters of choice. All the debate and choice in the world do not change whatever "natural" gender differences there may be; for instance no man has ever carried an embryo through gestation to produce a child as the result of cultural debate or personal choice, and the differences in brain structure (whatever they may turn out to amount to) between men and women do not go away as the result of any regimen of willful effort. Culturally determined gender roles, though, can be changed or modulated. Similarly, if a particular ethnic group shows consistently lower birth weights or higher rates of incarceration, and if we discover that this is a result of historical and social contingencies rather than genetics, the cultural forces that create those conditions can be addressed and the group's traits changed. All the will and cultural change in the world, though, will not suddenly cause Japanese babies to be born with precisely the same enzymes, hormones, bone and tissue structure, and skin color as Italian babies. Culturally determined traits, then, are proper subjects for public debate and private choice; facts about nature are far more recalcitrant and more often require accommodation and acquiescence. To mistake cultural artifacts for natural facts gives culture an appearance of inevitability that it does not merit and undermines the freedom to think, feel, and choose.[21]

By the same measure, if scientists had discovered the things mental health care professionals claims are facts about nature, we would have to accommodate those facts. For example, if uncovering childhood conflicts that have been buried under years of repression and distortion were a necessary condition for resolving certain problems, good therapy for those problems would have to be psychoanalytic. If such notions about the origins and cure of these problems are not facts about nature, but artifacts of a certain culture of healing, they may be no more necessary than any other cultural practice. *Perhaps* patients need be no more concerned about their Oedipal issues than women need be concerned about ring-around-the-collar.

If schools of care are indeed best understood as cultures, a substantial portion of their beliefs and practices are optional. Nature does not require them. As we shall see, the schools of care

---

[21] The historian Carl Degler has written a wonderful, highly readable book, *In Search of Human Nature: The Decline and Rise of Darwinism in American Social Thought* (1991), that (among other things) explains the distinction between culture and nature and explores the politics (and science) behind changing fashions in American social science.

we now possess do not rest on discoveries of the sort, "This is how this particular psychopathology must be understood and treated." The beliefs of the schools of care are not analogous to discoveries about how to become pregnant or dissolve a kidney stone. When mental health professionals make statements about good mental health, they are *not* making statements analogous to a cardiologist's statements about a healthy heart. They are making statements more nearly analogous to a politician's description of traditional American values or someone's mom or Uncle Joe telling her how to get on with life.

This has another side: If schools of care had genuinely identified what it means to be psychologically healthy, we could use them to know what to aspire to—we would know that their visions of health are attainable and good for us. With cultures of healing, though, as with cultures generally, it is a bit different: Cultures sometimes demand of persons what is not possible, what constricts their development, or what has less to do with current reality than with the needs or interests of some bygone time and its archaic purposes. We can be about as certain that what cultures of healing promise us is possible and beneficial as that America can be whatever the current political hero tells us it can—and that we would be well off if it were.

For patients, to say that a school of care is a culture means that one's understanding of one's problems and their solution (and, presumably, some significant portion of one's life) will be determined by beliefs and practices that have more to do with the culture of healing into whose province one wanders than with reliable truths about human nature. *Culture* (it should go without saying) does not mean *cult:* Enculturation of patients and practitioners is not inherently nefarious. It does mean, though, that to be a patient of one sort of psychotherapist rather than another is to become a member of a different group, to believe differently, and thus to have a different life than one would have with some other sort of therapist. Such divergence is not because givers of care differ in their closeness to the truth, but because they are emissaries of different cultures. How one understands oneself and one's world, and so how one lives, differs because of the culture of healing one joins.

How to Think About Cultures of Healing

If schools of mental health care are best understood as cultures, we have to think about them differently than we generally do. We have to think about them as we think about any other culturally determined ideas and practices—as social and cultural critics.

To say that the ideas and practices of the cultures of healing substantially lack scientific validity is not to say that their views are false. Nor is it to say that, whether true or false, they are useless. It is only to say that they do not have the credentials they claim—something like having gotten the job with a false résumé. If our thesis is correct, though, no one with the right résumé exists; the scientific image of mental health care is simply not anything that anyone can fulfill, at present. So we cannot simply fire the mental health professionals and get someone else to do the job. Rather, we need to change the job description. We need to change the status of the mental health professions and how we listen to them.

If our thesis is correct, we need to take the stance that the cultures of healing offer a variety of visions of how the world works, what life is like, and how persons are supposed to be. We must be very careful about accepting any claims that those notions deserve the authority of scientific validity. We should see them as urging upon all of us culturally created ways of looking at life and its problems. We should see them as players in the moral discourse that constitutes the life of (and the lives in) our society. We would expect them to own up to this. That would mean that mental health professionals would talk to us—and among themselves—in a language appropriate to choosing how to live and choosing ideals to pursue. They would offer their recommendations in the language of moral and cultural choice more than the language of scientific discovery.

That does not mean we would ask the cultures of healing to give up the quest for a science of psychopathology and healing. Though certainly many critics of mental health care (and critics of science in general) would urge such a change, nothing we will see in the course of this book necessitates our giving up hope for that kind of care. But since the cultures of healing have yet to attain that, we will no longer give them authority based on the presumption that they have, but we will pay close attention to such science as they produce.

If our thesis is correct, we should regard the mental health professions differently than we do and they should occupy a different status than we have given them. The status to which the cultures of healing could, in principle, lay claim is that of *professions of the best guess*. Mental health professionals do devote themselves full-time to trying to understand human suffering and its relief, and there is more scientific work used in this endeavor than in many other efforts to relieve the sufferings of individuals. Theirs would be the *authority* of the best guess.

This is the authority of folk wisdom and craft raised to the level of full-time professions. In these professions, folk wisdom and craft are disciplined by standards of logic and evidence acquired through an extensive education devoted to pursuing truth by the best methods currently available. Mental health professionals who have succeeded at such an education, who continue to spend their time learning, who devote themselves to the craft of sitting with a suffering patient and offering the best they have in adroit and skillful ways—such people, I think, can say that they know as much as can be known about psychopathology at present. *What* they know, and how reliable it is, does not usually rise to the level of established science. Most of it is much more local and provisional. Each culture is a mélange of some things that may be essential to human life, some things imported from the values of the surrounding society, some of its members' disgruntlement with the surrounding society, and some singular imaginings about what makes life good.

When we think this through, we realize that the authority of the best guess is a severely restricted one. For much of what we need to know if we are to guess wisely falls outside the purview of current training for mental health care. Mental health professionals have no particular expertise about our society and its needs, for instance. They have no claim to special insight into the sociological realities that affect people's lives and that their own activities affect. Valuing—for another example—seems to be better understood by poets and philosophers (among intellectuals), and as well understood by all sorts of individuals, as by mental health professionals.

While those of us who spend our lives treating psychopathology have a special perspective to bring to the conversation, its peculiarities create limitations on what we can see. Others may have valuable things to say that would never occur to us, precisely *because* they do not labor under the need for a workable perspective with which to conduct mental health care. Precisely because they have no investment in the perspectives by which we orient our activities, they may be freer to recognize provinciality and bias. Precisely because they do not identify their personal worth with the ideas that govern our work—our self-esteem, after all, does turn, in part, on whether we think we are doing good—they have the freedom to see its less salutary effects. The best guess is still a guess, and other guesses may turn out to be closer to the truth.

To think about each culture, we can usefully distinguish between its descriptive and explanatory claims, on the one hand, and its evaluative claims, on the other. "Descriptive and explanatory claims" are simply putative descriptions of facts and explanations of how those facts work. "Evaluative claims" are evaluations of what, given those facts, we would be well advised to do. These do not come neatly separated; many evaluative claims, as we shall see, get smuggled in as descriptive and explanatory claims. When we try to evaluate a culture, though, we must try to tease out how it is recommending that we live—usually embodied in its claims about what is "healthy." In an ideal world, descriptive and explanatory claims would be matters of science, while evaluative claims would be subject to social and cultural criticism. That is not the world our cultures of healing populate.

With the current paucity of scientific knowledge, even the descriptive and explanatory claims of the cultures of healing should be a matter for social and cultural criticism. Where we know ideas to be true—where we have sound science—we have no choice but to believe them. Where we have to choose what to believe, without adequate evidence, what choice to make turns on considerations other than truth, such as "What would be the effects on life of *believing* this?" So in the current situation, social and cultural criticism has to be applied to the descriptive and explanatory notions that constitute a culture of healing's account of life, the world, and the particulars they comprise.

Not only mental health professionals and their patients have a legitimate stake in the conversation that determines what gets believed and taught by a culture of healing. The cultures of healing affect the lives of persons who never become patients and of our society as a whole. Spouses, children, friends, employers, and so forth all have an interest in what goes on in the cultures of healing. Where these cultures are not delivering ideas that are clearly true, everyone affected by the ideas has a legitimate role in evaluating the candidates for belief. The way it is now, ministers of care seem to believe that anyone else affected by the changes they work upon patients simply *must* accommodate those changes because they are "healthy." This is wrong; we do not know these changes to be healthy in any objective sense that should command the assent of all truth-respecting persons.

We see, then, two very different roles for social, cultural, and moral discourse in the cultures of healing. One is straightforward critique and reform of their evaluative claims. The other is participating in the conversation that determines even the descriptive and explanatory claims that the cultures promulgate. This is not to say that moral and cultural evaluation has any special privilege. Critics have to make their best guess, too, and the effects of holding various beliefs are matters of conjecture. Yet this sort of conjecture is what, I believe, we have to live with (and by), and we would do well to be honest about it.

In choosing what to believe and do about mental health, the general criterion we all—mental health professionals, patients and prospective patients, friends and families of patients, and anyone concerned with how the cultures of healing shape life in our society—need to use, for now, is not scientific validity so much as wisdom. To invoke wisdom as the criterion for belief and practice provides clarity less than it evokes a noble ideal. The problem with wisdom as a criterion, of course, is that it cannot be objectified, codified, and enshrined in regulations. Wisdom offers no univocal deliverance of truth. Training requirements and legal descriptions cannot call it into being or give anyone a monopoly over it. If wisdom is the best criterion we can adopt, we may be settling for something other than we had wanted. Yet, it seems to me, what we want is not possible, for now.

What We Might Wish For

None of this is to say that we should abandon the ideal of scientifically based mental health care. *Wanting* a science of psychopathology is probably a good thing. As we shall see, the explosion of medical and technological knowledge in the late nineteenth century raised hopes that mental and emotional problems would soon be as well understood and treated as physical problems. The mature medical sciences have succeeded spectacularly; in general, people in the industrialized countries no longer die of infectious disease (except for AIDS), for instance. The wish for an equally powerful science of psychopathology is not, in principle, inconceivable or obviously ridiculous.

When we talk about "health," we are talking about an organism functioning as it should. A healthy liver does certain things; if it does not do those things, it is unhealthy. When we speak of someone's being "in good health," we mean that person's body is working as it should. Presumably, when we speak of "mental health," we mean the same thing: The mind is as it should be. When we speak of mental disorders, obviously enough, it would seem that we mean that the mind, like an unhealthy liver, is failing at its essential functions.

Conceivably, as with the clearly mature medical sciences, the complaints of patients that really *deserve* to be classed as disease might involve failures of essential functions of being a person. The idea of "essential functions of being a person" scares a fair number of people—as well it should, since the idea so easily becomes a way of enforcing a particular society's notions of how people ought to be. "How a mind should be" easily slips from the "should" of "fitness to design" into the moral "should." A good many critics of mental health care have claimed that "mental health" is mostly a way of medicalizing our society's values. While there is much to this charge—we will see quite a bit of it in the course of this book—the *idea* of a science of psychology and a corollary science of psychopathology is quite the opposite. If we really had such science, mistaking a certain culture's values and habits for the way people are supposed to be would no longer be possible. A good science of nutrition tells us a great deal about what human bodies have to have to be healthy, but it does not tell us what dishes we must prepare and enjoy. It does not tell us that one country's cuisine is the right one and no other can be chosen. Even so, a science of psychopathology would not enshrine one society's ways of life as healthy.

A science explicating such important facts of nature—essential functions of mind and the consequences of their impairment—seems a worthy goal. Certainly this is the sort of science Freud thought he was creating, the sort that others who proclaim a scientific basis for mental health care either implicitly or explicitly lay claim to. We need to be clear, though, what a large goal this is. *Believing* that we *could* have professions based on such a science requires several large leaps of faith, and the whole idea of mental "health" is fair game for skeptics who do not want to take them. To start with, the very idea of a science of mental health requires us to believe that there are indeed essential characteristics of human psychological life, analogous to essential functions of livers, kidneys, hearts, and so forth. Then we have to believe that deficiencies in those functions cause serious distress—presumably the distress that people bring to mental health professionals for treatment. We also have to believe that fulfilling those traits (or compensating in some way for deficiencies) would alleviate patients' distress. Finally, we have to believe that science can discover both those traits and ways to remedy deficits. Perhaps one or more of these ideas is illusory.

People who believe there cannot be any such science will certainly agree with one strand of the thesis of this book: that our image of mental health care as scientific is wrong. They will say more: that science can never provide such knowledge, so care can never be scientific. That seems a rather strong position to take, and a dangerous one: Science is forever managing to do what critics have gravely pronounced it cannot.

Some problems of some patients (schizophrenics, manic-depressives, agoraphobics, and the like) obviously *seem* to be deficits relative to essential traits. Whether other problems (the problems of most patients) merit a similar appraisal is less obvious. One result of a good science of psychopathology might be to shrink radically the number of people who should be receiving mental health care. If that is so, we have to hope for something else: that people other than mental health professionals take charge of research. For mental health professionals are unlikely to get around to discovering that the market for their services should be shrunk. Quite conceivably, the need of the mental health professions to expand their market may be part of the reason that we lack an adequate science of psychopathology; the professions themselves may have managed to blur the issues in their quest for more patients and a larger stake in society. Perhaps by claiming too much the mental health professions have made sure they know too little. Perhaps by claiming that an extraordinary range of complaints result from mental and emotional disorders, and by offering their peculiar kind of expertise as the remedy for that whole range of unease, they have included in the definition of "disorder" all sorts of things that have nothing to do with failures in essential human traits. That, we may well suppose, would make it very difficult to discern from the population of patients just what the normal and abnormal traits of persons are. We may reasonably suppose that it would also give the institutions of mental health care a strong incentive not to find a more accurate way of demarcating psychopathology from the distress that healthy humans are prey to.

We might even hope that a good science of psychopathology would give our society precisely this demarcation. We might hope to be able to know which of our difficulties reflect something wrong with us and which we simply have to find ways to cope with. We might want to know which of the demands our family, friends, and compatriots place upon us in the name of mental health should be acceded to and which we can deal with some other way. We might want to see the creation of professions that help us with nonpathological emotional distress and confusion about life, without conferring the stigma of mental illness.

That might be nice: a profession that does for our perfectly healthy psychological needs what engineers and architects do for our need for shelter. Of course, health insurance might not pay for that kind of thing—so perhaps some of us would not want to see successful demarcation between pathological and ordinary distress.

Hoping for a science of psychopathology and its cure is legitimate. Recognizing what is involved in this large hope will help us put the current status of mental health care in perspective.

Where We Will Come Out

Understanding schools of care as cultures will not resolve the very real problems that currently exist in mental health care, but it will give us a way to think about our current situation more wisely.

As we rethink the image of mental health care, the perplexities posed by the diverse cultures of healing take on a different appearance. If we stop thinking that the disparate visions of these cultures amount to scientific discoveries about human nature, the mere existence of diversity will not seem like a refutation of the (revised) claims of mental health professions. Diversity will simply seem like a reflection of the multiple possibilities that need to be considered. The conundrum posed by the effectiveness of such incommensurate schools also takes on a different aspect. If a culture manages to get itself into existence, we may assume that it captures something that some significant number of people find helpful. This does not mean that one is "as good as another," nor does it mean we have to value all effective forms of practice. Perhaps some ways of getting over depression (for example) cost us too much, as persons and a society. Perhaps some cultures consist of some good practices and some bad ideas—they may try to trick up from some effective practices an entire system of thought that, in its erroneous effort at universality, leads us into blind alleys. Diverse cultures each need to be evaluated, but how we evaluate them will be different than the evaluations appropriate against the backdrop of the scientific image of care.

The diversity of cultures probably has a great deal to do with the different temperaments and the intellectual and personal styles of the persons who have developed and populate them. The time may come when a science of psychopathology makes clear some one general view that all givers of legitimate care should adopt; that view, whatever it might be, could prove uncongenial to a great many people who now find providing care to be a very meaningful and fulfilling way to make a living. If it turns out that mental health care is principally to be a matter of medication, humanistic types are not going to be happy as mental health care professionals. If it turns out that humanistic types are closer to right, behaviorists will be unable to abide these ways of making a living. For now, though, we can really make no objection to persons pursuing what they love in a manner that suits who they are, so long as they are honest about what they do and do not know.

If we are going to have professions of mental health care in the absence of mature science, we probably do well to have different groups pursuing different possibilities. We do not yet know from which of the current cultures, if any, a comprehensive school of care would emerge. Perhaps none of our current cultures offer much that would someday appear in a comprehensive school of care; but that is all the more reason to hope for new cultures to arise. The competition between scientists for priority in discovery is one of the significant engines of progress. Thus, we have a positive reason to support the existence of a multitude of competing cultures.

If we are going to have mental health care at all, we also have a good reason to support cultures, rather than having every therapist make up her own version of care. (Unfortunately, we have too much of that going on at present, anyway, usually in the guise of eclecticism. We will consider that issue in the last chapter). *At least* cultures of care constitute *communities* of inquiry; *something* approximating mutual aid and peer review is possible within each culture. Having givers of care trained in and responsible to some culture that has managed to survive seems to increase the likelihood that pure idiosyncrasy will not govern the therapist's work. Too, persons who think in similar terms and share a common history will be available, in print and in person, to help the therapist think and learn. For all the reasons that community is preferable to isolation, cultures of healing are preferable to a host of therapists making up things on their own.

Since, then, there are good reasons to see cultures as beneficial and good reasons to think that multiple perspectives are to be desired at present, it would seem a good thing that we have multiple cultures. For this to be a good thing, though, we need to learn to think of them *as* cultures. We have to learn to think of them *without* imparting to them the authority of scientific truth. We have to look at each pragmatically, morally, and culturally to see whether it offers beliefs and practices that seem good. If we can think of the schools of care as cultures, we can choose among, rather than submit to, what they would have us believe and do.

If we can recognize that the schools of care for psychopathology constitute cultures, and if we can learn to think of them in terms of social and cultural criticism, we will be far less likely to believe and do what "experts say" we should believe and do. "Experts" will think of themselves and talk to others differently— more humbly, we may hope, more conversationally, listening as much as pronouncing. We will *all*—professionals in the field, patients, observers, policy makers—have a richer repertoire once we recognize these beliefs and practices to be the results of culture, not necessity. We may have also less faith in our healers— and that could be a problem. We will return to that topic in the final chapter.

Persons suffer, and the cultures of healing try to help them. But the cultures, and the particular therapists who populate and are formed by them, do much more than this. The cultures build up institutions, claim legitimacy and prestige and authority in society, find ways to secure their livelihoods, do things to reassure themselves of their value, and generally seek to satisfy all the most mundane and primordial needs of humans creating lives for themselves. The cultures of healing are joint creations of our society and of the persons (both practitioners and patients) who live within each culture. To understand mental health care, so that we can participate in its reform, we need to understand the social needs and dynamics that gave birth to the cultures of healing. We need to understand the multiple needs the cultures serve—and how some of those needs have little to do with the care of patients. We need to understand the traditions and institutions—and their habits of mind and action—that make care what it is. Since cultures are inherently historical entities, shaped by and living out of their histories, we must understand their histories to understand what moves their current life. Thus, we turn to an historical look at how we came to have cultures of healing at all.

Chapter Two

PROBLEMS AND PATIENTS, 1844–1963

IN NEURASTHENIA ONE SEES MIRRORED THE MORE GENERAL APPREHENSION OF THE MIDDLE CLASS VIS-À-VIS MODERNITY. . . .
DOCTORS IN THE VICTORIAN AGE SEEMED UNAWARE THAT THEY FREQUENTLY FAILED TO SEPARATE MORALITY FROM MEDICINE. . . . [I]N HIS THEORIZING [THE DOCTOR] BLINDLY BROUGHT TO THE BEDSIDE . . . HIS OWN COMMERCIAL VIRTUES OF SOBRIETY, HARD WORK, WILL POWER, DOMINATION OF THE EXTERNAL WORLD—ALL THE CHARACTERISTICS THAT HAD HELPED HIM PLOD FORWARD AND BECOME A MIDDLE CLASS DOCTOR.

—*George Drinka*
The Birth of Neurosis

LIKE MEDICAL RESEARCH, PSYCHIATRY HAD EMERGED FROM WORLD WAR II WITH AN ENHANCED PUBLIC IMAGE. BUT WHEREAS THE ACHIEVEMENTS OF MEDICAL RESEARCH HAD LED TO RECOGNITION, THE RECOGNITION OF PSYCHIATRY DURING THE WAR WAS, QUITE LIKELY, ITS GREATEST ACHIEVEMENT.

—*Paul Starr*
The Social Transformation of American Medicine

AMERICANS, INCLUDING PROFESSIONALS in mental health care, have never agreed for any substantial period of time on what counts as a problem requiring care, who is likely to have such problems, what causes these problems, or who is fit to treat them—and how. Professional care for mental health has evolved from giving "moral therapy" to the clearly deranged to claiming to offer, in the name of scientific advance, access to life reasonably free from emotional distress. The energizing notion underlying the fragmented, often chaotic, history of mental health care has been the wish that normal life need not involve too much misery. This is a social and cultural notion—which has shown itself in all of our technological and political efforts of the last two centuries to make life more pleasant and free from harshness—and the general culture of mental health care has been vouchedsafe stewardship over its psychological dimension.[22]

Psychiatrists developed the first organized medical specialty in America, in 1844. By 1955, mental health care had become a pervasive national concern, as evidenced by the creation by Congress of the Joint Commission on Mental Illness and Health in that year. In 1963, the Community Mental Health Centers Act was passed, institutionalizing this concern as a matter of the welfare

[22] No general history of mental health care in America has, to my knowledge, ever been written. There exists, though, an excellent body of history on the insane asylums and mental hospitals; Gerald Grob's *The Mad Among Us: A History of the Care of America's Mentally Ill* is an excellent book for the lay audience. Paul Starr's *The Social Transformation of American Medicine* contains excellent sections on the evolution of psychiatry. Nathan Hale, Jr.'s, *Freud and the Americans* is an extraordinary record of mental health care in the late nineteenth and early twentieth centuries. George Drinka's *The Birth of Neurosis* covers European developments more than American ones but nonetheless has excellent sections on the latter. Elliot Valenstein's *Great and Desperate Cures* gives an excellent account of the "radical" cures and their historical contexts. John M. Reisman's *A History of Clinical Psychology* (2d ed.) is very valuable. Jay Ehrenwald has edited a compendium of various writings, with comments on the place of each in the history of care, called *The History of Psychotherapy*. While the commentary is not very good history, the book has its uses as a compilation of texts.

of the nation. Notions of mental illness and health, and the attendant professions of care, bore little or no resemblance to the 1844 versions. In 1844, physicians who cared for mental illness presided over artificial communities—asylums—in rural settings, providing restorative care for the clearly insane. In 1963, mental health care pervaded—or aimed to pervade—the lives of ordinary persons in ordinary communities. Mental health care evolved from a peripheral vocation (offering asylum to the insane) to a central place in contemporary society (offering to lead ordinary people to mentally healthy life).

In the process, the entire notion of mental illness has been transformed. Most people who visit givers of care today would not have been considered candidates for care in 1844, nor would their peers have thought that they suffered from mental illness. Now huge numbers of people explain almost everything, from problems at work to problems at home to failed love affairs, in terms of psychopathology—generally, of course, the psychopathology of others.

We need to understand several strands of America's history with what we now call psychopathology if we are to understand the current state of mental health care. We need to see how insanity—which is a folk term long predating the idea of psychopathology—came to be seen as an illness and how it came under the care of medicine. We also need to understand how the *other* problems of life that now constitute the bulk of the mental health care market—what came to be called neuroses (though the term has been officially dropped from psychiatry in the last decade)— came to be seen as psychopathology. We need to understand how the various mental health professions arose. The overarching question is this: How did we get into the confused place we now occupy, with so many different types of professions partaking in mental health care?

Insanity, the Asylums, and the First Medical Specialty

Not much more than two centuries ago, there was, so far as anyone knew, no such thing as psychopathology, and no such thing as a psychiatrist, psychologist, psychiatric social worker, or mental health counselor. Some persons were insane or lunatic: "afflicted" with debilitating problems and behaviors, "deprived of their reason." Such persons were certainly problems—and obligations. They were people who, for differing lengths of time and to differing degrees, could not care for themselves; they had to be cared for by the community in which they lived. Where families were unable to care for such persons, they customarily fell under the care of their hometown. Explanations of their difficulties varied, and attitudes ranged from superstitious fear to righteous condemnation to loving kindness. Insanity was an intrusive occurrence in the life of a family and community, which forced attention by its very obviousness.

As America, like other Western societies, changed in the late eighteenth and nineteenth centuries, persons who could not care for themselves became a different kind of problem than they had been in more communal times. The rising individualism of the nineteenth century, the decline in community cohesion under the influence of urbanization and economic mobility, and the Protestant ethos of the Great Revivalism of that century made each person responsible for him or herself. At the same time, the spreading influence of the Enlightenment made common the notion of secular perfectibility and the image of a normal person as a rational, free, progressive individual. These Enlightenment beliefs bolstered the idea that problems with being an independent, rational, responsible person were defects relative to human nature—shortcomings. Rising individualism, Protestant meliorism and perfectibility, and the Enlightenment ideal of normal persons as rational individuals coalesced in American culture. The implication for the insane was that such persons were defective, relative to what a person is naturally.

To think of someone as suffering and therefore in need of care, or problematic and therefore in need of management, is quite different from thinking of a person as defective and therefore in need of remediation. Moreover, we can think of people as defective and in need of remediation in any of a variety of ways—for instance, morally defective or spiritually defective and therefore in need of improvements in character and religious devotion. Thinking of certain kinds of mental and emotional suffering as due to defects *relative to human nature* is a crucial turn in the development of the idea of psychopathology. Exemplifying the essential traits of one's nature is a different thing than being morally or spiritually just; the latter have always been considered accomplishments, not a matter of the natural state of being human. Relieving suffering is one thing, and achieving some transcendent rightness is another. Restoring a person to a normal state is a different matter altogether. The search for normalcy and the assumption that it is the job of the mental health worker to restore a defective person to a normal state are crucial elements of most cultures of healing.

Thus, the founding ideas of mental health care derived from viewing insanity—as psychopathology—under the influences of nineteenth century culture.

Doctors for the Insane

Insanity was neither discovered nor defined by the persons into whose care the insane fell: Insanity was fundamentally a folk term, and the insane were already identified as a social category long before doctors began caring for them.[23] The malady was not clearly defined in any explicit way; in a homogeneous culture, in which prevailing norms are considered right, in some absolute or transcendently justified sense, deviations substantial enough to merit the label of "insanity" were assumed to be obvious.

There was no intrinsic reason for care for the insane to fall to physicians in the nineteenth century; that they came under the care of doctors is as much a matter of historical accident as professional aptitude. Actually, humane care for the insane was

---

[23] Some historians, failing to note that "insanity" was a folk term, commit the anachronism of pointing out that many of the persons cared for in asylums were "really" suffering from organic illnesses, such as epilepsy, Alzheimer's, retardation, or the like, with the implication that such persons were under psychiatric care by error or ignorance. Insane people were, though, simply those who manifested obstreperous, persistent, or intense modes of thinking and behavior that were, by someone's measure, delusional or out of touch with what was taken to be reality. To impose contemporary medical definitions of psychosis on nineteenth-century folk notions of insanity is simply a conceptual error.

pioneered by religious organizations, and doctors in need of work took advantage of opportunities created by religious and philanthropic organizations. By the time that persons "deprived of their reason" came to be seen as defective persons and by the time that the social dynamics in America had shifted sufficiently that communities and families no longer accepted such persons as obligations to be taken care of, American medicine was generally in disrepute.

Before the late nineteenth century, Americans placed no more confidence in physicians, whatever their background and training (and a fair number had some sort of legitimate medical training, some in Europe), than they did in a variety of other forms of healing. Indeed, in the nineteenth century physicians became objects of contempt: Their "heroic" measures of bloodletting, blistering, and medicating with potent and noxious minerals and chemicals had shown no obvious therapeutic superiority over folk, botanical, and other forms of healing, while they obviously inflicted much more suffering. American doctors in general were neither especially well educated nor well trained. Even the most prestigious medical schools, such as Harvard and the University of Pennsylvania, did not require that their students have prior college educations, and the curriculum consisted of two four-month terms of lectures—with little or no laboratory or clinical training. Most physicians trained, if at all, in far less prestigious institutions—many of them commercial, proprietary schools—or as apprentices. Many states repealed licensure laws in the first two or three decades of the nineteenth century, on the grounds that there was no profession of medicine worthy of state sanction. Folk remedies, homeopathy, and a variety of other styles of healing rivaled or surpassed medicine in public patronage.

Medical men had difficulty making a living. At mid-century, the average doctor's income was about that of a skilled laborer, distinctly lower middle class, and young doctors generally had a hard time establishing a practice that gave them even that level of income. When states and charities began creating asylums for the humane care of the insane, some of these medical men found in them an opportunity for steady employment and full-time work. Positions as superintendents of the new asylums offered young physicians a steady income several times greater than they could expect if they tried to survive in the medical market, as well as living quarters, authority over a substantial institution, and respectability in the religious and philanthropic circles that sponsored the first asylums. Little wonder that a number of physicians saw the asylums as an excellent career opportunity.

The early asylums served two distinct purposes: providing society respite from the disorder and difficulties imposed by the insane, and providing the insane respite—asylum—from the demands of social life. Care in asylums followed, for the most part, regimens of "moral treatment" developed by Phillipe Pinel, a French physician, and William Tuke, an English merchant and devout Quaker with strong ties to American Quakers. Both Pinel and Tuke were dismissive of attempts to deal with insanity through medical means then available in Europe; neither found any value in the various nostrums and technologies deployed in the name of medicine. Both saw the road to recovery as a moral road: Insane persons needed opportunities to develop, sheltered from the demands of a world that was too much for them to bear. Contrary to the image of asylums that eventually became part of popular consciousness—as snakes pits, in which patients were chained in crowded, filthy dungeons and subjected to abuse—the early American asylums aimed, and to a substantial extent succeeded, at providing humane care for the insane. The superintendents of these institutions gave personal, kindly, supportive attention to patients, and staff were chosen with an eye to their character and willingness to work with the insane in helpful ways (and to submit to the authority of the superintendent). Moral treatment consisted of carefully orchestrated schedules of productive labor, spiritual and cultural improvement, socializing, entertainment, education, nutrition, and exercise. In short, moral treatment consisted of regimens designed to let insane people become what, it was assumed, all persons ought to, and presumably could, become. Asylums aimed to be restorative communities.

We must understand that physicians taking charge of hospitals and asylums was not a usual practice before this. Asylums, like hospitals, did not originally exist as medical institutions. Hospitals originated as places of refuge for the indigent, infirm, and dependent. Both asylums and hospitals were designed to offer care for persons who could not care for themselves, and both antedate by centuries the medical functions with which they came to be identified late in the nineteenth century. We generally do not realize today that prior to the very end of the nineteenth century, hospitals were highly feared places of contagion, not healing centers. The denizens of hospitals were rife with disease. Physicians had no special charge there, merely visiting hospitals and asylums to give such care as they could—without charge—to the people who lived there. That a class of physicians should come to identify themselves with care for the insane was initially a function of this peculiar development: that a class of doctors came to have their livelihood associated with taking charge of insane asylums. Such was the birth of the profession of psychiatry. Psychiatry did not originate with medical discoveries taken into humanitarian fields, but with humanitarian ideals over which certain medical men came to exercise stewardship for economic and social reasons.

American medical men in the nineteenth century wanted to achieve the prestige and power of Old World physicians. In Europe, physicians were generally highly educated (in England, for instance, members of the Royal Society of Physicians were graduates of Oxford or Cambridge), presided over a corps of subordinate surgeons and apothecaries, and were received into polite society. American physicians longed for similar standing in society. The medical men who came to oversee asylums were no different. In 1844—two years prior to the formation of the American Medical Association—thirteen of them gathered to form the Association of Medical Superintendents of American Institutions for the Insane (AMSAII). Thus, care for insanity became the first organized medical specialty in America.

The AMSAII undertook a vigorous, effective—and, we may fairly say, fraudulent—campaign to promote medical control over asylums and to ensure that their own views of care would be promulgated among the public and followed in other asylums.[24] The

---

[24] For a detailed account of the AMSAII, see Constance M. McGovern, *Masters of Madness* (1985).

original thirteen members maintained tight control over the offices and committees of the association to ensure uniformity of policy. The superintendents published annual reports, distributing them widely to libraries, policy makers, journalists, and anyone else with a possible interest in the asylums. In these reports, they extolled their own virtues at length, excoriated alternative forms of treatment, and boasted grossly inflated cure rates based on consciously manipulated statistics. (Statistical tricks included, for example, calculating cure rates on the basis of the percentage *released* who were deemed cured, leaving out of account all who stayed behind and ignoring relapses among those who had been deemed cured—or counting them as new and distinct cases.) Journalists were invited to the association's meetings; an official photographer was hired to record its activities. As the association succeeded at making itself the publicly recognized authority on care of the insane, its officers also became highly influential in determining who received appointments as superintendents, as their views were usually sought on nominees. In choosing persons to recommend, they considered political savvy and ability to deal with the public to be vital qualifications; no matter how highly regarded the work of some assistant physician might be, if he was not regarded as politically able he would not receive the endorsement of the association's elders. The association took as one of its principal tasks the shaping of public policy toward, and state regulation of, asylums. Within a few years of its founding, the AMSAII made itself the principal force in care for the insane.

For the most part, this influence was benevolent enough. The association assiduously guarded the highest principles of moral treatment and vigorously opposed all use of unnecessary restraints, bloodletting, harsh medication, treatment by any form of physical or emotional shock, and punishment.

The AMSAII effectively made care for the insane a principally medical specialty, though there was little the superintendents did that required any special scientific or medical knowledge. Nonmedical superintendents of asylums, no matter how influential or esteemed, were excluded from participation in the organization, and only medical persons were recommended for superintendencies by the association. Even the most famous nonmedical advocates of humane care for the insane, such as Dorothea Dix, were never allowed to join the organization, even in honorary positions. This creation of a new medical field created a body of medical professionals who had personal and professional interests in sustaining the field of psychiatry—and keeping others out of it. Once the medical superintendents had created this profession, more and more physicians sought employment in it, so that there was an increasing constituency within the medical profession for preserving medical privilege in care for the insane.

The association's more obviously detrimental effects included obstructing the development of more scientific approaches to treatment for the insane. Little or no scientific research, or even attempts at it, were done by the ruling elders of the association—one does not find the names of any of the superintendents among the pioneers in observing and categorizing the phenomena of mental illness. The conservative, nonscientific orthodoxy of the association would have significant ramifications by the end of the century and well into the next, when psychiatry would find itself held in low regard by practitioners of the emerging scientific medicine.

Moreover, the emphasis of the association on institutionalization worked to the detriment of psychiatrists, in a variety of ways. Insanity was never very well defined by psychiatrists, and persons who were problems to their families or society for all sorts of reasons were committed to institutions. Many state commitment laws, for instance, allowed husbands to commit their wives summarily. Though some of these persons would no doubt, by today's standards, have been in need of some kind of care, the rather indiscriminate classification of problematic persons as insane, followed by involuntary confinement to asylums, did much to discredit the psychiatrists. Beginning in the mid-1860s, cases of sane (however troublesome) persons committed by those to whom they were aggravations came to public attention. Such cases, to be sure, were the small minority of commitments, but they made good reading and received wide publicity. At the opposite end of the patient population, the chronically mentally ill, old persons suffering from senility, persons in the advanced stages of syphilis, the mentally retarded, and a host of other incurables came into the asylums, where they remained for years. In the first years of the asylums, a mix of these serious cases and those who were temporarily deranged or despondent or truculent encouraged the illusion that substantial numbers were being helped. As the sufferers of transitory problems left, and the chronically ill stayed, the asylums quickly became primarily custodial institutions. The claims of the psychiatrists to be able to cure mental illness came to be seen as quite obviously false; no amount of falsifying statistics could hide the fact that huge numbers of people who entered the asylums were staying for years. The crushing load of the chronically ill became a disincentive for young doctors to pursue a career in psychiatry. So little was known of how to help such people, who were so often difficult to deal with, that psychiatry became less appealing as other medical specialties developed in the nineteenth century.

Institutionalization as the principal—indeed, the only—mode of care also precluded care for persons who were troubled but functional or well supported by families. Inherent in the notion of moral treatment was isolation from society for a period of time sufficient to allow for a moral reordering of the patient's life. For persons who were genuinely suffering, but who were not without loving families or social ties (and whose problems were not so noxious that their intimates wanted to be rid of them), institutionalization for a substantial period of time was not necessarily an attractive option. Nor did institutionalization make sense for those whose difficulties were not far advanced. The superintendents' view of care for mental problems was analogous to insisting that no one could ever get care for an illness unless it were life threatening—as if, for instance, one never treated, say, bronchitis unless it became a serious case of pneumonia. Since the care offered in asylums was not particularly effective, we may doubt whether this was a great loss to potential patients. However, we can be sure that it was a great loss to physicians, who were thereby cut off from studying the sorts of problems that would come to dominate mental health care.

The hegemony of the medical superintendents lasted less than twenty years. By the mid-1860s, the asylums were overburdened with the chronically ill, public suspicion of the psychiatrists and their institutions had reached a significant level, and the states— growing wary of the dictatorial authority that the medical superintendents exercised within the asylums—began appointing boards of charity to oversee them, taking control out of the hands of the medical men. As we shall see shortly, new approaches to dealing with psychopathology were developing, and the medical superintendents and their assistant physicians failed to learn from these new approaches—or perhaps more accurately, they failed both to participate in such enterprises and to go along with the faith that such approaches would someday lead to scientific understanding and control of psychopathology. By 1875, the superintendents were being harshly criticized by other physicians, legal authorities, the religious and philanthropic organizations to which they owed their origins, and the public. The AMSAII was reduced to impotent fulminating (in the form of various formal resolutions to which no one outside the organization paid attention) against the controls that were being exercised upon them—and the loss of power and prestige that this entailed.

The profession also suffered from the clash of its rigidity with the effects of its own successes. The second generation of doctors who joined the profession were in many cases interested in contemporary advances in scientific medicine, but they found that interest unwelcome in the association. As the old guard died off and the younger doctors gained influence in the profession, internal tensions led the association into a period of confusion of purpose. Until the younger men assumed control early in the twentieth century, the association became an ineffective, divided shadow of its former self. While other doctors began to usurp the prerogative of treating the mentally discomfited, especially those who did not desire institutionalization, and as general hospitals began to achieve respectability and to offer psychiatric care without submitting to the authority of the association, younger members were confined to more or less decorous but vain attempts to make the profession more dynamic.

The difficulties of the association show themselves in a series of events in the mid- to late 1880s. The first problem had to do with the issue of membership for assistant physicians in the organization. There were, by 1880, more assistant physicians than superintendents. Most were younger, many were better trained, most had more direct patient contact than the superintendents (who had become, for all practical purposes, administrators of huge custodial institutions, rarely engaged in direct patient care), and a fair number had some interest in the emerging sciences. They were not eligible for membership in the organization that was the only game in town for physicians working in the asylums. A series of debates on the issue in the 1880s resulted in *ex officio* membership for the assistant physicians. It was not until 1892, when the name and avowed purpose of the organization changed, that assistant physicians became eligible for associate membership, followed by eligibility for full membership after three years' experience.

In 1887, a committee of the AMSAII recommended a variety of changes in the "propositions" that had governed association orthodoxy and the activities of asylums. Though the committee report emphasized the administrative role of the profession and did not challenge the authority of the superintendents, it did call for future appointments of superintendents who were competent scientists. The resolutions were defeated by the full body, but so was an attempt to reaffirm the old principles. The paralysis of the organization stood forth in bold relief.

The change of the organization's name, in 1892, to the American Medico-Psychological Association (AMPA), was accompanied by a new statement of purpose: to study all things pertaining to mental disease. The change was more expressive of hope than indicative of reality; for the psychiatrists were already far behind the medical community at large, and neurologists in particular, in moving toward a scientific basis (or self-image) for mental health care. Indeed, psychiatry declined from the first, most secure medical profession to a marginalized specialty, generally looked down on by other physicians. Yet the change of name and purpose indicated a release from old moorings, if not yet a passage to new seas.

Nerve Doctors, a New Disease, and the Dream of Science

One of the first groups to begin usurping the role of the psychiatrists was the neurologists—we shall call them "nerve doctors" here, to distinguish the practitioners who called themselves neurologists from the scientists who investigated the structure and functions of the nervous system. Nerve doctors addressed patient populations ignored by the psychiatrists—including all those who needed care but not institutionalization—and participated actively in the medical and nascent scientific communities. Study of the nervous system began to have significant success in Europe by the mid-nineteenth century, and the substantial number of head injuries resulting from the Civil War prompted acute interest in neurology. By 1875, there were enough medical men specializing in neurology for the founding of the American Neurological Association.

Before scientific medicine arose, when medicine was still an offshoot of philosophy, explanations for disease followed the classical model of philosophical explanation: to reduce the phenomena to "first principles," in which all phenomena were understood as due to the operation of one unified system. Disease and health were understood to be manifestations of such systems. Whether the system was the balance of bodily humors, heat and cold, solids and fluids, or the tension of blood in the vessels, diseases and health were assumed to be manifestations of a single set of principles.[25] Once nerves began to be isolated by anatomists in the seventeenth century, various medical theorists began to take states of the nerves as the underlying principles of their systems of natural philosophy, and the ancient illnesses were subsumed under the heading of "nervousness"—latinized to "neurosis" by William Cullen in the eighteenth century.[26] To see the eighteenth-century theorists of nervousness as forerunners of neurologists would be a bit misleading. Of the many systems of explanation available to

---

[25] The notion of health as a function of the "balance" of bodily substances is an example of how archaic ideas linger and inform later thought. As late as the mid-twentieth century, a fair number of neuroscientists assumed they would find brains working according to balanced systems—sympathetic balanced by parasympathetic, one chemical having a corollary in a counterfunction, and the like. That has turned out not to be true. Among the nonscientific cognoscenti who think themselves *au courant*, one frequently hears these days that scientists are discovering that this, that, or the other is due to a "chemical imbalance in the brain." In fact, what little is known about the neurophysiology of mental illness has nothing to do with balances at all. Yet Western thinking has so long assumed a balance of first principles that this way of thinking continues to carry a specious credibility.

[26] See Norman Dain, *Concepts of Insanity in the United States, 1789–1865* (1964).

eighteenth-century physicians, those based on nerve states were one set among many, and the men who formulated them chose the nerves because they were new and therefore interesting—not because of what was known about them. Since there were few known functions of the nerves until well into the nineteenth century, the nerve theories of the eighteenth and early nineteenth centuries were highly speculative. For the most part, they translated older philosophical theories into newer anatomic terms. To see these eighteenth- and early nineteenth-century nerve theorists as forward thinking would probably be an error. They just happened to speculate about structures that would eventually be found to be central to mental functioning. They bet on the right horse.

Though these theories played little or no role in the development of neurology, they set the tone for the late nineteenth-century nerve doctors. The eighteenth-century nerve theorists all postulated (in various forms and with diverse rationales) that nervous problems resulted from the stresses and strains of civilized life. Spicy foods, debauchery, masturbation, overwork, excessive thinking, and a host of other quintessentially civilized (in the eyes of these theorists) activities were thought to abrade or weaken the nerves in one way or another. This would come to be the principal doctrine of the late nineteenth-century nerve doctors.

The accomplishments of scientific neurology in the mid- to late eighteenth century included identification of the reflex arc (by Marshall Hull), locating parts of the brain that controlled certain bodily functions (by such luminaries as Paul Broca and Carl Wernicke), and discovering that the nervous system is made up of millions of discrete neurons (as formulated by H.W. Waldeyer). Though neurology proper did not yield any therapeutic progress in the nineteenth century, neurologists succeeded in showing that mental functions were related to the nerves in specifiable ways.

These neurological advances took place in a context of astounding scientific achievement. The last half of the nineteenth century saw the sciences leap ahead by orders of magnitude. This dramatic change in the body of human knowledge included sciences pertinent to health—medicine as we know it had its birth here. The germ theory of disease led to discoveries of a great many pathogens and, with the invention of antisepsis, to the control of many diseases that had hitherto been public scourges. Antisepsis and, a few years later, asepsis, made surgery a much safer procedure than the deadly gamble it had always been. Combined with the development of anaesthesia, sterile operating conditions made surgery in the last decades of the century a stunningly progressive field. Surgeons could take their time rather than rush through operations on patients who were not anesthetized. Infection was rarer, so surgery became more therapeutic, less a matter of desperate measures in dire cases. These developments, together with new technologies, made it possible to explore new surgical procedures and to develop surgical treatments for many conditions (such as appendicitis and gall bladder problems) that had previously been untreatable or left to the vagaries of systemic medications. Surgery bolstered the therapeutic success of medicine.

The heady days of scientific advance in the last half of the nineteenth century produced the illusion that nature was about to give up all its mysteries. Technology leapt forward, and the discovery of electromagnetism and the harnessing of electricity for productive work captured the public imagination. When it was proved that the nervous system is electrical, and when Helmholtz succeeded in measuring the speed of electrical transmission along the nerves, the stage was set for the nerve doctors to produce their own version of neurotic etiology and cure. In the general intoxication with the wonders of the new sciences, it took little to give the nerve doctors credibility. Unlike the psychiatrists, who drew both their ideological and institutional bases from religious and philanthropic notions, the nerve doctors identified themselves, in both their self-image and the image they presented to the public, with the most current scientific investigations.

If the nerve doctors were to find firm footing within the emerging scientific medicine, they would have to make good on their claim to cure diseases of mind. To do that, they needed to identify those diseases. Unlike the psychiatrists, who worked with a patient population defined by a social problem they did not discover, nerve doctors purported to discover diseases hitherto unrecognized. In so doing, they began the process of constructing a culture: defining for patients the nature of their reality and prescribing the activities that were, within this culture, believed to be appropriate to that reality. The culture of the nerve doctors differed from the culture of the psychiatrists in many ways, but two are most important for our purposes: They created from whole cloth a culture that had not existed before (rather than taking over folk notions and elaborating or altering them), and they justified and legitimized themselves by claiming to be men of science. In this, they are paradigmatic of what care for mental suffering was to become in the twentieth century.

The nerve doctors combined the ancient and venerable approach of the eighteenth-century theorists—philosophers, really—of neurosis with notions borrowed from the emerging science of neurology. They put forth the doctrine that mental problems were the result of disorders of "nerve force." Almost universally, these disorders were considered issues of depleted or weakened nerve force, and thus the disease that nerve doctors "discovered" was dubbed *neurasthenia*. Neurasthenics did not present themselves to doctors as deranged or suffering any obvious signs of insanity; rather, they presented with a host of physical and moral complaints. Headache, insomnia, lassitude, confusion of purpose, vague depression, phobias mild and severe, and a host of other complaints became grounds for a diagnosis of neurasthenia. Neurasthenia was something new under the sun: a disease of mind that did not result in obvious derangement, that might show itself in symptoms that were not obviously mental deficits at all.

Such gains as scientific neurology had made did not include any significant understanding of disease processes or any therapeutic measures. This did not stop the nerve doctors from saying an immense amount, nor were they reluctant to prescribe all sorts of activities and therapies to increase or conserve the diminished stores of nerve force. Bed rest and massage, special diets, exercise, and treatments with low voltages of electricity passed through various parts of the body were among the most popular. For the nerve doctors, the importance of the new sciences did not lie in any information they provided, but in an aura of authority, legitimacy, and public acceptance—and in providing the profession with an ethos of, if not an actual knowledge base from, science. This, too, was paradigmatic of how the medical cultures of healing would function: borrowing prestige from sciences that, in fact, shed little light on the problems that were claimed to have been discovered, understood, and treated.[27]

Within three years of the founding of the American Neurological Association, the neurologists and nerve doctors made a full-out attack against the psychiatrists—aiming to discredit their scientific competence, therapeutic efficacy, and administrative integrity—and the very idea of asylums. Their goal was to reduce psychiatry to a branch of neurology and to end the control of the asylum superintendents over the treatment of insanity. The neurologists contended that institutions for the treatment of insanity (which, they thought, would be mostly for the poor and those without families) should be organized as general hospitals, with a corps of visiting physicians, rather than as self-contained fiefdoms under the dictatorship of a superintendent.

The attacks of the neurologists on the psychiatrists' provenance over insanity tell us more about the atmosphere of the era than about any new knowledge. Not only had neurology accomplished little in understanding and treating disease processes, but neither the neurologists nor the nerve doctors had any significant amount of experience with the insane. Because the superintendents had established a monopoly over care for the insane, the

---

[27] The story of neurasthenia and its colorful "discoverer," George Beard, is told in many places, including Drinka's *The Birth of Neurosis* (1984). For a very helpful scholarly study of the place of the disease in medicine and society, see F.G. Gosling, *Before Freud: Neurasthenia and the American Medical Community, 1870–1910* (1987). As an interesting aside, I might note that S. Weir Mitchell, one of the two most important nerve doctors, originally conceived of his popular treatment regimen based on a theory that neurotic problems had to do with the fat content of blood. When Beard succeeded in promulgating the theory of neurasthenia, Mitchell simply reinterpreted his work in electrical terms. How we explain what we do frequently has little to do with what we do; this is an excellent example of that fact.

nerve doctors had been effectively prevented from studying them. The persons they saw—in their private practices and in general hospitals—did not resemble asylum patients in the severity or nature of their problems. The claim of the neurologists to be better qualified than the psychiatrists to deal with the insane spoke more of the scientific hubris of the age than of any body of knowledge, scientific or pragmatic.

We should note, in passing, that nerve doctors were not the only physicians who claimed to be able to treat neurasthenia.[28] As the concept spread through the medical community, general practitioners believed themselves competent to recognize and treat it. More disturbing, other medical specialties developing in the late nineteenth century—most alarmingly, gynecology— claimed to be able to treat mental and behavioral problems.

The notion that women suffer frail, nervous constitutions was part of general culture in nineteenth-century America, as elsewhere. That this was because they were controlled by their reproductive organs was dogma of ancient origin. For centuries, hysteria was assumed to be a disease of women caused by the "wandering" or other malady of the uterus. Gynecologists, anxious to profit from the idea that many problems of life were mental in origin, claimed as their province care for the nervous diseases of women. This claim was altogether logical, relative to the culture of the times. Besides prescribing various nostrums and activities to cure inferred lesions, tenderness, and "congestion" of the female reproductive organs, gynecologists performed various surgeries to relieve neurasthenia. At its worst, this medical

---

[28] Nor should we lose sight of the fact that psychiatrists and neurologists were not by any means the only nineteenth-century figures offering help for the problems the nerve doctors treated, some of which would, by the end of the twentieth century, be seen as psychopathology. A variety of spiritual and moral movements arose in the late nineteenth century, analogous to current "New Age" thought, to address the ills that plagued an emerging industrial, individualistic society. Herbalists, homeopaths, and mesmerists all claimed substantial followings among the distressed. The mainline churches, of course, continued to interpret many of the problems that would eventually be seen as psychopathology along traditional religious lines and to prescribe religious devotion and moral living as antidotes.

mythology led to hysterectomies and the absolutely outrageous practice of ovariorectomy—the removal of reproductive organs in order to restore "normal" mental functioning in "nervous" women. Popularized by Robert Battey in the 1870s, this procedure found a fair number of adherents. To their credit, the psychiatrists generally rejected this procedure; most ovariorectomies were done by private doctors, on willing patients. Gynecologists, and especially surgeons, were sensitive to criticism of their procedures, so they did better-than-average studies of removed tissue and follow-up exams of patients subjected to these procedures. They did, indeed, find all sorts of abnormalities in the uteruses and ovaries that had been removed—abnormalities we now know to be altogether ordinary or minor, but which were taken by the surgeons as clear proof of the postulated link between neurasthenia and "female problems." The reported follow-ups showed a high rate of improvement and cure (as would continue to be true of follow-up studies of radical psychosurgery and related invasions throughout their history, as we shall see).

Urbanizing Psychiatry and Expanding Its Scope

By the end of the nineteenth century, the transformation of American medicine from a maligned and suspect trade to a profession based on science (in intention and myth, if not in reality), and the transformation of the hospital from a refuge for society's marginal souls to a hygienic site of healing for all of the ill, were well under way. The asylums had become principally custodial institutions for the hopelessly infirm—including huge numbers of the aged suffering from various forms of senility. The scene of mental health care shifted toward general hospitals, outpatient clinics, and private practices—not because of changes in what was known, but because this was absolutely essential if the profession was to continue as part of the increasingly urban medical profession. The shift away from asylum care brought with it a decline in the prestige and influence of psychiatry as it had previously been practiced, an impetus to transform the profession, and the rise of competing givers of care.

By 1900, the doctors of the mind found themselves with hardly any clearly defined diseases or known causes of anything. Neurasthenia had fallen from favor because no one had been able to find any of the lesions or deficiencies of nerve force that it postulated. Only one putative mental disease had been isolated: general paresis, a particular kind of general paralysis that was found to be the tertiary stage of syphilis. The irony is fitting: Doctors of the mind knew about nothing but general paralysis.

Attempts to classify as diseases the vast range of problems that brought patients to see them led the doctors to create a host of incompatible nosologies. Therapeutic efforts were equally chaotic and often bizarre. In the early decades of the century, therapies for mental illness included not only the usual panoply of electrical stimulation, water baths, emetics, and the like, but also pulling of all a patient's teeth, colectomy, and colostomy.

This was not a promising situation for the doctors of the mind. If they were to become more than objects of medical derision, they had to make serious efforts to participate in the emerging scientific medicine. During the first three decades of the twentieth century, they attempted to emulate the successes of their medical colleagues, trying to put care for mental problems on a scientific footing. Psychopathic hospitals and research institutes were founded in a number of states. Psychopathic hospitals were few in number but large in visibility; they were designed for short-term assessment and treatment of acute cases of insanity and noninsane mental disturbance. The importance of these institutions lay in the fact that they gave concrete embodiment, and thus the appearance of institutional legitimacy, to the *idea* that mental problems could be cared for by doctors, outside the asylum system, in a relatively brief period of time. Though little they accomplished by way of theoretical or scientific work had a lasting impact, they kept the mental health enterprise moving in the direction of contemporary forms.

Among the more curious but effective vehicles for establishing the legitimacy of medical definitions of psychopathology—and expanding its scope to a wide range of problems that would not previously have been considered candidates for medical, especially psychiatric, attention—was the National Committee for

Mental Hygiene. Formed in 1909 and opening its permanent headquarters in New York in 1912, the NCMH was the brain-child of a highly influential former mental patient, Clifford Beers. Beers' 1908 book, *A Mind that Found Itself,* told the story of his treatment in various mental institutions and called for the reform and expansion of mental care. Beers wanted to start an organization devoted to the reform of asylums. However, at the urging of Adolph Meyer, the Swiss-trained neurologist who had become this country's most prestigious psychiatrist, Beers changed his focus to prevention of mental illness and promotion of "mental hygiene." Though Beers and Meyer would part ways in 1910 (over Beers' refusal to give physicians generally, and Meyer in particular, control over his work), Meyer's participation in the foundation was instrumental in Beers' prominence. Although Beers might well have succeeded without Meyer's initial help—William James was a strong supporter, and Beers had many lay admirers—the psychiatrist's participation helped him gain the cooperation of many physicians who would stay within the NCMH after Meyer's departure.

Thomas Salmon, who would become president of the American Psychiatric Association (the name taken by the AMPA, formerly the AMSAII, in 1921), led the NCMH during the second decade of this century. The NCMH fostered both traditional psychiatric concerns and the expansion of the concept of psychopathology beyond all previous bounds—indeed, some psychiatrists became alarmed that the committee promised psychiatric cures for problems psychiatrists had no idea how to deal with. On the orthodox side, the NCMH worked successfully with the AMPA to design a standard nosology that would allow uniform statistics on mental illness to be gathered—a nosology adopted by the U.S. Census Bureau—and conducted traditional surveys of conditions in mental hospitals. However, the committee also did much more, undertaking social surveys to discover how many social problems were due to mental illness. Since there existed no independent measure of mental illness, the surveys had the effect of declaring these problems to be psychopathological. Juvenile delinquency, prostitution, alcoholism, mental retardation, and a variety of other problems became issues of mental hygiene for the NCMH. One issue that received substantial attention was "dependency"—the inability to take care of oneself. Dependency became an indicator of inability to cope with life, and this became a matter not of social dynamics or misfortune but of psychopathology.

Meanwhile, psychiatrists in general were moving toward a new clientele and new practice. Many mental hospitals opened outpatient departments, and many general hospitals added mental health care to their services. Since the emerging scientific medicine was mostly urban in focus, the traditional mental hospital, with its bucolic rural setting, became something of an anachronism. Psychiatrists had to find a way to treat urban populations so that they could affiliate themselves with the general hospitals and medical schools that had become the centers of scientific medicine in America. The outpatient departments served quite a different clientele than that of the traditional hospital, of course. Most of the patients were referred by social agencies and schools, for disorderly conduct, failures to meet expected norms, and putative signs of "incipient mental disease." Of course, no epidemiological or longitudinal studies had ever been done to establish which sorts of things were signs of incipient mental disease. Nor were there any independent measures of mental health with which to decipher whether disorderly conduct was a manifestation of mental disease. No matter. Psychiatrists had begun to claim stewardship over the mental health of the entire community, and it followed that community problems were ripe for interpretation as mental problems.

By the 1930s, psychiatry had shifted its focus away from the traditional mental hospital and treatment of the insane. The new psychiatry, like the rest of the new scientific medicine, aimed at the treatment of urban, functional persons. This set the scene for the blossoming of American psychoanalysis, which got its start in America late in the first decade of the century.

The role of psychoanalysis in legitimating mental health care for the sane—and thus, for most of the patients whom most mental health professionals treat today—cannot be overestimated. Psychoanalysis was ideally suited to the treatment of highly functional, highly educated urbanites who were the chief market for the new scientific medicine—and it provided them with a coherent, comprehensive picture of human life that seemed more illuminating and more valid than any other extant theory of mental problems. Moreover, it made "the psychopathology of everyday life," to borrow one of Freud's titles, a legitimate arena for concern, for both patients and mental health professionals. Psychoanalysis was the first theory of mental illness that captured the public imagination (especially the imagination of the opinion makers and intellectual elite) that offered a way of understanding life in general that people could make use of, on their own, whether or not they had substantial mental problems. (There were, then as now, far more playwrights and theatergoers, novelists and literati, journalists and readers, social reformers, academic social scientists, and students who were influenced by Freud than there were psychoanalysts and patients.) With the influx of European psychoanalysts fleeing Hitler in the 1930s, America became the world center of psychoanalysis. The European psychoanalysts brought with them not only the state of the art in psychoanalysis, but also the prestige of European science and medicine.

Society itself was well prepared to receive psychoanalysis. Freud was part of a larger social and intellectual movement, exemplified as well by Havelock Ellis, toward reform of sexual and social morals and generally toward greater emotional freedom. The American intelligentsia brought Freud to the culture at large. In the same way that nineteenth-century psychiatrists took over religious and humanitarian notions that far outran any medical knowledge or therapeutic prowess, twentieth-century psychiatrists and their nonmedical colleagues took over a host of hopes and dreams inspired in the culture at large by a variety of social and intellectual influences. The place of psychoanalysis in mental health care did not begin with medical miracles, or with a record of successful cures, but with larger social forces.

The rise of psychoanalysis coincided with a pivotal moment in psychiatry's struggle to legitimate itself as a branch of medicine. Prior to the 1920s, there were almost no departments of psychiatry in American medical schools, and in the 1930s, the war between neurology and psychiatry for hegemony over care for mental troubles was at something of a standoff. The psychiatrists tended to emphasize "functional" theories—that is, theories that postulated deficits not in some identifiable biological organ or other entity, but in some "function" of the person, without specifying any organic basis for the functional deficiency. This was necessary to show that they were doing something different from the neurologists, who had held a superior position within the American Medical Association since the last third of the nineteenth century and were the principal opponents of the establishment of psychiatry as an independent discipline. Neurology lost ground in the AMA as neurosurgery developed into a substantial specialty from the 1920s through the 1940s, and its claim to superiority over psychiatry carried less weight as its own turf shrank. The rise of neurosurgery crippled neurology as a competitor in the delivery of care for psychopathology.[29] Psychoanalysis quickly established itself as the dominant functionalist theory. The confluence of psychoanalytic hegemony over other functionalist approaches, the need of psychiatry to make itself functionalist to establish itself, and the decline of clinical neurology made of American psychiatry in the 1930s and well into the early 1970s, a powerful and principally psychoanalytic discipline. By the end of World War II, psychiatry had firmly taken over nonsurgical treatment of psychopathology in American medicine, and the psychoanalysts had taken over psychiatry.

To insist on the importance of psychoanalysis in legitimating the new ambitions of psychiatry, and to point out its power to capture the imagination of the public and the emerging social sciences, is not to say that the new psychiatry was readily accepted within medicine. To the contrary, psychiatry was generally looked upon by most medical men as lacking a scientific basis, and its claims to therapeutic efficacy were widely doubted. Psychoanalysis, to medical men of a scientific bent, was seen as a form of metaphysics.[30] Not until after World War II would psy-

---

[29] Elliot S. Valenstein, *Great and Desperate Cures* (1986).

[30] For an interesting account of one episode, see the University of Chicago's chilly reception of the eminent Franz Alexander, described in Susan Quinn's excellent biography of Karen Horney, *A Mind of Her Own* (1988).

chiatry become more than marginal in the medical community. Nonetheless, the change began in the first decades of the century, and the shift to treating an urban, functional clientele, and to promising cures for social and community problems, were central to its eventual success.

While this change in focus was crucial in allowing mental health care to benefit from the medical community's consolidation of cultural authority and social power, it had a variety of consequences that would be problematic. For our purposes, the most important consequence was a problem for doctors rather than patients: The shift in clientele opened the way for the development of new mental health professions that would compete with doctors for the right to treat psychopathology.

The Rise of New Mental Health Professions

Asylums, as we have seen, had generally been located in rural areas, away from the stresses of urban life. The general hospitals, outpatient clinics, and private practices were generally urban. As care for the mentally ill in general hospitals and outpatient clinics was generally relatively short-term, psychiatrists perceived a need for managed aftercare of recovered or improved patients who had been discharged. Social workers, who had assumed stewardship over the waves of immigrants from Europe at the end of the century, were already expert at studying urban conditions, and they had in place a tradition of visiting families and helping to improve their circumstances. Thus, they were able to assume the role of managing aftercare. Equally important was the fact that American psychiatry, under the influence of Adolph Meyer and the burgeoning forces of community mental health, was going through one of its periods of interest in the social conditions *conducive to* mental illness. The ideology of the day was influenced by the American response to the wave of immigration from Eastern and Southern Europe: that mental illness, which was believed to be more prevalent among the immigrants, had to be addressed by changing the ways of life of the communities in which people lived. The social workers, again, were ideally suited for the task, and they were employed to gather information for the new doctors—to study the family arrangements and social situations of patients. The initial rationale never included any notion that anyone but physicians would actually deliver care. Physicians simply believed that they could give better care if they were provided with good information, which they had no intention of gathering themselves. The result, though, was to involve social workers actively in the concrete conditions of life to which the ideology of the day ascribed causal significance. From this, it was a small step for social workers to become primary givers of care—for they were, in fact, more conversant with, and had more direct effect upon, these conditions.

Psychiatric social workers did not long remain content with the role of physician's ancillary. In fact, they were delivering care, and they saw themselves as full players in the mental health enterprise. In 1920, the Psychiatric Social Workers Club was formed; by 1926, it had gone through several changes to emerge as the American Association of Psychiatric Social Workers (AAPSW), with the express purpose of formalizing psychiatric social work as a full-fledged profession. The AAPSW set high standards of education and training—membership required at least a bachelor's degree and a year of experience. (At this time, entrance into medical school still did not require a college degree, though some of the better schools were requiring one or two years of college.)

The AAPSW intended to work closely with the American Psychiatric Association, and initially psychiatric social workers found substantial support from some leading psychiatrists. However, the psychiatrists had always intended to remain dominant over the social workers, and they resisted both the professionalization of the field and the raising of educational standards. After all, they did not necessarily want to pay for well-trained workers, and they had no desire for a profession whose members would be demonstrably as well educated as many physicians. Equally important was the fact that social work was almost entirely an occupation for women. Nineteenth-century notions of the "woman's sphere," which included home and family and the moral uplift of the community, made social work an acceptable line of work for women, but less so for men. If psychiatrists were to agree that social workers—women—were capable of achieving professional status, doing the same sort of work as they, the profession of psychiatry would suffer a substantial loss of prestige.

Psychiatrists resisted mightily the social workers' efforts toward professionalization and primary care delivery. Yet the resistance to professional social work as an equal participant in mental health care delivery was quite without any rational basis, other than the physicians' wish to dominate the emerging field of mental health care. In terms of the leading ideology of the day (social conditions causing pathology), social workers had at least as sound a knowledge base for the delivery of care as physicians. Physicians refused to recognize this, and the fact that social work was pragmatic and empirical (rather than based in the emerging sciences, as psychiatry allegedly was), provided them with a rationale for repudiating the legitimate claims of social work.

Unlike the social workers, psychologists emerged to compete with physicians in defining and delivering mental health care from outside the medical system, but with at least as strong a commitment to the new scientific ethos. The questions of psychology, at least since the time of Descartes, had been dealt with by philosophers. The discipline of psychology arose as an academic enterprise out of a wish to deal with these questions in a sound scientific manner. Initially, some psychiatrists welcomed the discoveries of the new scientists of mind; as long as psychologists were content to engage in research only, they had no conflicts with the psychiatrists. Early psychologists, who were generally more interested in establishing a science than in instituting therapies or practical care, usually were not only content to engage in research but tended to oppose premature attempts to create a clinical psychology. The field was too new, they thought, for applied work, which would risk discrediting the emerging discipline. There were only a couple of dozen clinical psychologists in 1917, when the American Association of Clinical Psychologists was formed. This organization lasted only two years: The American Psychological Association, recognizing the claims of clinical psychologists to professional legitimacy, accepted the clinicians back into the APA and gave them their own "section" of the organization. The APA's move was politically prudent; the rapid growth of clinical psychology during World War I would otherwise have swelled the ranks of the AACP sufficiently to undermine the APA's position as the principal organization of psychologists.

Clinical psychology originated in the 1890s, not from concern for psychopathology but for the problems of children—especially educational and learning problems. Yet, as we have seen, psychiatrists themselves moved the problems of children into the arena of psychopathology early in the twentieth century by claiming that many such problems were the result of mental illness. Within the second or third decade of the existence of clinical psychology, its practitioners had begun giving attention to psychopathology. Most did not consider themselves, initially, in competition with the psychiatrists. They were not trying to "cure" anything but to help the disturbed to attain better "social adjustment" by learning new habits. Yet by the 1920s, some psychologists had begun to note that "psychiatric" problems looked a great deal like problems of adjustment, learning, and habit formation, and some of the successes of clinical psychologists looked a lot like cures.

For all the medical talk of neurological problems and other bodily ills underlying psychopathology, no scientific work had located any such physical malfunctions. By the first decade of this century, some psychologists had begun to construct a science of "abnormal" mental phenomena without filtering it through the prevailing dogmas about unknown, and hitherto undiscovered, bodily pathologies. That psychologists would begin to study aberrant mental states was more or less inevitable, since such phenomena are so strikingly interesting. Psychologists had at least as much to say about mental illness as the physicians, and the difficulties in psychological functioning were obviously real— an advantage over the mythical somatic maladies psychiatrists were forever proclaiming and never finding. In fact, by most any legitimate measure, psychologists knew more about the human mind than the psychiatrists did. Yet psychology was something new under the sun; thus, it lacked any tradition of cultural legiti-macy—the sort of legitimacy conferred by the European rever-ence for physicians. It also lacked an independent institutional base in either asylums or general hospitals. Psychologists were at a decided disadvantage to physicians in the delivery of mental health care, and the psychiatrists have done their political best to ensure that the advantage would remain legally guarded as their own.

Psychology got a significant boost during World War I, when psychologists were employed by the federal government to do extraordinary and extensive testing on hundred of thousands of soldiers. Since its origins, psychology had tried to develop valid, reliable tests to determine intelligence and a variety of other capacities. The massive mobilization of forces after 1917 required some basis for organizing the troops and selecting candidates for various tasks. To this end, the fledgling science was put to use. This research resulted in one of the most substantial bodies of knowledge about mental functioning ever to come into existence. Though its results were widely criticized and its methods may be arguable, the psychologists had succeeded in doing more than had ever been done to create a body of scientific knowledge about mental functioning. The very fact that the studies were so widely debated had a substantial impact, raising the visibility of the field and stimulating the interest of an increased number of bright students. In 1917, there were only a couple of dozen clinical psychologists in the entire country; by 1930, there were eight hundred.

In the first four decades of this century, anthropology and sociology were also developing as legitimate disciplines, and the psychologists were heavily influenced by these new ways of looking at human life. If the problems of life were personality problems, as they were coming to be viewed, and if personality was shaped by society and culture, then it followed that the problems of life were themselves results of socialization and enculturation. "Nurture" rather than nature—that is, social and environmental factors rather than genetic or innate factors—came to be seen as the salient determinants of mental health and illness. Medicine was principally the study of bodily ills. The shift toward the social sciences and personality and the idea of nurture as central to understanding mental functioning, did not augur well for psychiatry.

Though psychologists had at least as good a claim as physicians to scientific authority, and though the *zeitgeist* was turning away from somatic and constitutional explanations of psychopathology, the psychiatrists were quick to attack. By 1921, they were actively opposing certification and licensure of psychologists and attempting to preclude clinical psychologists from delivering mental health care. Not until 1945 were psychologists licensed in any state to deliver primary care. This battle continues to this day: Though by now psychologists have gained rights of licensure in all fifty states, few hospitals allow them admitting privileges or the right to oversee patient care. The licensing laws of all states delineate certain activities that psychiatrists, but not psychologists, may undertake. Such battles are pitched in the persiflage of providing the best care for patients, but they generally have more to do with protecting professional privilege and income. Psychologists continue to have at least as good a claim as psychiatrists on scientific legitimacy.

One element in psychology's gaining recognition as a legitimate clinical discipline was the fact that psychiatry itself came to be dominated by psychoanalysis. As psychoanalysis became the treatment of choice, psychologists were able to make the convincing point that psychoanalysis—as Freud insisted—required no medical knowledge and could be done by psychologists as well as physicians. Indeed, psychoanalysis had become a major presence in academic psychology, and the academicians were demonstrably furthering psychoanalytically inspired modes of understanding. Moreover, psychoanalysis gave prominence to issues such as motivation, ideation, emotion, personality, and the influence of childhood experiences on adult functioning—matters that psychologists had been studying since the emergence of the field. Psychoanalysis also brought about a revolution that would eventually undo the idea that psychopathology indicates physical pathology, for the Freudian view—as we shall see in the next chapter—required no such notion. Freud saw the problems of the mentally ill as due to altogether explicable functioning of *normal* physical processes. So it was that Freud himself came to see psychoanalysis as belonging to psychology rather than medicine.

Psychology in general, and clinical psychology in particular, was dominated in the 1930s by psychoanalysis and behaviorism, with Gestalt psychology as a powerful third force. Since psychologists were coming to do more and more of the assessment and evaluation even in hospitals, the impact of these schools of thought on care for mental problems coalesced into psychotherapy in something like the forms that we know it today—though the psychologists were not doing the bulk of the psychotherapy. Under the influence of psychoanalysis, personality testing became a prime concern, and psychotherapy was seen as aiming to change personality. Psychologists did testing, assessment, treatment planning, and "remedial education," but the care that their testing and planning indicated was delivered primarily by physicians.

Neither social workers nor psychologists succeeded in establishing independent institutional bases to rival the emerging medical institutions in the first half of this century. Neither possessed any social or cultural authority for "correcting" anything, so both depended on their alliances with medicine to participate in such authority. Physicians were not willing to share it generously or without severe limitations; yet the shift they had themselves instituted made the participation of psychologists and social workers an altogether rational development. In the needs of the psychiatric profession to establish itself on a wider base than care for the hopelessly insane lay the dynamics of the medical profession's later loss of monopoly. Every revolution, it is said, contains the seeds of its own destruction; so it was with changing the idea of mental illness from the idea of insanity to the ideas of neurosis, social maladjustment, and personality problems.

The response of the medical profession to the rise of nonmedical competitors in mental health care was to attempt to create monopolies. In 1934, the American Board of Psychiatry and Neurology was formed to attempt to legitimate the idea that care for mental problems required a specific set of medical skills and information. More important, the American Psychoanalytic Association succeeded, in spite of intense pressure from Freud and the International Psychoanalytic Association, at preventing nonphysicians from receiving accredited psychoanalytic training—with the help of outright lying: They claimed that U.S. law restricted mental health care to physicians, which was simply a fabrication. The importance of this is best understood in light of the central role that psychoanalysis played in legitimating mental health care: By transitive logic, if one had to be a physician to be a psychoanalyst, psychiatry was the legitimate profession for dealing with mental health problems. Unfortunately for psychiatry, the logic had another possible outcome, with only one altogether reasonable change in premises: If psychoanalysis is the correct way to deliver care, and if one need not be a psychiatrist to do psychoanalysis, psychiatry has no special claim on mental health treatment. The latter position would eventually win out, but the psychiatrists' efforts to monopolize psychoanalysis at least served to bring psychoanalysis within the burgeoning power of the medical profession and so served a useful function.

The claim that care for mental health required medical knowledge was not without substantial benefits to the culture of healing generally. If the cultures of care were to have any authority over the complaints of individuals, it would be through the cultural authority of medicine, for there were no other social institutions in place, other than the church, with the kind of authority of medicine. After World War II, the prestige and power of medicine would increase exponentially, and mental health care would share in the resulting public faith—and public money. Virtue by association, we might call it.

Though a good many mental health professionals today decry "the medical model" of mental health and illness, the fact is that the medical model created the field of professional mental health care. The idea of defects relative to normal, natural health gave birth to the culture of healing, and it was to medicine that implementation of this Enlightenment ideal was entrusted. Other mental health professions have ridden on the cultural and social coattails of the medical model. Indeed, the whole idea that there are sciences for dealing with psychopathology is parasitic on the success of other branches of medical care in which, in fact, there are sciences for dealing with pathology. The penumbra of medical science spread to psychiatry, despite its lack of basic science or therapeutic surety, simply by its association with other branches of medicine. To decry the medical model of psychopathology is to betray the history that created the discipline. Perhaps it is not always necessary to "dance with the one who brought you." It is generally a good idea, though, to know who that was, so that one may understand a variety of consequences if one chooses to dance with someone else.

Treating Insanity: Bastion of Medicine

One area where the authority of medicine was never significantly questioned was care for psychotics, the genuinely insane. The oddities of the mental processes of the insane, together with the near impossibility of curing them, encouraged the view that they, unlike the new class of neurotics, *were* different in kind from normal people. Thus, the idea that their brains must work differently—and defectively—remained intuitively credible, and doctors, as the stewards of bodily health, maintained control over care that involved physical processes. The late 1920s through the early 1950s brought a flurry of therapeutic activity in the asylums, activity that resulted in the only Nobel prizes ever awarded for care of the mentally troubled. These forms of therapy were troubling to a good many of the ethically astute or just humanly sensitive, but within medical circles they became widespread and heralded.

The one more or less unquestioned area of success came in the treatment of general paresis. By the early 1920s, it had been proven beyond doubt that a great many cases of general paresis were the result of tertiary syphilis, and by 1922, the syphilis spirochete had been isolated from the brains of paretics, clinching the finding that had been building toward conclusiveness for over two decades. Treatment of paresis took place on two fronts: specific drugs to kill the spirochete, and general stimulation of the immune system so the body itself could fight off the infection. The former mode found a silver bullet in Salvarsan. The latter, which led to a Nobel prize for Julius Wagner von Jauregg, is the

■ ■ ■

more interesting and, in some ways, horrifying story. Von Jauregg had noticed that some paretics who contracted malaria showed a substantial improvement in their paresis when the malaria was overcome. He began infecting paretics with malaria by injecting them with blood from persons with malaria. His results were significant, and many patients who did not respond to Salvarsan responded to induced malaria with improvement in paresis. There were, of course, several ethical problems with this: Some patients died of malaria, for instance. More troubling, there were not enough malaria victims in proximity to paretics, especially in America, to provide a supply of infected blood. Thus, physicians began taking the blood from one malaria-infected paretic and injecting it into another. Unfortunately, not all paresis was the result of syphilis, so nonsyphilitic paretics who received the blood of syphilitic paretics became infected with syphilis. Nonetheless, the plight of paretics generally led to a permissive attitude: These people were doomed anyway, so anything that *might* help was worth a shot, even if it introduced another pathogen into their hopeless systems.

What then happened—and this pattern was to repeat itself many times in the next decades—was that inducing fevered infections in mental patients, whether or not they were paretic, became more or less a general practice. Moreover, all sorts of other fevers besides malaria were tried. The successful treatment of syphilitic paretics with malaria evolved into the treatment of schizophrenics, manic depressives, and others with various infections (including rat bite fever). There was no scientific logic to this: There was no evidence whatsoever that schizophrenia or manic depression resulted from bacterial infection, or that the various fevers induced were fit to cause an appropriate stimulation of the immune system. But these therapies gave the physicians something to do and some appearance of expertise, and it gave the field the appearance of progress.

Von Jauregg had at least based his work on a sound empirical observation: that malarial paretics sometimes showed significant improvement in their paresis. Shock treatment—the second major development in this period—got its start, in the early 1930s, from a bizarre piece of reasoning based on an observation that has no obvious relevance to anything. J. L. von Meduna, a Hungarian physician, noticed that very few epileptics were schizophrenic and very few schizophrenics were epileptic. For reasons that escape detection, he decided that the two diseases were antagonistic: that a person could not have both. Why he should have leapt to this conclusion is a matter for biographers to divine; the absence of any concomitance between two diseases that are both present in only a very small proportion of the population proves absolutely nothing—von Meduna might as well have concluded that Bright's disease and Crohn's disease are antagonistic. (He also happens to have been wrong; a person can in fact be both epileptic and schizophrenic.) Von Meduna examined the brains of corpses of both epileptics and schizophrenics and convinced himself that he had found subtle differences in nerve cells—a finding that has not withstood further study. He then reasoned that if he could induce epileptic seizures he might be able to cure schizophrenia. His notion that the seizure (rather than some other element of epilepsy, such as neurological structure or chemical process) would be the element antagonistic to schizophrenia was another leap in logic, especially since he claimed to have found tissue differences. Nonetheless, he set out to find chemicals that would induce such seizures, and he reported substantial successes in his therapy.

Despite the fact that a great many physicians pointed out immediately that this form of treatment made no sense—its rationale was illogical and it bore no relation to any known bodily or disease process—shock treatment, as it came to be called, spread like wildfire. Around the same time, Manfred Joshua Sakel, a Polish Jew who claimed to be a direct descendent of Moses Maimonides, reported having discovered, in accidents involving diabetic mental patients, the effectiveness of insulin comas in curing both drug addiction and schizophrenia. Within a few years, Ugo Cerletti, an Italian polymath, and his assistant, Lucio Bini, discovered electroconvulsive shock treatment. Their work followed from an esoteric theory of Cerletti's based on *his* work with epileptics. He noticed that schizophrenics who *are* epileptic sometimes show fewer schizophrenic symptoms after a convulsion. He believed that the body produced a "vitalizing substance," which he called "acro-amines," in response to the convulsion. Three types of shock came to be standard: metrazol, insulin, and electroconvulsive. To this day, no one has any idea why some forms of shock treatment do some good—though almost exclusively in the treatment of severe depression, not schizophrenia or drug addiction. In the 1930s and 1940s, though, successes (that are no longer reproducible) in treating schizophrenia and drug addiction were widely reported. What was going on then, that so many successes with so many diseases were being reported, is anyone's guess. One guess that would probably be wrong would be that the shock treatments themselves actually effected the reported improvements in disorders other than depression. In any case, the practitioners produced speculative explanations of the supposed effectiveness of the treatments, speculations that provided rationales for continuing the practice. These speculations allowed the practitioners to believe they were doing something defensible.

The development of leucotomy, or lobotomy as it came to be called in the United States—though it has come to be synonymous with psychiatric evil in our time—was hailed as a stunning leap forward in the treatment of mental illness, both within the medical profession and in the popular press. Popular mythology has it that lobotomy was practiced principally on social outcasts squirreled away in state hospitals, but the reality is that it was a procedure of high prestige, and many of its victims, who were mutilated in leading hospitals of the day, were members of socially prominent families.

First developed by Egas Moniz, a Portuguese neurologist who received the Nobel prize for the procedure, lobotomy was introduced into the United States in the late 1930s and had its heyday in the 1940s and early 1950s, under the evangelistic promotion of Walter Freeman and James Watts. Lobotomy seemed to combine two of the most prestigious enterprises of the day: neurology and surgery. That it was based on murky neurology and crude surgery seemed to escape public notice. Though absolutely nothing was known about what regions of the brain were involved in what mental illnesses, or how, Moniz and his successors believed that by destroying parts of the brain they could alleviate symptoms.

The procedure consisted of boring holes in the skull, inserting an instrument resembling an ice pick, and wiggling it around, blindly, with no observation whatsoever of what was being destroyed. Eventually, boring holes would cease to be a routine part of the procedure; instead, the ice pick was hammered into the brain through seams in the skull just above the eye sockets. Though physicians realized that they needed specialized looking instruments to carry off the mythology that they were performing a scientific procedure, Freeman occasionally performed lobotomies with an ordinary hammer and ice pick—much to the embarrassment of his colleagues.

Until the advent of Thorazine and other drugs in the 1950s, the insane were generally at the ineffective mercy of the multiple imaginings of the medical profession. In the popular press, various of these unfounded practices were hailed as great good news.

The Great Transformation: Post-World War II Crusades for Mental Health

World War II radically altered mental health care, in the popular and professional minds and in actual practice, as it altered so much of American life. The war gave a huge impetus to the very idea of mental illness: Over a million potential draftees were rejected as mentally unfit, and around 850,000 soldiers were diagnosed with mental problems. Moreover, dozens of millions of Americans were given psychological tests during the war, in the effort to organize the military and its support industries. Over 1700 psychologists served in the armed forces as testers, evaluators, designers of psychologically appropriate equipment, and as counselors and therapists. In 1940, there were only forty armed services doctors assigned to psychiatric work; by 1945, an additional 2400 had been assigned. Countless social workers were enlisted by draft boards to gather information on the mental and family histories of potential draftees. The war thus legitimated the idea of expertise in mental diagnosis *and* the idea that huge numbers of Americans needed care, and it brought into being and gave government sanction to a large number of practitioners. After the war, these professions of healing would not quietly go away, nor would Americans forget the importance that the war effort had attached to mental issues. Over two million students would study psychology between 1945 and 1950; the number of graduate programs would jump from about twenty to about 150 in roughly the same period. In 1946, President Truman signed into law the National Mental Health Act, which created the National Institute of Mental Health. Postwar funding for mental health care would drastically outdistance earlier efforts.

By the early 1960s, the idea that mental health care should be ubiquitous in American communities would be enshrined in federal legislation and the profession's ethos. Psychiatrists, psychologists, social workers, and other mental health professionals proclaimed themselves expert in the social and personal conditions needed for mental health. Never mind that they lacked any special knowledge of social conditions, any scientific research identifying the difference between illness and health, or any coherent rationale for their claim to hegemony in defining what makes life good. They had decided that their mission was to make life good through mental health, and they convinced a willing public (and its government) that they should be given the authority and means to carry it out. The mental health professions (especially under the direction of the National Institute of Mental Health) did a brilliant job of arguing in their own behalf—and it seems they believed their own public relations, which is always a treacherous illusion.

An interesting historical accident played a significant role in the rise of mental health care after World War II—and solidified the extraordinary position that psychoanalysis came to hold in the 1950s through the 1970s: the influence of Will and Karl Menninger. William Menninger had headed the Army's military psychiatric service at the end of World War II and, in recognition of his extraordinary accomplishments, was promoted to Brigadier General, the first psychiatrist to achieve that rank in this century. In the 1930s, Karl had written bestsellers on psychiatry, popularizing a rather optimistic version of psychoanalysis, as well as making significant contributions to the literature of the psychiatric profession. The brothers, together with their father, had founded the Menninger Clinic, which was one of the highly regarded elite mental hospitals, providing care, of limited in-patient duration, for the affluent. After World War II, Karl took the lead nationally in arguing that wartime diagnosis and testing had shown vast numbers of Americans to need psychiatric care.[31]

Karl was widely seen as *the* great eminence on matters psychiatric. He succeeded in pulling off one of the amazing accomplishments of medical politics and administration: He convinced the Veterans Administration to turn over one of its hospitals to the Menningers to found a school of psychiatry, and in the first year the Menninger School of Psychiatry took in over a hundred psychiatric residents—more than had trained in the entire country in the previous year. The school became perhaps the most influential single psychiatric training facility in the country—and it taught its residents psychoanalysis and gathered together some of the finest psychoanalytic minds in the world. The roster of Menninger faculty and residents includes a virtual Who's Who of American psychiatry and psychoanalytic psychology for the rest of the twentieth century, including David Rappaport, Merton Gill, Roy Schafer, George Klein, Lester Luborsky, Robert Holt, Murray Bowen, and Otto Kernberg.

While Karl was overseeing the creation of a virtual missionary corps of psychoanalysts (Menninger graduates, more than the graduates of any other program, tended to go into teaching and public service jobs rather than exclusive private practice, thus magnifying Menninger's influence throughout the country), William was becoming an important—perhaps the most important—leader within the major organizations of American medicine and psychiatry. Though William never showed himself to be the intellectual giant or the restless and curious innovator that Karl was, he possessed an administrative and organizational acumen, and driven energy, that gave stable substance to the Menningers' joint efforts, as it had to the Army's psychiatric corps.

---

[31] For the story of the Menningers, see Lawrence J. Friedman, *Menninger: The Family and the Clinic* (1990).

Between the two, and the pivotal positions they held in the mental health care community and the public mind, the Menningers deserve substantial credit for the ascendancy of psychoanalysis in the 1950s. They commanded respect and authority in the public mind, eminence and influence with the principal sources of funding for mental health care and training, institutional support from the federal government, preeminence within the profession, and their own internationally recognized elite clinic—a combination no one else came close to achieving. Perhaps the American public would have been sold on mental health care, and on psychoanalysis as the therapy of choice, without them; but it had them, and their influence was substantial. We might note, as well, that the Menningers trained psychologists and social workers (and clergy) in psychoanalysis and included them in treatment delivery. At a time when the American Psychoanalytic Association was most adamant in enforcing its ban on psychoanalysis by nonphysicians (a policy Karl had supported, for political reasons[32]), Menninger psychologists trained, and practiced, as psychoanalysts—and as perhaps the best researchers with an interest in psychoanalysis in the country.

Perhaps most important, the war and its aftermath changed notions of what counts as a good life. Individualism and social mobility as social norms accelerated dramatically. Various social dynamics contributed to this, including new technologies and forms of industrial production, radically expanded access to higher education, and the advance of women into the workplace. Combined with the hyperdemocratic ideology of World War II and the Cold War, these forces reshaped popular ideas of good and evil—and thus changed what was considered pathological and what was considered healthy. Community and family allegiance suffered extreme erosion. "Social adjustment," which had been the overriding concern of psychotherapists prior to the war, gave way to the autonomy and dignity of the free individual. Social

---

[32] Karl was also politically active in opposing non-Freudian developments in psychoanalysis. See Helen Swick Perry, *Psychiatrist of America: The Life of Harry Stack Sullivan* (1982).

adjustedness itself came to be suspect, as antagonistic to individual development. Society needed to orient itself toward individual well-being, not the other, older way around. Concomitantly, inability to tolerate the autonomy of others became a corollary psychopathology. Failures of egalitarianism were soon to be seen as sure indicators of psychopathology.

When critics of current care fulminate against the evil effects on society of the selfishness promoted by psychotherapy, they have it exactly backwards. The contemporary emphasis on the sovereignty and happiness of the individual was imported into mental health care from the larger culture and represents the fidelity of the cultures of care to the larger culture that created them. Both conservative and liberal social, political, and economic agendas have furthered the development of individualism and the corrosion of community cohesion. Without a commensurate emphasis on individualism, the cultures of healing would never had been viable within contemporary society. It is not too much to say that the mental health professions were principal avenues by which society brought about the shift toward individualism.

For good or ill, though, this turn toward autonomy and individuality has had the effect of fostering the proliferation of diverse forms of care. No longer is there a set of social structures and cultural values sufficiently cohesive to dictate some problems as clearly pathological and some feelings and behaviors as clearly normal. The *idea* of such norms has not vanished, but there are about as many modes of care as persons wanting help or practitioners wanting to offer some particular vision of what life is about.

The period from 1945 to 1955 saw not only the acceptance of mental health care into mainstream culture and the proliferation of a huge number of alternate notions of health, illness, and care, but—paradoxically enough—the first serious studies of the effectiveness of the various modes of care. These showed that most of the psychotherapies and many of the somatic treatments had, at best, no demonstrable effectiveness.[33] Some practitioners,

---

[33] The various studies were summarized in various controversial articles by Hans Eysenck, beginning in 1952. See his 1966 monograph, *The Effects of Psychotherapy*. One need not share his dire conclusions to appreciate the weight of the evidence he presents.

scientists, and critics concluded that care was, in fact, ineffective—a conclusion bolstered by a variety of studies showing that control groups receiving no care improved about as much as groups that received care. Others merely concluded that no one knew as yet just what constituted effective care. Only in the 1980s would serious studies begin to show clearly that psychotherapy is beneficial. This paradox, of the proliferation and institutionalization of modes of care while little or nothing was known about whether or how they are effective, bespeaks how deeply felt has been the need for cultures of healing. The mental health professions did not simply dupe an unsuspecting public. Rather, they answered to deep unrest and distress in the rapidly changing populace, offering to provide what was wanted: professions based on a science of mental health that would offer a happy life to people in general.

Though the range of patients and therapies has varied widely, we can see several dynamics that underlie American mental health care since its earliest days.

What is usually called the "medical model" of mental illness did not have its origins in medicine. Rather, it resulted from the confluence of five social influences. The Enlightenment ideal taught that individuals are naturally rational and free, moving toward full realization of their "nature." Protestant theology of the nineteenth century taught a progressive meliorism, in which individuals could work toward their salvation. Urbanization and modernization dissolved communal ties and shifted the locus of responsibility for the management of life to individuals, who were presumed to be capable of self-sufficient independence. The social status of physicians led them to assume care over the insane, in the service of philanthropic and humanitarian institutions. Finally, the rise of nineteenth-century science, together with the rise of modern medicine, created the idea that a wide range of distress could be relieved through scientific efforts. These five strands of thought came together in the idea that individual distress may be a matter of defects relative to human nature, and that these could be corrected by doctors using the tools of modern science. To call this a medical model is accurate enough, but had it not been for the historical coincidences we have canvassed, it could as easily have been a "psychological model," or a "religious-humanitarian model," or something else. Because of the historical primacy of medicine, the mental health care professions have had to contend with severe turf wars that have at least as much to do with the needs of the respective professions as with delivery of adequate care.

By claiming to be able to identify and correct defects relative to what humans can expect normal life to be like, the culture of care for psychopathology has inherited the cultural authority of religious and moral institutions to define and shape life. Further, with this devolution of authority to naturalistic institutions and the secularization of religious ideals, an important shift took place: a reasonably happy, distress-free life came to be seen as normal, rather than as the result of attaining to a moral or spiritual rightness. Distress became illness, not a sign of further spiritual or moral work to be accomplished.

The professions have needs of their own, beyond competence at offering care. Since the mid-nineteenth century, the mental health professions have consistently expanded their area of putative jurisdiction, claiming ever more problems to be psychopathology. Ever more people who, in times past, would have been considered normal—if troublesome or unhappy or unlucky or even evil—are considered candidates for the ministrations of psychotherapeutic professions. The professions have also needed to convince themselves and society that they are doing what we ask of them, to ensure themselves social standing. Since the latter part of the nineteenth century, the authority of science has always been called upon to justify the authority and activities of the givers of care, though at every moment the claims of the practitioners have far outrun the findings of the relevant sciences.

The professional needs of practitioners and the development of new markets for their services have fed each other in creating the culture of healing. Expanding markets have had as much to do with the needs of the profession to participate in changes in society and in the medical profession as with new discoveries about psychopathology. Difficulties and miseries get classed as

■ ■ ■

psychopathology when there is a market that will pay professionals to try to get rid of them.

Thus, society has set the conditions for the creation of the cultures of healing, and the cultures, once extant, have had to create the conditions necessary for their viability and success. In the absence of a science of psychopathology, these mutually-supporting dynamics allow both professionals and the laity to interpret all sorts of things as shortcomings relative to "normal" or "healthy" human life. That is how we came to our current confused state in mental health care.

Chapter Three

THE FADED GLORY OF
PSYCHOANALYSIS

✳

THIS SWIFT, IF LIMITED, SUCCESS [OF PSYCHO-
ANALYSIS IN AMERICA, BETWEEN 1908 AND 1911]
RESULTED FROM THE COMMITMENT OF A FEW
PHYSICIANS, SOME OF THEM INFLUENTIAL, WHO
DEVOTED UNUSUAL ZEAL AND ENERGY TO THE
SPREAD OF THEIR NEW BELIEFS. SUCH A DEGREE
OF CONVICTION WAS NOT AN ABSTRACT PROCESS
OF COOLLY APPRAISING A NEW SCIENTIFIC THE-
ORY. RATHER, IT INVOLVED A DEEPLY FELT CON-
VERSION . . . THOSE WHO CAME TO CONSIDER
THEMSELVES 'PSYCHOANALYSTS' EXPERIENCED
THE HEAT OF A NEW FAITH . . .

> —*Nathan Hale, Jr.*
> Freud and the Americans

THERE IS SOME TRUTH IN PSYCHOANALYSIS, AS
THERE WAS IN MESMERISM AND IN PHRENOL-
OGY . . . BUT, CONSIDERED IN ITS ENTIRETY, PSY-
CHOANALYSIS WON'T DO. . . . NO BETTER THEORY
CAN EVER BE ERECTED ON ITS RUINS, WHICH
WILL REMAIN FOREVER ONE OF THE SADDEST
AND STRANGEST OF ALL LANDMARKS IN THE
HISTORY OF TWENTIETH-CENTURY THOUGHT.

> —*Sir Peter Medawar*
> Quoted in Hans Eysenck, Decline and Fall of the Freudian Empire

✳ THE FIGURE OF FREUD haunts the field of mental health care as the figures of Moses and Christ haunt the Western imagination. Freud has been both lawgiver and messiah for those who concern themselves with psychopathology, and no figure looms larger in the history and imagination of the mental health community. As we have seen, his influence helped create the field as it now exists; even those mental health professionals who detest his work owe the field of their endeavors in part to him. In recent years, a number of works have shown that most of Freud's ideas were present in the intellectual climate of Europe prior to his writing, as if to minimize his importance. Perhaps demythologizing Freud, showing that his work did not spring full-blown from the brow of Zeus, serves a useful purpose. The fact remains that Freud's synthetic genius, eloquent writing style, and political acumen made him a figure of prepotent importance. He would probably see the move to minimize his originality as a confirmation of his views: The father takes on supernatural power in the minds of his offspring and must be cut down to size in the course of their maturation.[34]

Freud began his career as a conventional scientist, doing research with some of the leading brain anatomists and physiologists. Freud produced a number of well-regarded papers in neurology, studying the nervous system of eels; he also wrote a

---

[34] Janet Malcolm's *Psychoanalysis: The Impossible Profession* is a good popular introduction to the world of orthodox psychoanalysis. Peter Gay's *Freud: A Life for Our Times* is well worth reading. Three fairly readable professional books, taken together, constitute a good overview of psychoanalysis: Stephen J. Ellman's *Freud's Technique Papers: A Contemporary Perspective*, Martin S. Bergmann and Frank R. Hartman's (eds.) *The Evolution of Psychoanalytic Technique*, and Morris N. Eagle's *Recent Developments in Psychoanalysis: A Critical Evaluation*. The Ellman book is especially good; it contains Freud's own papers on technique, with marginal notes by Ellman comparing Freud's position with contemporary Freudian perspectives. Introductory and comparative essays place each paper within Freud's opus.

well-regarded monograph on aphasias. Bench science lost its allure, however, and he became more interested in the grand, exotic work of Jean-Martin Charcot, the great French hypnotist and authority on hysteria. Unlike Charcot (who believed that hysteria resulted from the untoward life experiences of persons with "degenerate" brains), Freud became skeptical that organic pathology plays a role in psychopathology. He developed a novel synthesis: that an organically healthy nervous system underlies psychopathology, which develops through one's life experience.

Freud was nonetheless a thoroughgoing materialist; he believed that psychological phenomena would ultimately be shown to have their basis in biological reality.[35] Yet, believing that the problems of the mentally ill resulted from vicissitudes of a healthy nervous system encountering the problems of life, he had no real reason to remain within the confines of neurology. In fact, he had a passable rationale for bypassing it altogether: If the neurotic and the healthy person are not distinguished from each other by neurological problems (since organically healthy persons are capable of being neurotic), studying psychology directly should tell us what we need to know about psychopathology.

Whatever we may think of Freud's abandoning hard science, there *was* no science of psychopathology when he began his work, and Freud intended to create one. Psychoanalysts have generally been dismissive of complaints that psychoanalysis is unscientific, precisely because they believe that psychoanalysis *is* a science, a science possessed of and created through a method Freud discovered. To dismiss the discoveries of psychoanalytic method because they cannot be discovered by *other* methods is, psychoanalysts have generally thought, to miss the whole point of why psychoanalysis is important. Part of the appeal of psychoanalysis is that, in theory, it provides a method of studying that which is inaccessible to other methods.

Psychoanalysis dominated care for psychopathology in America from the late 1940s well into the 1970s. Psychiatric training

---

[35] For the development of Freud's early ideas, see Raymond E. Fancher (no relation to this author), *Psychoanalytic Psychology* (1973).

in medical schools tended to be psychoanalytically oriented—in the popular mind "psychiatrist" and "psychoanalyst" seem frequently to have been synonymous. "Real" psychoanalysts—persons eligible for membership in the American Psychoanalytic Association—had to undergo a minimum of three years' training in a psychoanalytic institute after completing their medical residencies. Outside of medicine, psychologists, social workers, and clergy could—after finishing their graduate degrees—train in psychoanalytic institutes that were not accredited by the American Psychoanalytic Association. Institute training required a "training analysis"—the trainee had to be analyzed, usually for a minimum of 300 hours. In no case was psychoanalytic training required by states for licensure to practice; the willingness of mental health professionals to commit themselves to the lengthy (and expensive) additional training was a function of the prestige of the discipline.

How the mighty have fallen! In the 1950s, psychiatrists who were not much impressed with psychoanalysis, or who had to minister to patients not capable of the esoteric self-reflection demanded by the psychoanalytic process, began to have success with pharmaceutical treatments for severe mental illness. These seemed to be effective and to work more quickly and cost much less than psychoanalysis. They bolstered the idea that psychopathology is organic in origin, not the manifestation of repressed wishes and distorted personality structures. In the 1960s, psychoanalysis came under attack for arrogating to itself the right to define what is normal and what is sick—and trenchant critics exposed with savage intensity how psychoanalysis purveys values and judgments under the guise of "analyzing" personalities. From the 1970s on, astounding advances in brain science and genetics raised hopes for a truly scientific study of psychopathology and suggested that treasured psychoanalytic principles were either wrong or superfluous.

Meanwhile, psychologists—psychiatry's main competitors in providing secular care for human suffering—gained their own powerful armamentarium with the rise of sophisticated versions of behaviorism in the late 1950s, and of the cognitive sciences and social and cognitive psychologies. With the rise of scientific psychologies that addressed the same sorts of human problems as psychoanalysis, psychologists could stop being the poor relations of psychoanalysts. Psychoanalysis was not at all helped by the proliferation of heretical psychoanalytic sects.[36] It seems that, using the psychoanalytic method, one can discover all sorts of radically incompatible things. This does not inspire confidence in the probity of a method that claims to serve the purposes of science.

Defining Psychoanalysis

Freud invented psychoanalysis and coined the term, and he and his devoted followers (represented in the United States by the American Psychoanalytic Association—the APA—which is frequently said to be "more Freudian than Freud") created the institutions that brought the profession into existence. Conceivably, the Freudian agenda is fundamentally misguided, and perhaps conscientious intellectuals should reject it. Yet it is Freudian psychoanalysis that established the field, made the claims to scientific legitimacy that conferred authority on the discipline, and led the way in making the "psychopathology of everyday life" a legitimate area for treatment.

All sorts of people call themselves psychoanalysts, many of whom do things quite at odds with Freud's perspective, and psychoanalysis as a field has become so many Balkan states. Several national associations have been formed in competition with the APA, but none has ever rivaled the APA in institutional power, public influence, or membership. This multitude of psychoanalytic subcultures exists amidst institutions and a public reputation created by classical psychoanalysis. Each of them draws central features of its culture from the orthodoxy from which it dissents, and several would make interesting cultural studies in their own right. Our focus on orthodox psychoanalysis

---

[36] See Arnold A. Rogow, *The Psychiatrists* (1970), for an account of splits in psychoanalysis in the 1950s and 1960s.

does not mean that the dissenting schools of thought are unimportant or lack unique elements. The point is to understand the orthodox culture by which even the dissenters have been shaped.

Everyone (at least, everyone likely to be reading this book) knows that psychoanalysis concerns itself with the unconscious, childhood memories, sex, and aggression. Everyone has some passing familiarity with phrases like repression, inhibition, the id, ego, and superego, Freudian slip, the oral and anal phases, the Oedipal complex, and so on. How these various notions hang together to make up psychoanalytic psychology is extraordinarily complicated—the Standard Edition of Freud's own writings fills twenty-four large volumes, and thousands of books and tens of thousands of articles by other classical analysts embroider, elaborate, and modify the picture. Achieving some clarity is possible, though, even within the confines of a single chapter.

First, we need to understand that underlying the Byzantine complexities of psychoanalysis is a fairly simple and interesting concept: Some things about life no one can avoid. Yet some of them, for some people, are highly problematic. Trying to cope with these inescapable, problematic realities leads to distortions and convolutions of the personality that constitute psychopathology. For psychoanalysts, what cannot possibly be escaped are *bodily imperatives* and *the presence of the past.*

Freud and the most orthodox psychoanalysts focused on two bodily imperatives: libido and aggression. Later analysts have focused on other inherent drives, like the need for relationships and attachment, which do, in fact, seem to be hard wired into our biology. No one has a choice about these matters; they come with the body. We can change where we work and live, we can change how we dress, we can change our hobbies, we can change our friends; but according to psychoanalysis, we cannot change the biological facts that we want sensual pleasure, the protection of our resources and existence, and intimate affiliations with other persons.

Nor can we change the fact that we are creatures who remember. Psychoanalysts believe that what originated in the past *continues to function in the present.* When nonanalytic therapists say things like, "We are more interested in the present than the past," they betray a failure to understand the psychoanalytic account of the present, namely, that it is very much constituted by dynamics comprising the past.

The second thing we need to understand, in order to get some clarity on the complexities of psychoanalysis, is that psychoanalysis consists of three distinct elements: the psychoanalytic method of investigation, psychoanalytic psychology, and the psychoanalytic process of treatment. The method of investigation constitutes psychoanalysis' claim to scientific status. The psychology is the view of persons and their problems that supposedly emerges from using this method. The process of treatment aims to correct psychopathology. We will understand more about each of these elements in the course of this chapter, but to get started we need a sketch of each of them and how they hang together, and we need to see how they relate to the bodily imperatives and insistent memories that (for psychoanalysis) make up the unavoidable dimensions of life.

First, psychoanalytic psychology: Psychoanalysis rests on the belief that conscious thought, feeling, and behavior are governed by, and expressions of, unconscious dynamics. *Everyone*, according to psychoanalytic psychology, shares this characteristic—healthy persons no less than the troubled. In healthy persons, the unconscious dynamics pass easily and recognizably into the realm of conscious activity, so that the mind functions smoothly and efficiently, fulfilling its functions in the individual's life. For the healthy person, unrealistic unconscious activities can be corrected by conscious thought, since the unconscious passes easily into consciousness. The person with psychological problems is distinguished by a disjunction between conscious and unconscious dynamics; he has repudiated or repressed elements of his psychological makeup, trying to render them inactive. Nonetheless, libido, aggression, longing for attachment, and memory continue to function, shaping the person's thoughts, feelings, and behaviors. Since he refuses to acknowledge them, they cannot become conscious except in distorted forms, and he cannot think about them clearly and realistically.

The troubled person's ability to function is impaired in three ways. The first seems fairly obvious: He is unable to integrate conscious and unconscious dynamics, so that matters of great importance get determined without (and even counter to) conscious deliberation and choice. This obvious problem has a less obvious complication, according to psychoanalysis. Psychoanalysts claim to have discovered something very interesting about unconscious processes—namely, that they function according to *primary process thinking*. This is the sort of thinking we encounter fairly directly in dreams. Primary process thinking is, by ordinary standards, irrational: It is oblivious to distinctions between time, place, gender, and the like. Primary process thinking condenses disparate images, experiences, and feelings into bizarre amalgams, displacing passions and affections from one object to another regardless of the appropriateness of the second object for the affective connotations evoked by the first. Further, primary process thinking is incapable of distinguishing between fantasy and reality. Consciousness, by contrast, can function according to *secondary process thinking*, which is the sort of rationality we are all familiar with: logical, sensitive to distinctions, capable of reality testing, and the like. When a person attempts to repudiate inevitable aspects of being a person, he confines them to the jurisdiction of primary process thinking. The failure to bring them into conscious deliberation, then, does not merely mean they do not get thought about wisely; it means they get thought about very badly.

The second harmful consequence of trying to repudiate one's unavoidable characteristics is this: Psychoanalysts believe that unconscious dynamics of psychopathology are infantile in origin and nature—that is, the repudiation begins in childhood. Thus, childish wishes and needs get shunted out of interaction with reality, so that the person cannot shape them into mature forms. Infantile wishes, fears, and beliefs continue to determine (via the unconscious) how the adult relates to the world and to his own needs. Immature wishes and needs get thought about in irrational (primary process) ways, and these determine the person's overt thoughts, feelings, and actions.

The third way that repudiating realities of one's existence renders one decrepit is not especially obvious, but it is important: According to psychoanalysts, defending oneself against problematic dynamics requires a great deal of energy. Thus, a great deal of psychological energy is diverted from making a life into keeping the repudiated elements at bay. So we have a person whose immature wishes, thought about through unconscious primary processes, shape his life. Presumably, that has deleterious consequences itself. But one's efforts to keep these wishes and fantasies at bay enervate him, so that he has less energy than he otherwise might to cope with the consequences of his distorted habits of mind. The problem itself—repudiation—causes a diminished capacity to cope with its consequences.

Perhaps it seems odd that we have started our definition of psychoanalysis by looking at the psychology, rather than at the method of inquiry. After all, psychoanalysts claim to have discovered these notions through use of the psychoanalytic method, and the claim of psychoanalysis to scientific status lies in the power of the method. Wouldn't it have made more sense to present the method, then show how its use leads to discovery of the psychology? Unfortunately, the method only makes sense if the basic premises of the psychology are true. Unless one accepts the idea of a unified, determinative unconscious *prior* to observing the patient's presentations, there is no reason to take the patient's manifest behaviors at anything other than face value.

The psychoanalytic method consists (as we shall see in more detail later) of studying what *is* conscious in order to infer from that what is *not* conscious. If we assume that the mind is a unified system, integrated with the bodily imperatives of libido, aggression, and the like, then it makes sense to infer from observable actions and conscious phenomena to underlying activities that unify them. As Freud himself put it: ". . . the data of consciousness are exceedingly defective; both in healthy and in sick persons mental acts are often in process which can be explained only by presupposing other acts, of which consciousness yields no evidence. . . . All these conscious acts remain disconnected and unintelligible if we are determined to hold fast to the claim that every single mental act performed within us must be consciously experienced; on the other hand, they fall into a demonstrable connection if we interpolate the unconscious acts we infer."[37]

---

[37] Sigmund Freud, "The Unconscious," in *Collected Papers*, Volume IV.

The assumption of unconscious mentation requires the prior assumption that mind is unified. This assumption of unity justifies interpolating unconscious links between the obviously disjointed, apparently random, often contradictory phenomena of consciousness and overt action. However, that these unconscious links must be *mental* acts is a further assumption. It *could* be that conscious phenomena and overt action are analogous to light bulbs strung along a wire: The connection is neither light nor light bulbs. It could be that something other than thinking produces thoughts— different physiological processes might "light up" different regions of thinking and acting at different times, and these physiological processes might not be aptly characterized as mental acts. Or, to use a different analogy, consider a stereo system: Between the performance recorded and its reproduction at the speakers, there is no sound. Conscious acts could be related by energy that is nonmental in the same way that performance and playback are related by energy that is not acoustic. Freud, though, believed that trying to give a *purely psychological* account of mental phenomena justified postulating unconscious mental activity.[38]

Once this postulate is in place, psychoanalysts see the "dynamic unconscious" revealing itself in indirect and symbolic representations in conscious activity. We can decipher the unconscious by studying dreams, slips of the tongue and, perhaps most important, repetitive, patterned sequences of thought and behavior. These are (in psychopathology) the product of primary process thinking, with only an overlay of secondary process thinking. Deciphering the problematic dynamics requires that one go "below" the secondary process characteristics of what a patient says, to reach the primary process that formulated and continues to energize the patient's problems. That is the task of the *psychoanalytic method of inquiry.*

This method of inquiry consists of two dimensions: the patient's reporting to the analyst, insofar as possible, every thought and feeling she has while lying on the analyst's couch; and the psychoanalyst's studying these, together with the patient's

---

[38] Sigmund Freud, "A Note on the Unconscious in Psycho-analysis," in *Collected Papers,* Volume IV.

comportment toward her, to find patterned sequences that psychoanalysts assume are caused by the patient's unconscious dynamics.

The *psychoanalytic process of therapy* uses the method of inquiry, but with a specific purpose and specific features. The *investigative* task of psychoanalysis as a form of mental health care is to study the patient's manifest thoughts, feelings, and behaviors in order to infer from them the essential elements of life that have been repudiated and the internal mechanisms used to sustain this repudiation. The *therapeutic* task is to lead *the patient* to analyze the manifest contents of her life so that the patient herself is led ever closer to revealing and experiencing the repudiated elements of herself. As a result, these elements can be acknowledged, owned, and taken up directly into new ways of thinking, feeling, and acting. The patient can then develop ways of living that do not require the impossible effort to deny the facts about oneself and one's history—ways of living that are not infected with uncorrected infantile assumptions and fantasies. We will look at the psychoanalytic process in detail in the next section.

To understand psychoanalysis, we must keep in mind the central place it gives to fulfillment or repudiation of essential characteristics of being a person—characteristics that cannot be escaped because they come hard wired into the body, including libido, aggression, memory, and affiliative and attachment needs. The complexities of psychoanalytic psychology and the purposes of psychoanalytic treatment take shape from this fundamental orientation.

The Psychoanalytic Process

The fact that many of Freud's writings are easily accessible to any educated reader (and the vast influence exerted on our general culture by his work and the work of those who have been guided by his ideas) easily clouds the understanding of psychoanalysis *as a form of mental health care*. Reading Freud's writings, or studying the great intellectuals who have been influenced by him and his followers, gives one an understanding of the general principles of

Freudian psychology—and its applications to general social, cultural, and conceptual issues. It does not give one an understanding of the psychoanalytic process of treatment.

When a patient first encounters a psychoanalyst, it is usually for a "consultation." A psychoanalyst does not assume, on first hearing from a prospective patient, that the patient is "analyzable," so she usually will not agree to take on the patient until they have met a few times.

An "analyzable" patient is a person who possesses the potential for self-observation that constitutes psychoanalysis. There is more to this than might first meet the eye. The psychoanalytic process of self-observation is extremely rigorous, and the patient must be able to withstand the frustrations and deprivations inherent in the process. According to psychoanalytic doctrine, patients have developed all sorts of defensive maneuvers to avoid experiencing or knowing what they have repudiated. They have become masters at enlisting others in this self-ignoring. The psychoanalyst serves her role partly by refusing to play her role in the patient's usual defensive strategies. Thus, the patient will find that in psychoanalysis, he will often be in significant distress, without necessarily knowing exactly why. In general, the "why" will be that the patient has tried to enlist the psychoanalyst in some defensive maneuver, and the psychoanalyst has sidestepped the invitation. Since the patient's defensive effort has failed, he experiences some measure of what it was supposed to protect him from—which is distressing, since the repudiated element is wrapped in dire associations. Learning what the distress is about is a central task of the analysis, and the patient must be able to tolerate the distress in order to analyze it.

This distress has its peculiar features. Ever since childhood, the patient has associated some basic bodily imperative with something fearsome, or she has been trying to ward off some terrifying memory or fantasy. Basic longings and early memories have, for years, been elaborated upon by primary process thinking; terrible unconscious beliefs about those wishes and early experiences have become richly elaborated horror stories. As the various layers of defense dissolve, these unconscious fantasies and wishes emerge in all their horror. As if that were not bad enough, the patient gets confused; she thinks what she is experiencing in the therapy room is *about* what is going on *in* the therapy room. She will experience the analyst as she experienced the most fearsome persons of her past or the most feared parts of herself. Thus, the analyst becomes ominous and threatening. To be analyzable, the patient must be able to undergo such precarious experiences, while "recognizing" that her feelings are not "really" about the analyst or the analytic setting, but about herself or figures from her past.

The patient who cannot sustain these experiences and make these important distinctions is not analyzable. For instance, a patient whose infantile dynamics thoroughly overwhelm the mature dimensions of his mind will take the analyst as a dangerous figure from the very first. He will fail to recognize that what terrifies is his own unconscious wishes and ways of relating to certain people—authority figures, perhaps, or persons who supposedly offer help. Thus, he will flee the therapy and add his tale to the popular mythology about incompetent, destructive therapists.

If the analyst decides that a person is analyzable, she will offer to take him on as a patient. If the person agrees, he will be instructed in "the fundamental rule" of psychoanalysts—the rule of "free association," that he is to say whatever comes to mind, no matter how irrelevant or unacceptable it may seem. In classical analysis, the patient will be instructed to lie on a couch, and the psychoanalyst will sit behind him, out of sight. The reason for this follows from the fundamental assumption of psychoanalysis: that the patient's problematic thoughts, feelings, and actions are determined by the dynamic unconscious. With the patient on the couch and the psychoanalyst out of sight, interaction between the two will not distract from the patient's emerging dynamics. The psychoanalyst, as an invisible observer, will be able to study the patient's productions without playing a role in creating them.

The patient's job in psychoanalysis, then, is to say whatever comes to mind. The psychoanalyst's job is to listen with "evenly hovering attention," that is, without paying special attention to any element of the patient's presentation or trying deliberately to make sense of it. The analyst takes a "neutral stance." "Neutrality" has a specific technical meaning: The analyst shows no preferential interest in any particular dimension of what the patient says, nor does she take any position on how the patient might address what emerges. She does not offer advice, and she does not answer questions. When the patient asks questions or seeks advice, the analyst analyzes why the patient asks. Her job is to perceive, through evenly hovering attention. Since the psychoanalyst, using evenly hovering attention in her neutral stance, simply perceives what emerges from the patient's self-determined productions, the analysis is purported to be sound—that is, scientific.

We will assess this claim later in the chapter, but for now this much needs to be recognized: *At least* the psychoanalyst, unlike other practitioners of talk therapy, works primarily with what she is able to observe directly, rather than with patients' reports on their lives. The psychoanalyst assumes that the patient's reports are distorted by the pathological internal processes that need analysis and change. Thus, the psychoanalyst treats the "manifest content" of the session, including the patient's reports on his life, as distorted and erroneous except insofar as they are consonant with what the analyst is able to discern within the therapy room. Whatever the scientific shortcomings of psychoanalysis, at least the psychoanalyst *tries* to work with what she—the presumably competent scientist in the patient/therapist collaboration—actually observes, rather than taking the patient's naive and (one assumes) biased reports as reliable data.

Two sorts of patterns in what patients say and do—transference and resistance—are especially important, and perceiving these is the analyst's claim to expertise.

"Transference" is the patient's transferring elements of his inner life outward to the psychoanalyst. These may be images of important figures from out of his past, disowned elements of himself, or idealized visions of what he might become or might have experienced from others. The transference is unconsciously determined: the dynamic unconscious causes the patient to mistake the analyst to fit its own distorted notions of reality. Transference, essentially, is the fiction that the patient's unconscious dynamics construct out of the psychoanalytic encounter. Analyzing transference consists of unraveling this fiction and thereby inferring the unconscious dynamics that created it.

This is not, on the face of it, a preposterous notion: It is like any other kind of troubleshooting, in which what is manifest is taken to imply what is not obvious. A computer expert who is called in to fix a glitch in a system, for instance, will study the patterns of malfunction in order to infer what sort of problem it is—hardware, software, programming, or whatever—and then use her expert knowledge of the computer to identify the problem and fix it. Analyzing the patient's overt presentation as transference and inferring from this to the underlying problem is not (in principle) different from what the computer expert does.

Patients, though (unlike computers), actively desire *not to know* what the psychoanalyst has perceived—for she is perceiving what is disowned or otherwise defended against. Thus, the patient *resists* revealing or knowing the truth about himself and his past. "Resistance" is what the patient says and does to prevent the repudiated dynamics from coming to light in the analytic setting. (One of the most common forms of resistance is to deny that one is resisting. The patient who righteously proclaims how seriously he wants to get to the bottom of things, "no fooling around," is often using his virtuous show of compliance to seduce the analyst away from probing too deeply.)

"Analyzing the resistance" is at least as important as analyzing the transference. For one thing, the resistance displays the patient's manners of defense, which must be given up before any change can take place. For another, the resistance must be analyzed before the patient will be in a position to understand the internal matters he has repudiated, for the defensive measures keep him distant from them. Without analysis of the resistance, the patient simply will never believe the psychoanalyst's analysis of the transference—the analysis will be like a report from a land one has never seen and does not believe in. Finally, the patterns of resistance point the analyst toward what is being resisted: By observing when and how the patient resists, the analyst is able to formulate hypotheses about what underlies these various maneuvers—triangulating, as it were, on what is being hidden.

We must remember that according to psychoanalysis, the patient's problems originate in infancy and childhood. By the time the adult comes into treatment, the original difficulties lie masked under layers of defense and distortion. Thus, as the analysis proceeds, the analyst will interpret the patient's troubling experiences within analysis as *regression* into infantile conflicts. From the miseries that emerge in the treatment setting, the psychoanalyst infers what the patient's childhood was like. From this, together with her beliefs about child development, she can predict the further dynamics that will be discovered within the patient: If the patient had a certain kind of childhood, and people with that kind of childhood have certain kinds of psychological dynamics, she can infer that *this* patient has some version of those dynamics.

We need to be very clear when we speak of "what kind of childhood the patient had." Psychoanalysis, contrary to both popular opinion and current notions of "dysfunctional" families, does not "blame" the parents or the family. Psychoanalysts generally do not buy into the romantic notion of children as blissfully innocent; thus, they cannot possibly see them as simply innocent victims. Children have all sorts of nefarious and unsavory inclinations, according to psychoanalysts. Nor do psychoanalysts generally believe that the main purpose of parents is to provide a "perfect" environment for children. Furthermore, no classical psychoanalyst assumes that the patient's perceptions during childhood were accurate; he was, after all, a child, lacking in mature cognitive and emotional capabilities. The classical psychoanalyst, furthermore, believes that primary process plays a substantial role in shaping childhood perception, so that all sorts of disparate and unrelated elements coalesced for the patient to make childhood as difficult as it was. Generally, psychoanalysts assume that parents come in all flavors, and all sorts of parental characteristics that are really innocuous (or ordinary, if vexing) can be perceived by children as threatening. This is why psychoanalysts are not especially interested in finding out "what really happened" in a person's childhood. They just want to know how the patient perceived his childhood, since they believe that is what determined his psychological development. Most important, psychoanalysis sees *the patient* perpetuating his early experience in adulthood by his own failures to come to terms with it. Psychoanalysis calls for a morally heroic, awesome assumption of individual responsibility: The patient's own make-up must be faced with fear and trembling. Whatever did or did not happen in the past is no longer happening, except within the patient's mental life. What is happening *now* is *within* the patient, and that is what has to be addressed.

If the analysis goes well, analysis of resistance and transference moves the patient beneath her defenses and she confronts *in her experience of the psychoanalysis* what has been disowned. This has three therapeutic benefits. First, the patient no longer has to waste energy repressing or repudiating parts of herself. Second, she is able to see that her fear of these elements pertains to the past rather than to current circumstances, and she sees that she has been compromising her comportment toward reality in accordance with these early concoctions. Thus, she is able to place her troublesome feelings "where they belong"—in her memory of what is long since over—and to get on with discovering current reality free of the distortions she previously imposed. Finally (and most important), the patient is able to incorporate into her current functioning the drives, impulses, interests, and so forth that were previously circumscribed.

We can see psychoanalysis as fiercely and severely devoted to the truth of the patient's life—as psychoanalysis conceives it. We are all familiar with the human capacity to kid oneself—to make up stories about oneself and one's actions, one's feelings and wishes, even to hide from oneself truths that we find unpleasant, forbidden, or embarrassing. All of us can, at times and to some extent, recognize when another person is deceiving himself and asking us to join in with his self-deception. Psychoanalysis has raised this basic human activity of detecting diminished candor, as it were, to an extraordinarily elaborate and subtle art. Psychoanalysis calls the patient to face the truth in order to become one with himself—as psychoanalysis conceives of this.

Psychoanalytic Enculturation

Classical psychoanalysis has always claimed that psychoanalysts listen with evenly hovering attention and simply perceive what emerges from the patient's unconscious. Still, we can be sure—

and some analysts now admit—that psychoanalysts, like all other persons, perceive according to their own categories of mind. Entry into psychoanalytic culture requires that the patient come to share implicitly the psychoanalytic categories of mind and some version of one of the stories psychoanalysts tell in those terms. More important, the patient must come to believe not only the general psychoanalytic version of how life works; he must believe that psychopathology fits into that story in the ways psychoanalysts claim. This may seem like a subtle distinction, but it *is* important. It is one thing to buy into the general psychoanalytic account of how life works; it is altogether another thing to believe that psychopathology works the way psychoanalysts say it does.

Remember, from chapter two, that Robert Battey and his followers, who removed ovaries to cure psychopathology, found histological and structural abnormalities in the ovaries they removed. That proved to them that neurosis was due to such abnormalities. Yet the presence of abnormalities in the putative cause of neurosis is not, in itself, evidence that such abnormalities cause the psychopathology in question. If a theory says, "Abnormalities in x cause y," and abnormalities are found in x, the causal hypothesis still remains to be proved. The abnormalities may have nothing to do with the pathology, or both the pathology and the abnormalities may be caused by some third factor. Conceivably, by listening to the tortured tales of their patients, psychoanalysts have learned a great deal about life but not much about psychopathology. Patients may spend years in psychoanalysis learning interesting things (or at least plausible stories) about themselves, and these may have nothing to do with the problems that brought them into treatment.

In case there is any doubt that psychoanalysts do, in fact, enculturate patients, let us look at the issue directly. Consider the "fundamental rule" of psychoanalysis: that the patient say everything that comes to mind. Even the most orthodox psychoanalysts would certainly admit that they give the patient overt instructions in this rule. By giving the patient this instruction, and by interpreting deviations from it as having significance, they enculturate her into several beliefs and practices. They lead her to think of her inner life as a monologue to which she can have introspective access. They lead her to think of her inner life as something she observes and reports, rather in the manner one describes the passing countryside as one looks out the window of a moving train—to use an image of Freud's. They also lead her to think that whatever goes on subjectively *can* be put into words. Even the fundamental rule, then, involves substantive beliefs about what it is to have an inner life.

Consider further the fact that psychoanalysts find significance in the sequences and patterns of "free associations"—namely, they find that the associations are not free at all, but causally determined by something outside of awareness. They say things to patients like, "The sequence of your associations suggests . . . " or "I noticed that you associated from . . . to . . . . There must be some connection there." The patient is then supposed to associate to the analyst's "observation," and these associations are intrepreted as following causally from unconscious dynamics. Thus, the patient is taught to think that his inner life has a unity underlying its apparent randomness. When randomness seems to occur, the patient is taught to suspend judgment, waiting for further associations to "reveal" the underlying dynamic that unites the "superficially" random associations. Since thinking and talking often appear to most of us random, with rapid changes of topic, the patient learns that how mind "really" happens is different from how it ordinarily appears. The idea of an underlying, causally determinative unity, to which one need not have direct or ready access, is one of the central features of analytic culture.

By interpreting halting or intermittent verbal production or "drawing a blank" as resistance or suppression, psychoanalysts teach the patient that the inner monologue is "normally"—i.e., when not interrupted by unconscious dynamics—a continuous stream. They also teach her to *look for* the unconscious interrupter of this stream and to interpret some plausible suspect as, indeed, the culprit. By attributing her words and actions in the therapy room to her internal, unconscious dynamics, they teach her that internal dynamics (more than interpersonal or interactive dynamics) determine thought, feeling, and conversation. By using certain vocabulary in their interpretations, they teach the patient a certain repertoire of self-interpretation. By calling attention to some patterns rather than others, they teach the patient that patterns differ in significance precisely as they evaluate that significance.

Consider the fact that *nobody* enters psychoanalysis to discuss his relationship with the analyst—since prior to entering, he has no relationship with that analyst at all. Patients enter analysis to discuss the problems in their lives. By analyzing the transference, the psychoanalyst transforms all ordinary understanding of life's problems. The patient learns to think of all of life as analogous to what takes place in the therapy room. Perhaps more important, she learns that what she *thinks* she is talking about is often *not at all* what she is really talking about—she thinks she is talking about work or romance or politics, only to "discover" that she is talking about, or undertaking some maneuver aimed at, the analyst. She learns that she is a stranger to herself and that her actions have long been determined by things so far outside of awareness that she does not even recognize them.

The sorts of things psychoanalysts generally *do not* include in their interpretations (or that they insist on interpreting as symbolic representations of deeper material—or even as resistances—when the patient talks about them) constitute as important a part of the enculturation of patients as anything else. Among these are the patient's ethnicity, his social milieu outside the family (including his education, school chums, teachers, clubs and sports, and social customs such as racism or class or other discrimination, and so forth), social or political beliefs and passions, and ethical commitments. Because psychoanalysts give fundamental weight to the internal life of the person (as shaped by the drama inside the family), sociological, religious, ethical, and community issues do not have primary importance. At best, such matters may contribute to the superficial coloration of the family drama and to the individual's stock of images and concerns. Current, adult concerns with such issues may reflect (i.e., be derived from) one's personality structure and one's conflicts, but they do not shape one's pathology—or explain it.

Most people (and several other cultures of healing) would consider contemporary reality to be a potential cause of pathology. Psychoanalysis, by its own logic, has no room for the idea that contemporary reality can cause pathology. Once psychoanalysis interpreted pathological distress as the result of internal dynamics originating in childhood, and once the analysts made "successful adaptation to reality" an essential indicator of health, it followed, as night follows day, that they *could not* see contemporary reality as causing pathology. For pathological distress is, by definition, a failure to adapt to reality. Thus, despite our ordinary assumption that current reality may be the cause of our pain, psychoanalysts teach people that pathology is the recrudescence of unconscious dynamics originating in another time and place, long ago. That contemporary reality causes pathological distress is an idea no one would be heartily inclined to give up, unless his analyst resolutely refused to consider it a possibility.

Psychoanalysts do not talk about a great deal of what most people consider essential psychological phenomena. Psychoanalysis works with a drastically impoverished set of emotion terms, for instance: Joy, hope, disheartenment, pride, regret, and a host of other apparently important emotions almost never appear in psychoanalytic writings and are *never* given an explanatory role. Pleasure and pain, anger and lust, anxiety and guilt—this is about the size of the psychoanalytic emotion vocabulary. Similarly, motivation terms are equally limited: Sexual longing, aggression, attachment, and defense against their negative dimensions are the fundamental motivations. Honor, grace, compassion, decency, and a host of other apparently important motives rarely appear, and, again, never as primary explanations. Whenever psychoanalysts confront what anyone else would consider ordinary emotions or motivations, analysts assume that they are at most surface derivatives of the fundamental emotions and motives related to libido, aggression, and attachment—if not, in fact, resistance to the analysis.

Nor do psychoanalysts seem ever to consider the contorting and disabling effects of rank ignorance about how life works. It would not seem farfetched to think that some people are sufficiently naïve, sheltered, or bequeathed backward beliefs by their origins that they cannot cope with important realities adequately. It would not seem farfetched to believe that at least some neurotic problems result from this. Not for psychoanalysts.

If a person has problems in his sex life, that cannot be because of debilitating ignorance or unworkable beliefs about relating to those he desires. It has to be a deep underlying conflict, probably about his lust for his mother and fear of his father.

That psychoanalysts enculturate patients, then, seems beyond peradventure. It simply cannot be the case that all of these characteristics of psychoanalytic interpretation, including refusals to interpret in many terms most people consider important, do not result in a set of canonical ways of thinking about one's self, to which one would not necessarily come without the psychoanalyst's influence.

Being a Person in Psychoanalytic Culture

By seeing all of the patient's productions as the result of a core set of internal dynamics, continuous since childhood, psychoanalysis imposes an extraordinary unity, complexity, and insularity on one's understanding of life. The most disparate and apparently unrelated items of thought, feeling, and behavior come to be seen as "manifestations" of the same underlying unconscious dynamic; this dynamic is seen as originating and enduring since the earliest years of life. One's manifold experiences, in the most diverse social contexts, do not touch it, change it, or render it inoperative. Psychoanalysts "shrink" the most diverse activities into manifestations of an underlying set of dynamics. One's self-understanding takes on a self-referential unity that makes factors outside one's self just so many patterns of camouflage and distraction.

The central psychoanalytic notion, that analysis is analysis of the transference, illustrates this self-referential unity at its starkest. There are two dimensions to this. First, social influences on one's personality are deemed negligible. If it were possible for one's social experiences or one's experiences after childhood to change one's inner dynamics, there would be no reason why, by the time a person enters analysis, drastic changes might not have been worked on the original dynamics. Thus, there would be no validity in inferring from the transference to the early "formative" years. Thus, one cannot give analysis of the transference any credence and simultaneously hold that social experiences play formative roles. Second, the analyst assumes that the issues that cause problems in the patient's life are precisely the issues active in the relationship with the analyst. The transference reveals the patient's pathological dynamics precisely because those dynamics are always and everywhere active, no matter with whom the patient interacts or under what circumstances. Without this assumption, analyzing the transference makes no sense at all. With it, transference is theoretically an elegant way to investigate directly what the analyst would otherwise never have occasion to see—namely, the dynamics that are active in the patient's life outside the therapy room.

This self-referential complexity may have its charms, but it is purchased at a price. This price surely includes devaluing variety of personality, randomness of experience, and adult social relationships as fundamental determinants of mental health. To understand the significance of this, consider an alternative notion of how life works. Suppose that personality is a fairly loose-knit conglomeration of habits and proclivities, open to change by the experiences one has through the course of one's life. Suppose that change may come about through the experiences one has with persons, institutions, books, works of art—whatever. Thus, the people and events one *happens* to run across in the course of life, the circumstances in which one happens to find one's self, and—in short—the luck one happens to have will be major factors in one's psychological changes. If we are taught to undervalue such things as sources of personal change and growth, we probably miss many opportunities for resolving our problems (or rendering them moot). We probably do not develop keen eyes and adroit skills for identifying and making use of such opportunities.

Suppose, in addition, that there is no inherent unity to personality: that we all have a variety of more or less coherent subsets of habits and predispositions, each subset operating more or less independently of the others, depending on the circumstances in which we find ourselves. Thus, we will think, feel, and act very differently in church, at the post office, at work, on vacation, in bed, with our children, etc. If we are taught to think of different domains as so many reflections of some underlying unity that must be ferreted out, we may not learn to exploit the flexibility of our own personalities. When we could be getting over our problems by learning where and when to deploy different dimensions of ourselves (or acquiring skills at doing so), we will probably instead be preoccupied with divining what our habits reveal about our unconscious processes.

The price to be paid for seeing oneself in terms of an underlying, unconscious unity may be even higher, itself causing or exacerbating psychopathology. The last few years have seen the consolidation (outside of psychoanalysis) of what is probably the most scientifically careful psychological explanation of depression (and a variety of other psychopathologies): the idea of "learned helplessness."[39] According to this view, depression results from a *depressive explanatory style,* in which one explains negative events that happen to one's self as the result of persistent, pervasive internal factors: "This happened to me because of something that is wrong with me, that is essential to who I am, that will pervade my further experience." According to the proponents of the idea of learned helplessness (and of therapy through learned optimism), this explanatory style is the result of certain cognitive mistakes, and the point of therapy is to give up this style of explanation. A patient needs to learn to see negative experiences as the result of transient, temporary factors, not necessarily located inside himself, which have no necessary implications for other experiences. *The psychoanalytic perspective consists precisely of the explanatory style that the learned helplessness advocates see as causing depression.* Psychoanalysts do, in fact, teach patients to think of their problems as the result of internal, persistent, pervasive factors. They see this *style* of thinking as appropriate, and they see the remedy as locating the internal factor and either changing it or coming to terms with its permanence.

Perhaps the psychoanalysts are right—these alternative views we have just sketched are not yet conclusively supported by science. (Even the learned helplessness/optimism model has a

---

[39] Christopher Peterson, Steven F. Maier, and Martin E.P. Seligman, *Learned Helplessness* (1993).

long way to go to merit such a claim, as its proponents clearly know and honestly state.) The point, though, is that this notion of self-referential unity is neither clearly true nor obviously unqualifiedly helpful. It is, though, the view into which practitioners and patients of psychoanalysis are enculturated.

Psychoanalysts and their patients also come to hold very specific, perhaps peculiar notions about the relations of consciousness and the unconscious. The dire view of the unconscious as oblivious to reality, dominated by primary process thinking, leads psychoanalysts to a vast overvaluing of consciousness. If the unconscious is so treacherous, so prone to infantile, wishful fantasy, we had best be sure that we discipline and control it by conscious mentation.

For psychoanalysts, conscious mentation means *verbal* ideation. Psychoanalysts believe that everything important can be put into words and that a failure to articulate signifies a failure of conscious awareness—and therefore the presence of a pathological distortion of the flow of consciousness. This has the effect of making psychoanalysts and their patients ardent devotees of what can be said and relatively oblivious to what cannot. Thus, psychoanalysts and their patients are extremely distrustful of any dimension of their lives for which they cannot give a coherent verbal account.

This has two consequences: the self-absorbed need of citizens of the psychoanalytic culture always to be articulating what is going on with them (and the frequently exasperating demand that their significant others should do the same) and a further shrinking of personality to fit the story that one is capable of articulating about oneself. The well-analyzed patient is precisely the one who has such a story, that he finds sufficiently complete that he is not driven back into analysis to revise it.[40]

---

[40] We should be clear that "having such a story" is sufficient, in psychoanalytic terms, only if the story *parses and interprets one's experience as it emerges in the psychoanalytic setting.* Simply being able to tell a story about one's life—simply having the words—does not effect change. A story may be just a type of intellectualization, a way of avoiding direct experience of one's self by substituting words for experience. This is why psychoanalysts are generally not impressed with self-help books and generally do not encourage patients to read psychoanalytic literature: Those are sources of intellectualization, not experiences of one's dynamics.

So psychoanalytic culture is a culture of introspective self-absorption, dominated by words, pervaded by a distrust of spontaneous inarticulate feeling and the trajectories of passions that do not fit the story one has about one's self. In general, large passions and colorful emotions are taken by analysts to be signs that further analysis is called for; a well analyzed person has a well-composed, even tempered, verbal account to give for anything she is feeling, rather than activity propelled forward by the trajectory of the feeling itself. At its best, this promotes a kind of reflective equanimity and personal quietude. Less optimally, the equanimity that characterizes a well-analyzed person is likely just to be a sort of formal, inhibited, unspontaneous lack of color.

Thus, to have feelings, passions, or spontaneous notions that one cannot give a verbal account of raises suspicion that one is not yet well enough analyzed, that one is therefore revealing latent pathology. This is rather ironic: Psychoanalysis originated from a vision of fundamental passions as the font of all health. The stoicism and verbalism of the well-analyzed analysand resembles nothing quite so much as the inhibited, highly civilized, unpassionate propriety that Freud himself railed against. How strange it is that the movement that began as a critique of social propriety should have evolved to the point where "appropriate" and "inappropriate" are its two most frequent terms of evaluation!

Psychoanalytic Values

Psychoanalysis involves a particular realm of values, beginning with the fundamental value it places on the patient's internal sensations, moods, feelings, thoughts, and so on. Psychoanalysts seem not to recognize that the value they place on the inner life is quite optional.

While psychoanalysis may not be overtly antipathetic to community life, social solidarity, and family ties, it certainly places no great value upon them. Indeed, it is not too much to say that psychoanalysis generally sees close family ties as evidence of reaction formation against murderous wishes, failure to complete individuation, dependency due to a faulty ego, or some other sort of pathology. Ties to one's fellows that might lead one to sacrifice one's own well-being, or to defer the advancement of one's own projects, are likewise suspect. Self-interest, defined in terms of one's ability to satisfy one's internal needs, remains the fundamental motivation; "appropriate" social relations are those in which one's pursuit of one's self-interest is sufficiently enlightened. Where it seems that healthy persons are pursuing social ideals, these are, in the psychoanalyst's view, sublimated ways of pursuing internal satisfactions.

We can illustrate the place of socialization in the psychoanalytic world by looking at a pair of common terms: "true self" and "false self."[41] The way the story goes, a child's development ought to be guided by discovery of her inner needs and interests. If she lives in a "good enough" environment, she will be able to explore the various forms her drives and wishes might take. She will develop a repertoire of actions and a character structure that is "true." The self she then experiences herself to be, which she presents to the environment in her social interactions, is a true self. Ideally, this true self will be in harmony with the social structure around her; her environment will have room for her needs and interests. However, if a child has to be guided primarily by the demands and structures of her environment, she will develop a repertoire and character structure based on that environment's expectations, and her own inner needs and inclinations will be subordinated. A person who is dominated by social expectations in this way is possessed of a "false self." Truth and falsity thus find their definition by reference to the values and motivations that have primacy in a person's life.

Psychoanalysts do not seem to recognize that there is no inherent reason why the satisfaction of instinctual needs and

---

[41] These are not terms of Freud's, but terms that developed out of the "object relations" school—the school that emphasizes the need for attachment. They are consistent with Freud's original views, I think, and most psychoanalysts have no great difficulty with this notion. It seems to me especially telling that the psychoanalytic sect that has most insisted on relatedness to others as a basic drive has developed these ideas of "true" and "false" selves—the sect that insists most strongly upon social relatedness gives us this idea of socialization as dangerous to health!

inclinations must necessarily be the measure of truth. There is no inherent reason why internal dynamics, rather than one's place in society, must be the principal source of health or illness. For most of history, in most civilized cultures, the kind of internal fulfillment that psychoanalysis values has been suspect, and fidelity to one's "station and its duties" has generally been a higher value. The psychoanalysts may offer a superior way to live, or a way of living that makes more sense in a highly mobile, modern society. What they are also doing, though, is promulgating a set of values that they rarely defend on moral or social grounds—though the moral and social ramifications of these values are immense. Their justification, instead—and this is one of the main problems with all mental health care—is that this is what "health" is.

These values, of course, are precisely the values of the larger culture that brought psychoanalysis to prominence. As we saw in chapter two, psychoanalysis took over the hopes and dreams of reformers, literary and creative types, and other forward-looking modernists for a society rebuilt around individual freedom. Psychoanalysis has not had to defend these values because it did not originate them. Psychoanalysis was granted stewardship over modernist values by a society that wanted to see these values as "naturally" superior to social and other obligations that place limitations on the free expression of the individual. In this, we can see psychoanalysis as an instrument of nineteenth-century liberalism's fruition in the twentieth century: the idea that "progress" in history is the unfolding and realization of individual freedom. Psychoanalysis took this old idea and rewrote it in microcosm, making the history in question the history of the individual herself.

What counts as "appropriate" individual freedom in psychoanalysis is, I think, also a reflection of a nineteenth-century ideal, that of the reflective intellectual gentleman. The value that psychoanalysis places on self-understanding of an introspective sort ranks as one of its more distinguishing features. Psychoanalytic culture expects of its members a degree of reflective self-awareness that exceeds what any other social institution expects of its members. How could it be that mental health requires a higher degree of introspective self-awareness than people commonly possess? The fact that psychoanalysis emphasizes self-awareness of basic passions makes this all the more curious: It seems doubtful that reflective, articulate self-awareness is universally, or even ordinarily, necessary for healthy experience of one's bodily drives. All species other than humans seem to manage their biological drives reasonably well without articulate self-reflection. It would not seem imprudent to hazard that most humans do, too.

This, of course, leads to a fundamental issue: Psychoanalysis purveys notions of health that transcend anything that has ever prevailed on Earth, if not in heaven. *If* there were a science of psychopathology, we might suppose it would have the potential to transform how we think life ought to go—in the same way that many genuinely scientific discoveries have transformed public hygiene, eating and exercise patterns, and the like. Indeed, one of the things we would like to have from a science of psychopathology is knowledge of what we can change to minimize distress and make for fuller lives. The problem with psychoanalysis is not that it tells us we need to live differently than we do. The problem (which we will see in the other cultures, as well) is that it tells us this, with the authority of science, though the image of life it would have us pursue is more a matter of specific values than of scientific validity.

The psychoanalytic notion of a well-integrated, healthy person is a transcendent ideal in service to modernism. Most patients who come for treatment initially want relief from distress, not reformation of their character structure. Psychoanalysis enculturates patients to think of their distress as symptomatic of deeper problems, which require for their cure reformation of the very structure of personality. This may not necessarily be a bad thing; character reformation may be altogether salutary, and the psychoanalytic vision of what it is to be a whole person may be a noble thing. What it is *not* is a restoration of "normal" or "essential" human attributes. To believe that the world would be a better place, or that appreciably fewer people would suffer psychopathology, if people attained to this ideal expresses the desires of psychoanalysts more than the findings of serious researchers.

The Scientific Poverty of Psychoanalysis

The credibility of psychoanalysis in scientific circles seems almost to have vanished. Conventional wisdom now has it that psychoanalysis is, for the most part, inherently untestable. Psychoanalysts have certainly not done much to test psychoanalytic psychology; but that is a different issue from whether psychoanalytic psychology *cannot* be tested. As we have said, psychoanalysis consists not only of a method of investigation and a method of treatment but of a specific psychology. It is one thing to say that its methods are unreliable; it is another thing to say that its psychology is in principle beyond the reach of scientific testing.

The notion that psychoanalytic psychology is untestable probably reflects practice, not principle; psychoanalytic psychology is untestable in the same sense that a heavily-guarded nuclear site is "uninspectable." The psychoanalytic community has shown an unwavering refusal to test its basic ideas and—more important—has exerted relentless efforts to protect its basic beliefs from testing. In practice, psychoanalysis allows for almost anything to be interpreted as a sign of almost anything. In psychoanalytic theory, the wish to kill one's father, for instance, can show itself as excessive aggression, excessive solicitude, homosexual wishes, or womanizing—to name a few. To be sure, psychoanalysts invoke very intricate theoretical notions to explain why the wish appears as one rather than another of these in a given situation. Since, in principle, such theoretical distinctions refer to distinct processes, *in principle* they could be tested. *In fact*, in psychoanalytic culture they are not tested. The psychoanalytic theory gets preserved no matter what happens. Non-analysts generally find psychoanalysts' ability to interpret everything extremely exasperating—and no wonder. In any debate, if one's opponents will not specify exactly what they are predicting and admit falsification when it fails to occur, debate cannot go anywhere. While it may not be true to say that the psychology is intrinsically untestable, it is certainly true that it has been impossible to get psychoanalysts to submit psychoanalysis to serious testing. That has infuriated non-analysts and probably explains their belief that psychoanalysis cannot be tested.

Psychoanalysts, of course, *believe* they have tested their views very thoroughly, by their own unique method. The claim of psychoanalysts to have developed their own scientific method carries little weight in the larger scientific community, though. This method always seemed suspect to many people—William James thought that its preoccupation with symbolism made it "a tumbling ground for whimsy." Several factors have probably combined to discredit it, but we need note only one: Psychoanalysts have always "discovered" the most wildly divergent things by using the psychoanalytic method. The way that Freud and his followers dealt with this was to pressure dissenters to see their disagreements with Freud as evidence of error or personal psychopathology. Those who did not relent—like Alfred Adler and Carl Jung—were booted out of the psychoanalytic movement.[42] As the number of mental health professionals using psychoanalysis grew, the Freudians lost control over the psychoanalytic community. The community is more splintered now than ever, with more widely divergent notions of what the psychoanalytic method "reveals." A method that does not yield reliable results—results that turn out the same no matter who is using the method—does not meet minimal standards for scientific objectivity.

Yet many psychoanalytic notions *have* been submitted to more standard methods of scientific appraisal—though primarily outside the accredited institutions of mainstream psychoanalysis. Psychoanalysts simply refuse to give much weight or pay much attention to such work. In a comprehensive, classic review over twenty-five years ago, Seymour Fisher and Roger P. Greenberg had this to say: "We have been amused by the fact that while there is the stereotyped conviction widely current that Freud's thinking is not amenable to scientific appraisal, the quantity of research data pertinent to it that has accumulated in the literature grossly exceeds that available for most other personality or developmental theories . . ." In trying to understand why few people seem to know of the immense research literature on psychoanalysis, Fisher and Greenberg had this to say: "Perhaps the negative attitude of the psychoanalytic establishment toward experimental

---

[42] See Phyllis Grosskurth, *The Secret Ring* (1991), for a very readable, dispassionate account of how Freud and his followers protected their orthodoxy.

observations has persuaded those most interested in Freud's ideas to wear blinders that shut out the very existence of a vast literature."[43] For our purposes, this antipathy toward scientific research is a critical element of psychoanalytic culture. The claim of psychoanalysis to scientific status has depended on an irrational aggrandizement of psychoanalytic method and a concomitant derogation of standard science.

Freud himself set the tone for this insistence on the primacy of psychoanalytic method and disdain for what others consider science. In a widely referenced episode, Freud received a friendly letter from a psychologist informing him of some experimental results that seemed to validate some psychoanalytic notions. His hostile letter in reply informed his well-wisher that psychoanalysis needed no such validation. Psychoanalytic institutes have made sure this view remains current—Leopold Bellack, for instance, tells the story of having to threaten to sue the New York Psychoanalytic Society to get it to rescind a rejection of his proposal to do an empirical study.[44]

For our purposes, we need to ask how psychoanalysis has fared in scientific testing, even if psychoanalysts have not taken such work very seriously. Fisher and Greenberg's sympathetic assessment reached conclusions similar to those of Paul Kline, who had conducted a similar sympathetic survey five years before: that some parts of Freudian theory have received some empirical support. Neither review claimed that any part of Freudian theory had been proven. Kline concluded that "the theory needs far more careful empirical analysis than it has yet received."[45]

Other reviewers of the literature have been less kind. Hans Eysenck, who is both an important scientist and perhaps the most tenacious critic of psychoanalysis, has examined every scientific study that seems to support Freudian views and has claimed to show them to be seriously lacking.[46] His overall conclusion is that

---

[43] Seymour Fisher and Roger P. Greenberg, *The Scientific Credibility of Freud's Theories and Therapy* (1977).

[44] Leopold Bellack, "Teaching Psychoanalysis as Science," in Gerd Fenchel, ed., *Psychoanalysis at 100* (1993).

[45] Paul Kline, *Fact and Fantasy in Freudian Theory* (1972). In 1984 he wrote a very nice introduction to the topic, *Psychology and Freudian Theory*.

[46] Hans Eysenck and Glenn D. Wilson, *The Experimental Study of Freudian Theories* (1973).

Freud "was, without doubt, a genius, not of rigorous proof, but of persuasion, not of the design of experiments but of literary art. His place is not, as he claimed, with Copernicus and Darwin, but with Hans Christian Anderson and the Brothers Grimm, tellers of fairy tales."[47]

For our purposes, deciding between these views is not very important. If the best that can be said for Freudian theory, by sympathetic reviewers, after eight decades of psychoanalysis, is that some parts of the theory have some support and more careful empirical appraisal is needed, our point is well made. The place of psychoanalysis in our culture, insofar as it rests on its claim to have provided scientific knowledge of psychopathology, health, and treatment, is not deserved.

A Culture in Chaos

Over the last four decades, a bewildering array of alternative schools of psychoanalysis has emerged as splits have developed in the psychoanalytic community. The various schools of thought generally agree with the Freudians on the central place of transference and analysis of resistance; they usually agree that unconscious internal dynamics revealed in the transference underlie the patient's problems. Most agree that early childhood experience shapes the unconscious dynamics. Most continue the emphasis on self-reflective awareness. Most continue to see the individual and his satisfaction as the basic unit of health or illness.

They tend to disagree on the contents of the unconscious, the formative forces (or at least, their relative weights) that shape psychodynamics, what an integrated personality looks like, and how to conduct analysis. Many of the alternative schools allow social factors a more significant role than the Freudians—this was the basis of the gigantic fight between the orthodox psychoanalysts and Karen Horney, Eric Fromm, and their allies in the 1950s. Some downplay sexuality; some play up aggression. Some concern themselves more with "what really happened" in childhood and develop

---

[47] Hans Eysenck, *The Decline and Fall of the Freudian Empire* (1985).

a host of theories about how childhood is supposed to go—and the effects of deviation from those ideals. Some pay attention to a wider range of emotions than classical analysts. Some—following the lead of Thomas French and Franz Alexander, famous analysts of the Chicago Institute—have come to see the work of the analysis as providing a "corrective emotional experience," in addition to a venue for increased awareness. In this view, as the patient experiences the repudiated dimensions of himself in treatment, the analyst serves in some role analogous to a good parent. Others emphasize the role of the analyst in catalyzing change by manipulating the transference, sometimes by provoking the patient's aggression. Most of them have gone to great pains to portray themselves as "true heirs" of the Freudian legacy.

As new schools develop, old ones do not go out of business. This is one of the ways that cultures work: Subcultures develop, offering new interpretations of old ideas and claiming the pedigree of the culture's values for whatever they come up with. The multiple claims to legitimacy lead to blurring of ideas and confusion of terms. That is not generally how sciences work. In science, alternative views are sharply defined as alternatives, and the differences are insisted upon. New findings tend to usurp old beliefs, and within a short time no one holds the old views anymore.

Some practitioners of psychodynamic therapy who retain a strong sense of psychoanalytic identity, and some psychoanalysts who feel bruised by the complaint that psychoanalysis is hidebound and moribund, point to the proliferation of psychodynamic therapies as a sign of "vitality" or "ferment" in psychoanalysis. They claim, on this basis, that psychoanalysis has changed. Certainly it is true that orthodox psychoanalysis has declined radically and the multitude of alternative versions of psychoanalysis have gained ground, even in formerly orthodox arenas. These changes have not come about because psychoanalysts have suddenly started doing science, replacing old dogma with new basic research. In sciences (and even in academic disciplines), we generally see ferment when some new set of basic principles or some new technological advance causes a rethinking of old data and an emergence of new hypotheses to solve extant problems. We would be hard pressed to identify such new developments underlying the rise of disparate ideas within psychoanalysis. The changes in psychoanalysis do not resemble growth in a discipline or progress in a science; they resemble a loss of coherence and loosening of social and cultural bonds in a declining society.

Two recent developments in the murky culture of contemporary psychoanalysis deserve specific attention. One is the growing popularity of a "hermeneutic" view of what goes on in analysis. The other is the proliferation of short-term psychodynamic therapies.

Hermeneutics, which is the study of methods of interpretation, is a discipline that originated from Biblical criticism in the nineteenth century; it has spread to become a general theory of the interpretation of texts and, recently, of persons. The central point of the psychoanalytic hermeneuticists is that psychoanalysis is not a process of uncovering one's actual dynamics but of *interpreting* oneself and experience. When we read a book, we have to decipher its meaning. A book may be open to many different interpretations; the book that has a single possible meaning is fairly rare. Hermeneuticists see the analytic encounter as analogous to a text that has to be deciphered. The words and actions that make up the patient's interaction with the therapist carry meaning, and the process of analysis consists of deriving from these an understanding of the patient's dynamics. The interpretations we place on these are not right or wrong in the sense that a scientific description is right or wrong. They are a way of reading the encounter. The point of doing this is to help the patient come to a workable interpretation of himself.[48]

---

[48] The literature on psychoanalysis as hermeneutics is already immense. Donald P. Spence's *Narrative Truth and Historical Truth* (1982) played an important role in winning it a place in American psychoanalysis. See also his *The Freudian Metaphor: Toward Paradigm Change in Psychoanalysis* (1987). Roy Schafer has also been important. See his *The Analytic Attitude* (1983) and his recent *Retelling a Life* (1993).

The turn toward hermeneutics may be an inadvertent construction of a Trojan horse that will undermine not only psychoanalysis but mental health care in general. Study of narrative has a substantial history outside American psychoanalysis, and its results are not entirely heartening. If the French poststructuralists, like Derrida, are correct in their analysis of narrative, the hermeneutic turn will end in the recognition that there is no unified or centered subject behind any text. Attention to narrative ends not in analysis of the self but in its absence. If, on the other hand, critical theorists like Habermas are correct, narrative dissolves into social discourse. One way or the other, hermeneutics ends not in constructing but in dissolving the self. The delight of American psychologists toward hermeneutics seems like the delight of a child bouncing blithely on the diving board above an empty concrete pool: Innocence, uncomprehending in its excitement, is bound to end in disaster.

Thus, what matters is not whether everyone literally has an Oedipal crisis, or literally fulfills some other psychoanalytic doctrine, but that those doctrines are useful tools for interpreting one's life to oneself. Psychoanalysts who thought they were confirming psychoanalytic doctrine in the treatment process were actually finding that patients' experiences can, in fact, be interpreted in terms of the psychoanalytic version of life. Psychoanalytic theory, then, is not so much a matter of scientific discovery as it is a system of of interpretive principles to which the patient's experience can be assimilated, and by which the patient can therefore gain a coherent sense of herself. The psychoanalytic process is a process of analyst and patient constructing together a narrative through which the patient makes sense of herself.

The importance of this development is that it takes psychoanalysis completely out of the realm of science, into the realm of literature. This parallels the career of psychoanalytic theory itself—as it has declined among scientific disciplines, it has grown in the literary disciplines. Seeing psychoanalysis as essentially a literary venture may be a good thing, but it strongly suggests that the original basis for doing psychoanalysis was simply wrong. The hermeneuticists' argument entails that psychoanalysis is not science. If we think that mental health care should be scientific, the appropriate response to the hermeneutical school would be to stop doing psychoanalysis. The other option is to give up the claim to the status and authority of scientific validity.

That the hermeneuticists see themselves as providing a new basis for psychoanalysis, rather than undermining it, suggests a maneuver typical of cultures but not of sciences—namely, finding a new rationale for continuing a cultural practice whose original justification has passed away. In science, proving the basic principles to be false undermines the science itself. Consider, for instance, geometrical optics. A condition for its very existence is the fact that, under average conditions, light travels in straight lines—that is why geometry is applicable to optics. If someone was able to prove that this was untrue, the science would have to cease to exist. The hermeneuticists claim to have done exactly an analogous thing. So why should this not be the death knell for, rather than reformation of, psychoanalysis? The answer, I think, is that the practices of psychoanalysis are ways of life that persons are not going to give up simply because (if the hermeneuticists are right) the reasons that brought them into existence are wrong. Cultures do not suddenly commit suicide when they realize their ideologies are defunct.

Psychoanalysts who recognize the scientific barrenness of the discipline but who do not want to give up their professions and the ways of thinking that constitute their world—that is, people who have been enculturated into the psychoanalytic way of understanding, for whom it constitutes the reality of their lives, but who are faced with the knowledge that the reasons they accepted this way of understanding are inadequate—will probably embrace hermeneutics in increasing numbers, as a way to keep going. Practitioners and patients who value literary speculation more than scientific soundness will find hermeneutics attractive. Persons devoted to scientific understanding of psychopathology and its cure are not likely to flock to it.

If psychoanalysis has any future within scientifically oriented care, it will probably come through one of the many recent efforts to develop a short-term "psychodynamic" psychotherapy. Leading contenders among these therapies have have developed at Vanderbilt University, the University of Pennsylvania, the University of California at San Francisco, New York's Beth Israel Hospital, and Harvard University (where two very different models have developed).

Psychoanalysis has lost favor as much because it takes so long—and costs so much—as because of its scientific shortcomings. Though some analysts—like Sandor Ferenzi—began trying to develop short-term therapies early in the history of psychoanalysis, such efforts found little popularity until competing cultures of care developed short-term treatments. Orthodox psychoanalysts generally insisted that the transference could not become richly apparent or resistance be successfully analyzed in short-term work. In the last decade, short-term psychodynamic therapies have moved from a suspect, little-respected place to command much attention.[49]

---

[49] A good overview may be found in Paul Crits-Christoph and Jacques P. Barber, eds., *Handbook of Short-Term Dynamic Psychotherapy* (1991).

These modes of care command our interest for at least four reasons. First, being short-term, they are more affordable and better suited to compete in the mental health marketplace. Second, most of them have developed out of universities and hospital departments of psychiatry, so they are not subject to the discipline of orthodox psychoanalytic institutes. Third, counter to the anti-research spirit of psychoanalysis, many of them do extensive scientific work. Finally, they allow therapists and patients to make use of the conceptual riches of psychoanalysis. Taken together, these four characteristics may allow these schools to make of psychoanalysis something scientifically sound and economically viable.

The short-term therapies generally continue the psychoanalytic emphasis on unconscious dynamics originating in childhood, and they continue to make analysis of the transference central. They continue the idea that the patient's problems are due to dynamic conflicts within himself. The therapist's role continues to be analyzing the dynamics, not giving advice or instruction. These therapists tend to be very selective in choosing patients; generally, each school develops criteria of what kinds of patients are capable of undergoing their mode of treatment. Short-term therapies generally differ from traditional psychoanalysis in two major ways. The therapist identifies an area to focus on in the first session or so, rather than letting the treatment unfold in an open-ended fashion, and she also takes a much more active role in probing the dynamics in service to this focus.

For our purposes, the respective doctrines of these schools are not highly relevant. None of them has risen to the level of a comprehensive or generally attractive school of care; we do not know whether any of them will be remembered a hundred—or even twenty—years from now. The important point for us is that they have not arisen because they have already discovered portions of psychoanalysis to be scientifically valid. They exist because the culture of psychoanalysis exists, in order to try to make something viable of the psychoanalytic heritage. Whether they will succeed, no one knows.

What is instructive, for our purposes, is the overriding nature of the research characterizing these briefer therapies: Virtually none of it aims to determine whether the psychological principles of psychodynamics are true or to delineate which of the competing psychodynamic schools is most accurate.

The creators of a new form of psychodynamic therapy generally construct their version of therapy, codify "manualized" prescriptions for how to conduct clinical work, then do outcome studies to see whether patients who are treated according to this regimen get better. "Getting better" is usually determined by a consensus of like-minded clinicians (members of the same culture) looking at some selection of clinical data. What does not seem to be recognized, though, is that the assessments by the "independent" or "objective" observers carry weight only for those who *already* accept the terms in which the observations are made. When the terms in which observations are made do not derive from validated psychological principles, agreement about the observations cannot possibly speak to the accuracy of the treatment school's assertions. At best, such research shows that the therapy has brought about the changes that the therapists of that particular school aimed to bring about—it enculturated the patient effectively—and that the patient is happy with it.

Another example of research that cannot establish the accuracy of the underlying psychodynamic hypotheses involves a group of like-minded clinicians looking at data from a session, analyzing it, and predicting what will happen next. If they make similar predictions and these come to pass, they assume that this validates the principles. The curious thing is that many different schools use this same research paradigm to validate substantially different versions of psychodynamic therapy—which would seem to show that it cannot select between hypotheses. That would seem to mean it lacks probative weight.

Perhaps what actually goes on in such research is this. A school of thought develops and fosters a number of members, all of whom learn to speak the same language. They learn to call certain clinical phenomena by certain names, and they connect the names in a conceptual picture bound together by a speculative theoretical system. They learn, as all of us do, that certain phenomena occur in certain regular patterns. When one phenomenon occurs, we expect its usual successor. (This requires no scientific insight; indeed, it is our ability to recognize such patterns that leads us to look for scientific explanations.) Imagine a long suspension bridge: It touches down to earth (and water) only at certain points, while above those points is suspended a complex of beams, wires, and other structures. The psychodynamic therapy being studied "touches down" to clinical reality at certain points, as well—namely, the points of clinical phenomena—and above those points we find the entire theoretical and ideological apparatus that weaves these observable phenomena into a conceptual structure. The observers observe—they see which of the clinical phenomena do in fact occur—and they interpret and evaluate them according to the vast bridgework that is *not* a matter of empirical observation. Since the people involved in a given research project are all members of the culture out of which the project emerged, they all live under the same bridge, as it were. From the fact that they agree concerning the clinical data we can only infer two things: that the clinical phenomena occurred according to pattern, and that the observers have all learned to spin out the same story about those phenomena.

That, I think, is why researchers at a university or hospital can make up their own version of psychodynamic therapy, give it an acronym (STAPP and TLP at Harvard, CRCC at Penn, TLDP at Vanderbilt, ISTDP at New York's Beth Israel, and so forth), do research, and then report back that their research shows them to be doing something sound—while the whole of it fails to add up to any general consensus, only to so many discrete projects addressing so many discrete programs. At best, the researchers learn ways to conduct *their* program more effectively. They do not present us with any findings that help us choose between programs, or even to decide whether the program studied has basic validity. Which variant of psychodynamic theory a given therapist works with (and thus the one by which her patients are taught to see themselves) has little to do with science. It has mainly to do with the medical school or psychology department to which she happened to get accepted or what workshop she attended when she was discouraged with her earlier training.

The turn toward research, and acceptance of the challenge to base therapy on science, is a much welcomed development. As psychoanalysis continues its senescence, we will probably see at least some of these cultures develop into more autonomous players in the larger culture of care—and thus in shaping our society. In care for psychopathology, the cultures that currently try to be scientifically rigorous offer such slim pickings, such thin ideas addressing such a restricted range of the problems patients bring to treatment, that the psychodynamic therapies offer to practitioners and patients the richest variety of ideas in which to vest faith. Thus, it will probably be the case that the *field* of psychodynamic therapies will continue to receive a great deal of attention. Some one or more of this disparate lot may eventually become a successor to psychoanalysis, if one of them manages to catalyze a compelling vision from the miasma of conflicting contenders for succession to psychoanalytic orthodoxy.

Classical psychoanalysis had a logic and a coherence that resembled the kind of theoretical consistency required for a science to develop. It had a method of investigation that seemed, on the face of it, valid enough. In its explanatory sweep—the range of phenomena it had something to say about—it was awesome. Perhaps more important, it answered to professional needs of the developing psychiatric community, the wishes of society at large for a comprehensive theory of mental health that could illuminate the "psychopathology of everyday life," and the modernist wish to place the inner life of the individual at the center of human concern.

The method of inquiry showed itself to be unreliable, however; and the process of creating psychoanalysis turned to fostering institutions that would teach the original theory and its attendant practices, rather than toward correcting the theory through sounder science. Differences of opinions led to splits and the founding of competing subcultures, not to the scientific testing of alternative hypotheses. The claim of psychoanalysis to scientific status no longer even persuades—we never read announcements, "Psychoanalysts have discovered that . . ." because no one even considers psychoanalysis capable of discovery.

The passing of psychoanalysis from prestige in mental health care is no occasion for unmitigated joy. For psychoanalysts, arguably more than any other ministers of care, have listened to massive volumes of richly detailed accounts of people's lives. They have had more opportunity to learn of life's travails, especially its dark underbelly, and of the vast gulf that separates the conditions of existence from socially approved versions of life. The greatest legacy of psychoanalysis is its highly developed art of listening for what is not being said, for self-deception that is being perpetrated, and for the wishes and terrors that patients cannot own honestly. When psychoanalysis functions at its best, it makes possible a level of honesty concerning what the patient is about unrivalled by any other institution in our society. Psychoanalysis may not be very good science, but at its best it has possessed a venerable speculative and literary, if not scientific, culture, that has been arguably more sophisticated and intricately elaborated than any other extant culture of healing.

The decline of psychoanalysis has at least as much to do with its own culture as with any inherent unworthiness of its basic project. In its success, psychoanalysis institutionalized the conditions for its demise: the resolute refusal to subject it claims to careful science, the blithe ignoring of other sciences, and the authoritarian tradition that compromises its credibility among persons committed to intellectual freedom and reform. The culture of psychoanalysis is a bit like the culture of organized crime—alluring, often rewarding, admirable in certain particulars, but ultimately corrupt.

Yet the legacy of psychoanalysis lives on, in our society and in the general culture of healing, as the legacy of English law lives on in the countries that were once its colonies. For good or ill we can count on revivals of interest and the tenacity of restorationists. Cultural beliefs, unlike disproved scientific hypotheses, do not die so much as fade into the background of our collective interpretive repertoire, to resurface when we want them. We will not see the resurgence of the cosmology that puts Earth at the center of the universe, nor are we likely ever again to believe that atoms are the fundamental units of matter. We will probably, from time to time, see the resurgence of psychoanalytic ideas. That happens, when belief is determined by the needs, wishes, and fashions of a culture rather than scientific validity.

Chapter Four

BEHAVIORISM'S FAILED IMPERIALISM

✳

IT IS NOT POSSIBLE WITH PRESENT TECHNOLOGY
TO TRACK HUMAN MEMORY ACCURATELY. . . .
A HUMAN'S CONDITIONED EMOTIONAL RESPONSE
CANNOT BE REDUCED TO AN ELEMENTARY ASSO-
CIATION. AN ABSOLUTELY MASSIVE BANK OF
MEMORIES MAY BE RECALLED BEFORE THE EMO-
TIONAL RESPONSE IS TRIGGERED. . . . SO DIVERSE
AND NUMEROUS ARE THE MEMORIES WITHIN A
SINGLE RECOGNITION EXPERIENCE THAT HOSTS OF
BRAIN REGIONS MUST PARTICIPATE IN THE
PROCESS.

> —*Daniel Alkon*
> Memory's Voice

PSYCHOANALYSIS ESSENTIALLY DEFINED the field of mental health care through the 1950s, despite multiple competitors and proliferating sects spinning off from psychoanalysis proper. In the late 1950s, though, behavior therapy developed as a distinct field, and within a decade it began to displace psychoanalysis in many quarters. The influence of behaviorism on our society may well equal that of psychoanalysis. We now refer to various psychological fields as "behavioral science," even when they have nothing to do with behaviorism (or even behavior). Talk of "changing behaviors," including "mental behaviors," is a commonplace of daily speech now—as it would not have been a couple of generations ago. All sorts of academic disciplines, such as economics, have been shaped by behaviorism, even as psychoanalysis had shaped such fields as anthropology. Whatever else behaviorism has or has not accomplished, it has successfully transformed received wisdom so that virtually all of us now accept the idea that study of behavior is central to the study of mind.

Behaviorism must be understood as two distinct entities: behavior science and behavior therapy. What the two share is a commitment to understanding human life in terms of overtly observable events of behavior and the observable conditions that sustain or extinguish them. Repeated behavior, according to both, is learned, and this learning takes place through processes of conditioning. Unobservable internal events, according to behaviorism, are myths of a prescientific age, akin to ghosts and demons. A science of human life should not appeal to such mythical notions, any more than a science of physics should appeal to poltergeists and the intervention of God.[50]

[50] B. F. Skinner's *Beyond Freedom and Dignity* and *About Behaviorism* remain the best popular accounts of what behaviorism is about. For clinical material, S. J. Rachman's *Fear and Courage* is very nice. Albert Bandura "wrote the book" on classical behaviorism, *Principles of Behavior Modification;* he later wrote the most sweeping revision of behaviorism in a cognitive direction, *Social Foundations of Thought and Action.* Hersen and Last have compiled an illuminating compendium of case reports, *Behavior Therapy Casebook.* Alan E. Kazdin's *Behavior Modification in Applied Settings (4th ed)*, is easily readable and reliable.

Behavior science had been around for several decades before clinicians used it to derive a unique form of therapy. Behavior science, also called "learning theory," developed as part of the effort to create a science to explain human life that would be separate from philosophy. Psychology as a discipline is usually dated from around 1879, when the first laboratory was founded by Wilhelm Wundt to study phenomena of mind rigorously. The early psychologists relied heavily on introspection—it was an indispensable part of virtually all their experiments. They labored mightily and produced volumes and volumes of rigorous, fairly uninformative results. Worse, it eventually became clear that *what* the experimental subjects saw when they cast their eyes inward was heavily influenced by what they knew they were supposed to see. Debates in the fledgling science of psychology were heated, multifarious, and (despite the effort to be empirical) hardly discernible from philosophy. In reaction, the early behaviorists proposed, in essence, *that there should be no science of mind.* They believed that mentalistic concepts were useless in explaining human life, and they proposed dropping from our system of explanation all those constructs that referred to mind. They offered an alternative explanatory program: to understand life in terms of stimulus and behavioral response. Behavior science took shape in the early decades of this century, and by the 1930s had the dominant position in psychology departments in America.

At various points in the 1930s through the early 1950s, psychologists (and a few psychiatrists) had used learning theory as a way of interpreting what went on in the standard, psychoanalytically oriented psychotherapy of the day. These were mostly academic exercises, aiming to show that learning theory could *encompass* the phenomena of psychodynamic therapy, and they consequently had little effect on what happened *in therapy.* Behavior therapy developed as an identifiable form of care in the 1950s, when a few people took an opposite tack—rather than interpreting standard therapy in behaviorist terms, they asked how therapy *ought to be done if* behaviorism were true. Thus, they came up with a substantially new way of doing therapy.

Like behavior science, behavior therapy began with the contention that terms of stimulus and behavioral response would be helpful in understanding and alleviating certain problems of life. Attempts to understand those problems in terms of internal mental processes, they believed, had failed. Like behavior scientists, behavior therapists believed that, since both stimulus and behavioral response are in principle observable, it should be possible to investigate scientifically just how patterns develop and what needs to be done to change them. They hypothesized the existence of lawful relations between stimuli and responses and, consequently, between stimuli and alterations of response. The conceptual program is elegant and, in principle, highly susceptible to rigorous execution (since everything is observable). Much of the initial appeal of behaviorism came from this conceptual elegance and susceptibility to empirical research.

Behavior therapy offered another very appealing promise: Instead of sitting around talking endlessly about one's mysterious inner workings, with a rather uncommunicative analyst, a patient could *do something* about his obvious problems under the *active* guidance of the therapist. Moreover, relief could be effected in a few sessions. Behavior therapy offered rapid, active cures based on expert prescriptions.

We can therefore easily understand why clinicians would look to behavior science for a model of therapy. Psychoanalysts were, for behavior therapists, horrible transgressors against careful scientific observation and testing, and the interminable muddle of psychoanalytic treatment offended the sense that therapy has to *do something*—and do it in ways that can be clearly understood. Using behaviorist terms and methods offered clinicians a way out of this morass: A behavior therapy, it seemed, would be clear, sound, methodical, and well defined.

Behaviorism also offered clinical psychologists emancipation from their servitude to psychiatrists. Behaviorism required no reference to anything medical, medical schools did not teach behavior science, and behavior science was already in control of psychology. Add to this the promise that a therapy derived from behavior science would have a stronger scientific justification than the psychiatrists' beloved psychoanalysis, and we can easily understand why American psychology found behavior therapy attractive. As always, hope for salvation precedes a leap of faith.

Many people fail to understand behaviorism's appeal because of its most controversial feature: its denial of all our ordinary notions of mind. To many people, behaviorism looks extremely threatening—a desiccated notion of life that robs us of all that matters. Behaviorists, though, are offering a contention about *what sorts of terms are useful in understanding life.* Behavior science was not, in principle, errant in proposing the possibility that a good science of human life will be profoundly counterintuitive— profoundly at odds with the sorts of terms we have ordinarily used to understand life. They were not undertaking a corrupt enterprise by ignoring the outcry from those who do not want to put the terms we ordinarily use at risk. Science frequently leads to new, deeply counterintuitive ways of understanding, and people frequently express outrage at sound scientific findings precisely because they do not like having their intuitions undermined. Conceivably, an adequate science of psychology—and psychopathology—may resemble our everyday accounts of how we experience ourselves, and what we *seem* like to ourselves, as little as physics resembles how we experience the physical world. The appropriate question is not whether a science matches up with our prescientific modes of description and explanation; what matters is that it *explains* nature to us. Despite the profoundly counterintuitive nature of physics (e.g., "If a tree falls in the forest, and there is no one there to hear it . . .), the evidence is so overwhelming and we gain so much in our understanding of the world (including our understanding of how our experience gets generated) that we eventually accommodate the paradoxical truths. Even so, it *could* have been that behaviorism would revolutionize our understanding of ourselves.

Principles of Behaviorism

Behaviorism generally recognizes two broad classes of conditioning: classical and operant. "Classical" conditioning is the sort we all learned about when we studied Pavlov's dogs in high school: A neutral object, paired with a stimulus, comes to elicit the response that initially occurred only to the unconditioned stimulus. Thus, dogs to whom a light and food are presented simultaneously learn to salivate to the light alone. "Operant" conditioning is the sort of conditioning associated with the work of B. F. Skinner: A behavior becomes associated with its consequences, so that behaviors that become associated with positive results are more likely to be repeated than behaviors that do not, and behaviors that meet with negative results are less likely to be repeated than ones that do not.[51] Reinforcers, like stimuli, may be natural or learned; where a naturally occurring reinforcer is paired with a salient concomitant, the concomitant may come to be a reinforcer itself, in the absence of the original reinforcer.

Notice that in *both* kinds of conditioning, behaviorists recognize a class of natural phenomena *not* caused by conditioning, namely, the response to an unconditioned stimulus, and the pleasure or pain found in the results of operant behaviors. Natural associations, so to speak, are necessary for behaviorism to get any kind of purchase on the world. Obviously, there could be no conditioned response without underlying mechanisms to generate the unconditioned responses that conditioning works upon. If dogs did not salivate to meat, they would never salivate to light presented along with meat, much less to light alone. Similarly, if children did not take pleasure in the warmth of touch or shrink from pain, or if they did not enjoy sugar and dislike receiving electric shocks, these reinforcers could not be used in operant conditioning. The behaviorist position is that innate mechanisms cannot explain much of human behavior: They are the necessary substratum of learning, and understanding them is essential to understanding learning, but most of human life must be understood in terms of *what* has been learned.

Behaviorism is the ultimate expression of the belief that nature, though real, is relatively impotent in the face of "nurture." The point is important: Behaviorists do not fail to recognize natural sources of pleasure and pain, but they *do not* make much of these. Psychoanalysis and behaviorism give radically different weight to

---

[51] Notice that there are three possibilities here, not two: behavior that elicits positive results, behavior that elicits negative results, and behavior that elicits no particularly noteworthy results. Behaviorism recognizes that some behaviors may not meet with reinforcers at all. It makes the empirical claim that repetition of such behaviors is a matter of chance, so that unreinforced behavior cannot account for repetitive, patterned problems.

the organism's innate preferences, pleasures, and aversions. Both recognize intrinsic forces, then, but they give to them radically opposite sorts of significance and functions.

Behavior therapists have generally come to recognize three sorts of internal mental process: stimulus generalization, higher order conditioning, and vicarious learning. These processes are at odds with the original assumptions of behavior science, but behavior therapists have been forced to recognize them, as "mediators" between stimulus and response: For behavior therapists, mind is a stimulus-response mediator. Stimulus generalization is the process by which some attribute of a conditioned stimulus or learned reinforcer is taken as salient, and that attribute becomes a pervasive stimulus or reinforcer. Thus, if a child who takes food without asking is harshly punished by his mother but not his father, the stimulus "woman" may generalize and the person may become fearful of eating in the presence of *any* woman. Higher order conditioning is a process of linking associations across different experiences, which leads the person to expect the conditioners in contexts other than those in which they were first learned. So, for instance, a person for whom women have become negative stimuli in the presence of food may come to see dresses, perfume, high-heeled shoes, or other stimuli characteristically associated with women as negative stimuli. Vicarious learning consists of acquiring information concerning stimuli and reinforcement by observing the learning experiences of others, as when a child learns that a new situation is dangerous or not by observing what happens to others in that situation. These three types of mental process may combine—one's own experience, what one observes from others, and what one infers on the basis of all this go together to make up a stimulus and reinforcement calculator, so to speak.

That is the basic behaviorist concept of mind. Notice that in this concept, mental activity is anchored in experiences with the external environment. This means that mind is always a *mediator* between stimulus and response. Moreover, mental health has to do primarily with what has gone on in one's environment, not with whether one's mind is working correctly. Never do behaviorists entertain the fundamental notion that psychoanalysts consider central to psychology and psychopathology: the smooth or conflicted operation of the internal apparatus of the organism. Behaviorists refuse to define mental health in terms of the proper internal functioning of the organism, and they refuse to develop a concept of the proper and pathological functioning of mind. Minds work the way minds work; problems have to do with interactions with the environment. *Minds* are not disordered, but experience can be so unfortunate that orderly minds generate problematic associations.

Behaviorists have no qualms about, and have a coherent enough (though perhaps false) theory to account for, symbol making as a mode of behavior. According to behaviorists, words and objects themselves may become conditioned stimuli and learned reinforcers. A symbol, according to behaviorists, is a word or object that has become a conditioned stimulus or learned reinforcer. Through higher-order conditioning and vicarious learning, symbols take on extensive scope in controlling systems of behavior. Thus language, in the behaviorist view, is learned like any other behavior, and words come to have psychological significance because of the situations with which they are associated. For example, the word "bad" may carry anticipation of punishment, so that when the word occurs to one, the conditioned consequences are anticipated and negative feelings aroused.[52] Thoughts—which behaviorists call "self statements" and "covert behaviors"—thus have their behavioral significance.

Behavior therapists believe that problematic states result from complex processes of conditioning and the mental processes that extend learning beyond the original situation. Here, though, is an interesting issue: In a great many cases, the patient's history does not show any events of the sort necessary to give a behaviorist account of the problem's etiology. Behaviorists have generally shifted away from claiming to account for the origins of problems to explaining what sustains and what can ameliorate them. They believe that what has been learned only continues to function if it continues to be reinforced—states that do not continue to be reinforced "extinguish." Thus, a behavioral analysis of a problem

---

[52] Howard Gardner includes a good account of the debate on behaviorist notions of language in *The Mind's New Science* (1985).

always focuses on the conditions that currently sustain a problematic state. A person's history, for behaviorists, is highly relevant, but only to give clues as to what keeps the problem going. By studying what the patient has learned through conditioning, reinforcement, and the mental processes we have described, the behavioral therapist undertakes to decipher the stimuli and reinforcers that keep the problematic state active. The reasoning is quite logical: If reinforcement determines behavior, and if a problematic state (behavior) exists, it is being reinforced. Remove the reinforcement, and the state will extinguish, no matter what happened in the past.

Behaviorists, for the most part, deny that the idea of "personality" has much scientific or explanatory validity. This makes sense, from their perspective: In a world in which behavior must be sustained by current reinforcement conditions, in which inner mental activity and innate proclivities do not have central determinative force, and in which change results from altering current interactions with the environment, the personality cannot be very important. Personality is relegated to the waste heap of prescientific ways of explaining life that, in the world of behaviorism, *must* be useless. Though the early English behaviorist Hans Eysenck developed a widely used personality test, most behaviorists have gone to great lengths to explain this as a vestige, a response to the mental health community's requirement that personality be seen as important. A substantial body of behaviorist research aims (and seems) to show that personality is not a useful predictor of behavior and, especially, that personality tests do not reveal any behavior of clinical or practical use.

To account for the fact that individuals do differ, and that the specific characteristics of the individual mediate stimulus and response (or action and reinforcement), behaviorists use the construct of "person variables." A person variable is a characteristic (such as temperament, taste, belief, habit, or whatever else) the individual brings to the party, as it were. Distinguishing between personality and person variables is not an academic, hairsplitting effort to smuggle personality in through the back door. For person variables do not add up to a personality "structure" for behaviorism. Person variables, in any situation that comes in for behavioral analysis, are simply discrete elements of the mix that has to be analyzed, and they are subject to alteration through reinforcement like any other characteristic. Person variables do not reflect any "true" self, and no assumption can be made that such variables will not change their values over time.

This position is dictated principally by the needs of the culture of behaviorism, though. The research purporting to show that personality is not a salient variable is fairly tendentious; certainly it has not deterred the vast industry of personality psychology, including personality testing and assessment. Intrinsic to behaviorists' rejection of personality theory is their insistence that for personality to be useful, it must help us *predict specific behaviors* and be clinically useful *in a behaviorist therapy program*— that is, personality must do what *behaviorists* want a good theory to do.

This is a good example of how a culture insists upon understanding things in its own terms, for its own purposes. Certainly, for psychoanalysts, the idea of personality does not make primary reference to behavior; personality evolves to regulate *internal* states. It seems at best ingenuous to expect a concept that was constructed to account for internal states to find its validity in overt behavior. In any case, the behaviorist rejection of the idea of personality is an example of a culture's translating an alien concept into its own terms, then declaring it false because the translation proves unhelpful within its culture. Curiously enough, there is now substantial evidence suggesting that personality traits, as measured by Eysenck's methods, show a high degree of genetic determination.[53] It seems that personality might, in fact, not only be real but be under significant genetic control. The behaviorists reject as uninformative a view of personality, and a method of ascertaining it, that continues to find new utility in other fields of investigation.[54]

---

[53] Robert Plomin, J.C. DeFries, and G.E. McClellan, *Behavioral Genetics: A Primer* (1990).

[54] Behaviorists have historically been very good at producing research that proves to them the nonexistence of psychological phenomena that turn out to be very important in other fields. Another example would be the Freudian notion of displacement, which behaviorists have argued does not exist. The problem is that, in elegantly controlled studies, rats not only show displacement but, as the Freudians would expect, the displacement measurably lowers stress-related disease. See Robert M. Sapolsky, *Why Zebras Don't Get Ulcers* (1994).

Behavior therapists have developed an extensive array of techniques for altering behaviors they have identified as problematic. Cataloging them here is beyond the purposes of this book, but we need to identify some representative methods. Perhaps the most widely used are the "exposure" techniques of systematic desensitization and flooding, relaxation techniques, and assertiveness training. In addition, as behaviorists have brought cognitive issues within their purview, they have developed techniques to change thought "habits." They have an array of "aversive techniques" to cause patients to associate negative outcomes with previously desired behaviors. These are ways of inflicting unpleasant experiences, like electric shock (though shock is less often used these days, in response to public dismay), in conjunction with behaviors that the therapist and patient have targeted for extinction. Behaviorists also train persons in social skills, especially conversation and communication.

The exposure treatments—systematic desensitization and flooding—take opposite approaches to achieving the same end: extinguishing conditioned anxiety or fear responses. Either may be done in imagination or "*in vivo*"—a fancy Latin term for "in real life." In systematic desensitization, the patient and therapist construct a "hierarchy" of possible situations leading up to direct exposure, in imagination or in fact, with the feared situation—the feared stimulus. Beginning with a fairly nonthreatening situation, the patient imagines, or actually encounters, some distant approximation to the feared situation. She learns to relax in the presence (in reality or in imagination) of this distant approximation. Once she can tolerate this encounter without anxiety, she moves up the hierarchy to encounter the slightly more threatening situation immediately above the one just mastered. This process continues until the person can be exposed directly to the most feared situation. The idea is that the patient will find that the most feared situation does not actually carry the negative consequences that have become associated with it, so that the conditioned response will extinguish and the person will no longer respond to it as if it did. Sometimes this method works; sometimes it does not. Research on when and with whom it works best is helpful but not entirely conclusive.

As an alternative, the method of flooding also sometimes works. Here, the patient confronts the most feared situation directly, in imagination or real life, and tolerates a high rate of anxiety until the anxiety abates. Flooding has a basis in something discovered in the course of systematic desensitization: Unless the patient goes through vivid imagery, or is kept from averting attention from the feared stimulus, the exposure, even in systematic desensitization, does not result in extinguishing the response. Flooding is designed to force vivid imagery or attentive perception by immersing the patient inescapably in the feared situation for a protracted period. Again, the idea is that the patient will learn that the feared situation does not, in fact, have the feared consequences that have become associated with it. The centrality of vivid imagery, or attentive perception, seems a bit surprising; it seems to suggest that internal mental events are essential to the effectiveness of even these most behaviorist of behavioral techniques.

Relaxation techniques often accompany the exposure methods, but they may also be used on their own. The relaxation techniques involve controlling one's breathing and one's awareness of one's body by contracting and relaxing different muscle groups one after another, so that one's physiological reaction to an anxiety-making stimulus is not allowed to rise to the level of an autonomic anxiety reaction. Autonomic reactions, once they start, pretty much run their own course; this we know from physiology. Developing awareness of cues that precede anxiety is essential to relaxation techniques; one learns to identify such cues and institute the relaxation techniques when they first appear.

Assertiveness training, which has received so much press over the years that most of us are familiar with it, relies on the assumption that patients have come to associate the seeking of rewards with negative reactions, and in response have adopted the habit of passively waiting on others to provide them with positive experiences. Assertiveness training aims to extinguish the association between seeking rewards and receiving negative reactions, such as punishment or various forms of domination. Part of this involves teaching patients to distinguish self-assertion from aggression towards others, on the assumption that aggression is less likely to be met with positive outcomes. In practice, assertiveness training involves a great deal of talk about rights and the legitimacy of one's actions, and it involves a great deal of coaching and exhortation from therapists that patients "stand up for themselves." Nowhere does behavior therapy resemble active indoctrination into a way of looking at one's place in relation to others more than in assertiveness training.

Behaviorists also undertake to teach patients various social skills, though it is not at all clear that what they teach has a great deal to do with stimulus and response. They teach patients to observe the content of discussions and transactions and their emotional tone, to react to them, to modulate their behavior with an eye to the response it is likely to induce, and the like. Good things to know, no doubt. Social skills training does seem to help some patients to enter into social situations with more confidence and less anxiety.

The way behaviorists try to change people's thought patterns varies, depending on how much the particular therapist has departed from behaviorism and moved toward cognitive therapy. What the various behaviorist methods share is an assumption that thoughts—which are treated as "silent verbal behavior"—are discrete events that recur and may be caused by conditioning to occur less frequently or more frequently. Thus, the basic strategy is to increase positive thoughts, or thoughts that lead to positive experiences, and to decrease the frequency of thoughts that carry negative connotations or lead to negative consequences. For behaviorists who have remained roughly consistent with behaviorist ideas, the strategy involves conditioning the person to decrease or increase certain silent verbal behaviors by extinguishing prior associations or instituting new ones. What distinguishes behaviorists who use cognitive methods from cognitive therapists is the assumption that thought itself is principally determined by conditioning. Thus, a person's thoughts are the result of his conditioning history, and changing them requires changing what he is conditioned to think. Some of the methods used are very direct. For instance, a patient may have either a heavy rubber band or an electric shock device attached to the wrist; she then reports her thoughts to the therapist, who snaps the rubber band or administers a shock whenever the sort of thought they are aiming to extinguish occurs. The patient will then be instructed to administer similar aversive experiences to herself whenever she has such thoughts.

In general, we must remember, behaviorists believe that any behavior, including thought, exists because it is sustained by current conditions. In principle, behaviorists do not believe that one changes thought *in order* to change overt behavior, but rather that acting according to a different hypothesis will lead to new experiences that will condition one to accept the new hypothesis and reject the old way of calculating contingencies. The source of conditioning, as always for behaviorism, is finally interaction with the environment.

The analytic work of a behavior therapist, when a patient presents herself for care, is to understand what the presenting problem really is, in behaviorist terms, to decipher the conditions that keep it in play, and to develop a treatment plan to alter or extinguish the problem. To do each of these tasks well requires extensive knowledge of the research literature and skill at making fine-grained differentiations between behaviors and between reinforcement or stimulus conditions. The behavior therapist, once she has decided what needs to be changed—the "target behaviors"—decides what techniques need to be used to extinguish the problematic behaviors or replace them with less distressing alternative behaviors. One of the accomplishments of behavior science, which has its applications and its analogues in behavior therapy, has been to discover a great deal about how, in fact, conditioning works. Contrary to the glib assumptions of many clinicians (and lay people) who have never bothered to read the behaviorist literature, behavior modification is not "just common sense." Quite the contrary. It turns out that learning often does not take place very effectively in the common-sense terms most parents, teachers, bosses, and others apply. Knowing exactly in what sorts of circumstances, and to what end, various sorts of conditioning and reinforcement works is an exacting study.

Behavioral analyses can be quite persuasive and even breathtaking in the exquisite attention given to reinforcements.

Behaviorists find all sorts of conditioning factors that one would never see if one were not trained to look for them, and if one did not have knowledge of the extensive research literature on behavioral learning. Especially interesting are cases in which, through history taking, the behaviorist decides that the problem the patient presents with is not the root cause, but rather an extrapolation from the root cause. Wolpe, for instance, has reported a case of a claustrophobic woman whose claustrophobia was successfully treated only after it was construed to be derived from her fear of her husband. Teaching her behavioral skills to stand up to her husband lessened her fear of him, and her claustrophobia disappeared.[55]

The behavior therapist may avail herself of many different procedures, and which one is chosen depends on the kind of behavior that has to be changed and the system of reinforcers taken to be currently in play. Two patients may present with similar complaints of sexual anxiety, for instance, and their anxieties may be completely different in origin and sustenance. What has to be done to give each relief may be radically different. One of them, for instance, may be suffering from a generalized expectation that women will reject and treat him badly if he expresses sexual wishes; this may originate in experiences he had with his mother or sisters or other women. For this patient, the therapist may decide to employ "discrimination learning" to teach the patient that not all women respond negatively to men's sexual wishes, but he may precede this with a course of systematic desensitization to lessen the patient's anxiety prior to exposure to women in sexual contexts. The other patient's anxiety may have less to do with sex than with awkwardness in social situations with women, perhaps because he does not have the social skills to interact comfortably in social, flirting, courtship, or seduction situations. His anxiety over sex may derive, through higher-order conditioning, from a more basic anxiety over courtship interactions with women. In this case, the therapist would be more likely

---

[55] Joseph Wolpe (1969), reported in K. Daniel O'Leary and G. Terence Wilson, *Behavior Therapy: Application and Outcome* (1975).

to prescribe acquisition of social skills, on the assumption that as the patient's anxiety with women diminishes, sexual anxiety will dissipate. In many, perhaps most, cases, behaviorists identify multiple behaviors that need attention and institute multiple discrete techniques of dealing with each.

Cultural Disparities

We can now understand a radical difference between behaviorist and psychoanalytic notions of problems and health: Behaviorists simply *do not aim to do what psychoanalysts do.* Psychoanalysts aim to reform personality, so that the patient can incorporate the full spectrum of his abilities, instincts, and resources into a life as full as reality allows. For behaviorists, cure consists of behavior change that ameliorates the patient's complaints. The behaviorists' frame of reference does not include notions of personality structures that inhibit fulfillment of basic instincts, drives, etc. Observable behavior change, leading to curtailment of complaints, is enough, for behaviorists—and for those of their patients who are satisfied with their treatment. Behaviorist comparisons of the effectiveness of behaviorism and psychoanalysis beg the question of what counts as effective therapy. Psychoanalysts do not deny that change in behavior eventuates from personality change, but they deny that looking at behavioral change is an accurate barometer of personality change. Far too many other factors, besides behavior, are involved in personality, on the psychoanalytic reading of what life is about. Behaviorists consistently point out that psychoanalysis does not do exactly what *psychoanalysts* would be the first to say they do not even *aim* to do. This is persuasive to behaviorists, in the same way that Republicans are much impressed with their own arguments against Democrats: Unless one already buys the behaviorist's position, the argument is simply beside the point.

The difference between psychoanalytic and behaviorist notions of health and illness is not an empty one. The psychoanalytic idea that differences in psychic functioning might not reveal themselves readily in behavioral difference is not inherently preposterous. A Porsche with a faulty fuel pump and worn suspension may perform on tests exactly as well as a perfectly functioning Pinto. That does not make it a perfectly functioning Porsche. Psychoanalysts can easily claim that persons, like cars, differ in their potentials. Thus, the possible truth of the psychoanalytic claim that behavior is not a good indicator of health is not beyond imagining. Behaviorists, in effect, claim that two cars that behave alike are alike.

We see here a fundamental cultural divide. Because the two schools conceive of things so differently, what one says about the other tends to miss the point. Members of the culture doing the criticizing are much impressed; members of the culture criticized are not. All the behavioral research in the world, so long as it takes place in behaviorist terms, will never impress psychoanalysts, precisely because it does not address the things psychoanalysts say are important. Conversely, psychoanalytic critiques of behaviorism, articulated in psychoanalytic terms, look to behaviorists like so much myth making and obfuscation. Whenever a school of care touts its scientific studies, one does well to ask whether those studies have begged important questions by using only their own terms.

The Behaviorist View of Life

With behaviorism, unlike psychoanalysis, we do not have to prove the point that patients are enculturated. Behaviorists make no pretense of neutrality; they know that they are actively teaching and changing the patient, and they go to great lengths to understand how to accomplish this.

Within the technical processes of behavior therapy, the role of the therapist could hardly be more different than the role of the psychoanalyst. The behavior therapist directs, informs, and assigns activities, supposedly based upon his expert knowledge of behavior analysis and techniques. He assigns homework, to get the patient to gather data on daily behaviors and to get her to institute new behaviors in ordinary life. Frequently, behavior therapists enlist significant persons in the patient's life as paraprofessionals (or teach the patient to enlist them): They are taught to gather data and to participate in altering behavior, and their role is usually seen as crucial to creating change. The behavior therapist is a source of intelligent analysis, information, direction, and orchestration of resources. He is not himself supposed to be the medium of change, either directly or in his relationship to the patient. Change requires new patterns of behavior and reinforcement, which means that the patient must enact new behaviors and receive new reinforcements in the daily environment that controls her behavior. The therapist tells her how to do this and instructs others on their roles in bringing it about. Since the environment's reaction to the patient's behavior controls reinforcement, the patient and the environment, not the therapist, ultimately determine the success or failure of treatment.

Behavior therapy enculturates patients into more than its overt techniques, however. In teaching patients that their problems and possibilities are to be understood and addressed according to the techniques of behaviorism, behaviorists teach patients distinctive ways of looking at how life works. To "do behaviorism" requires adopting the ways of approaching life that are implicit in what behavior therapists teach. As we shall now see, to learn to think of one's problems as amenable to behavior therapy is to acquire a very specific idea of what problems amount to—and how the world works.

The behaviorist view of life appeals, as we shall see, for a deeply humane reason: If life is a matter of emitting behaviors and meeting with reinforcements, if mind is a matter of calculating and anticipating routes of finding positive and avoiding negative reinforcements, and if there are no inherent drives and passions that may compel us or put us at odds with our environments, we should be able to have nice, manageable lives. What we need to do (what behavior therapists aim to help us do) is identify accurately what is going to work for us in our environments and to formulate symbolic rules and guidelines that let us anticipate correctly when to do what. In principle, what controls the quality of one's life is identifiable, and improving the quality of life is within one's grasp—if only one's activities are well crafted and one's thoughts well controlled.

Behaviorism is generally a fairly optimistic philosophy: Problems result from the formation of associations that are, in fact, erroneous. One anticipates problems where they are unlikely because of some fortuitous contingent correlation in the past. Whatever has been learned can be unlearned, behaviorists say. Thus, in principle, reconditioning should be possible, and the problems should disappear.

What makes this highly optimistic view of life possible is (among other things) the denial of intrinsic internal imperatives that determine the quality of life. Humans do not suffer raging passions, except insofar as we have some reason to expect they will do some good—and if we are wrong in our estimations, we can get that under control by changing the learning contingencies and their symbolic representations in self-statements. Humans are not subject to a battering, bewildering welter of imperious emotions, born of being a body at all or born of being the particular person that one happens to be. Individuals do not find themselves possessed of, and by, innate temperaments, needs, and proclivities that are hopelessly at odds with our environments—where the individual and the environment seem to be at odds, the individual can be brought to "more realistic" habits and expectations through behavior therapy. By learning to look at themselves as their behavior therapists teach them to do, patients learn *not* to think of themselves in terms of internal imperatives, imperious emotions, or innate needs. They learn to look for contingent associations between environmental occurrences.

Only slightly less important in sustaining behaviorism's optimism is its sanguine view that one's history is relatively ephemeral. Behaviorists look for the conditions that "currently sustain" problematic behavior. Here we have two amazing assumptions: that behavior has to be "sustained" in order to continue, and that what sustains it is current. The assumption that behavior only occurs if it is sustained amounts to an assertion that, once something happens, it will not continue to happen without a reason— an assertion that occurrences in life possess a natural evanescence. The assumption that behavior has to be sustained by something current, rather than memory or inertia or fantasy or meaning derived from one's history, amounts to an assumption of the omnipotence of the present. Together, these amount to a belief that an ephemeral present wields complete power over what happens in a person's life. In behavioral terms, the power of the past to override any satisfactions the present might offer, the compelling power of perplexity over one's past to render the present unimportant or insufficiently meaningful, the possibility that history may have meanings possessing a weight that cannot be undone by the fleeting unimportance of the present—these simply do not exist, except as confusions benighted, mistaken patients have been conditioned to believe.

The optimism of behaviorism could not exist, either, without its peculiar take on what constitutes a human's environment. Environments possess order—a simplicity in their components and articulation in the relations of those components—in behaviorism. Environments exist as compilations of identifiable events, with discernible (if complex) relations. They do not have to be comprehended, analyzed, categorized, and digested in order to *become* sources of gratification and displeasure. Accordingly, basic ways of parsing the world are not central to satisfaction and unhappiness. A person is not seen as possessing a basic, life-orienting worldview that may render him bewildered and inept if it is badly formed. Nor will he find himself in agony when his previously-workable worldview suffers challenges—the distress of having one's ownmost notions of life under siege and no clear way to move past confusion into a new and acceptable clarity. Patients of behaviorists concern themselves with identifying discrete contingency events, not with creating a coherent take on ambiguous reality.

Behaviorism, then, postulates a world of incredible discreteness—elements discrete in their existence and in their bearing upon each other. Stimuli and response each have, in the behaviorist world, a distinctness, and they pair in lawlike causal relationships. Life is no miasma or mèlange of inextricably interacting but only randomly related elements. Interactions between the elements of one's life do not fail to maintain discrete boundaries and meanings and impacts. Confusion, for behaviorists, arises not from the muddled collisions of disparate and ill-defined events, not from the inexorable melding of memories one into another, not from any impossible conflict of meanings that cannot be neatly resolved into coherence, but from failure to analyze carefully exactly which stimulus evokes which response, what reinforces what. The world of behaviorists resembles the artificial laboratory conditions of behavioral science more than it does a blooming buzz of confusion. They *believe* in their hearts that careful analysis can show, underlying apparent confusion, the lawlike working of paired stimuli and responses, actions and reinforcements, including workings that result in the "mediational" processes of "self-statements" and thoughts that govern behavior. Surely this is faith, not science: belief beyond anyone's observable experience!

The optimism of behaviorism stands in curious relation to its principle view of life's problems and their solution: fear and courage. Behaviorism sees neurotic and other problems principally in terms of anxiety and fear (with anxiety being seen as generalized fear). Fear is anticipation of negative events; courage consists of facing such events. Behaviorist ideology presupposes that the world is *not* an especially fearful place—that generalized fear is the result of conditioning, not of anything resembling a reasonable appraisal of how the world works. Desensitization, relaxation, and most of the thought-substitution techniques of behaviorism rest upon an assumption that, when reality is confronted, it is not so bad. This includes the reality of who one is; negative self-statements are assumed to be generally inaccurate. Many psychotherapists and patients of other therapeutic cultures attest that psychotherapy usually involves revealing and facing dimensions of one's history and character that are deeply shame-filled. Behaviorists do not seem to take such confessions as pointing toward any deep truths about what it is to be a person; they are, at worst, evidence that people get conditioned to take needlessly negative views.

Perhaps this optimism about the world (and the belief that fear is the greatest problem) accounts for the prevalence of assertiveness training in behaviorism—and the absence of, say, patience and humility training, or resignation to one's lot training, or loyalty training, or training in fidelity to one's station and its duties. Assertiveness is a good counter to fear. Patience and humility, resignation to one's lot, or any number of other possible stances toward life do not address fear, in any direct way. Assertiveness also carries with it an implicit premise that what one wants is there to be gotten, if one asserts one's self. Asserting one's self in the absence or impossibility of what one wants, or in the face of an implacably inhospitable environment, promises frustration and dismay, even repudiation by the environment of which the impossible is expected, not greater well-being. Without their faith in a generally hospitable environment, behaviorists could not view assertiveness in so positive a light.

We can understand how behaviorists and their patients come to understand life by looking at what, for behaviorism, life is *not*—what its views contrast with, deny, or negate.

To ask what makes up a life, for behaviorism, is almost to ask a question alien to its culture. For "a life" implies a continuity, a cumulative process, that behaviorists do not countenance. For behaviorists, change extinguishes things. A person's life has no inherent continuity, no coherent "flow," for behaviorism. A life is a collection of reinforcement events, leading to a succession of sets of behaviors. Behavior does not occur simply because some-where, for some reason, it *got started* and has not stopped, because it brings closer to fulfillment some basic life agenda, or because (being who one is) one can scarcely help doing it—these, each, would imply internal continuity and a determinative force for internal dynamics over and above the environment.

This is probably why behaviorist therapy comprises techniques that seem, to the more humanistically minded, artificial and gim-micky. (We should remind ourselves that the assumption of an inherent course to life, a coherence and direction that accu-mulates through one's history, is a basic assumption of literature, theater, and biography, not merely an idiosyncratic notion of some cultural fringe.) The feeling of gimmickry comes because, for non-behaviorists, these techniques look as if they are imposed upon a life, irrespective of that life's own organic flow. "Imposed" here means what it literally means, not some brute exercise of political domination: The techniques are placed into the flow from outside, not arising from the flow itself. Such imposition makes good *behaviorist* sense: Change only comes through a change in contingencies, so something has to intrude—"inter-vene"—upon habitual behaviors. For persons with a more humanistic sense of a life's contours and progressions, interjecting behaviorist techniques feels like an interruption, an alien event grafted willy-nilly into a life without respect for its logic and process. Behaviorists seem genuinely puzzled when their critics use terms like "imposed" and loudly declaim that behaviorism lacks respect for individuals. Behaviorists do not see themselves this way. But they do not see themselves this way because in *their* terms their techniques *are not* unmindful impositions. They do not think about, and thus do not attend to, what *others* take to be the *organic integrity* of an individual life—for they do not see lives as possessing such characteristics. Thus, their techniques, in their view, do not impinge upon such organic integrity. They may be right; the more humanistic view may be an artifact. In any case, behaviorists and their patients learn to look at life in a way incompatible with humanistic notions. *Being an individual* does not mean, in the culture of behaviorism, what it means in many other places.

Changing, for behaviorists, therefore, does not entail a substantial re-orientation of what has been accumulating. When behaviorists talk about change, they talk about future states being different from past states; they do not talk about changing the shape and direction of one's history. "One's history," for behaviorists, is not an entity requiring attention. Change, for behaviorists, does not entail that we have to give up our investment in what *has been;* we do not have to reinterpret what we have been about up until now. Behaviorism has no room to see hesitance to change as reluctance to abandon the projects that gave past events meaning. It has no room to see that grief over change is not merely confusion over where to find new gratifications when old ones pass but is instead sadness over lost meaning.

For behaviorists, life is not made principally of memory, hope, and the continuity they have with the present—that is, what most people mean by "meaning." Though behaviorists have (as is necessary in the nonbehaviorist context of contemporary care) taken to using the word "meaning," giving lip service to "what the stimulus means to the patient," they do not seem to understand the meaning of "meaning." They do not seem to understand that "meaning" consists, for those cultures that see it as primary, of the vast web of significance that an event, habit, or aim acquires *because* of its vital connection with events, habits, and aims beyond itself. "Meaning" is a construct that fundamentally denies the discreteness essential to behaviorist views of events, including problematic events.

The peculiar behaviorist account of hope and memory, which derives from its view of life as concatenation of discrete and changeable events, can appear as a dismal, deracinating reduction—or a relief from viewing problems under the weight of an accumulated life history. If we are behaviorists, we need not hold to unpleasant memories as defining who we are, nor need we assess foreseeable events in terms of their potential to fulfill projects we took on long ago, to complete trajectories that give our histories coherence and significance. Our more general ways of thinking are just strategies for mediating between stimulus and response, not the tasks whose fulfillment and frustration, realization and compromise, constitute who we are. Looking at life with this much simpler notion of hope and memory can relieve a host of cares.

Relief or not, this is obviously not a necessary way to conceive of hope, memory, mind, and life. We might, for instance, think that *behaviors* are mediational of our deeper agendas: Events are sought or avoided, evaluated or discounted, as they help us fulfill projects that are larger than the events themselves. Not so, for behaviorists. For them, memory, hope, meaning, and the like subserve the pursuit of positive and negative events. For behaviorism, experience of events is our principal motivation, with mental activity being mediational.

Behaviorist Values

Behaviorism, like any other school of thought, has its own norms for human life. First among them is the expectation that persons should be most concerned with the quality of immediate experience. Behaviorists, with their view of thoughts as mediational, expect patients to test their ideas against the real consequences of behavior in the present. They do not take this view out of any logical necessity, but because that is *how people are supposed to be,* for behaviorism—people are supposed to give greater weight to what they experience than to the beliefs by which those experiences are evaluated. Yet this is a view of belief and falsification that behaviorism itself defies. For whether or not we take experience to falsify a belief depends very much on our investment in that belief and its place in our overall view of life. Most of us, like behaviorists themselves, will go through all sorts of machinations and contortions to preserve our beliefs in the face of apparent contradiction.

Behaviorism also expects people to be changeable, and rather quickly so. Behaviorism can cite many cases of persons who have, by behaviorists' standards, changed significantly, very quickly, without going through a laborious process of dissolving internal mental structures. Behaviorists give substantial weight to this, and it does not surprise them; that is what we can normally expect life to be like, they believe. Unlike psychoanalysts, who see such changes as superficial and relatively inconsequential, behaviorists take such changes as indicative of what it is to be a person: changeable. The famous behaviorist myth, that whatever has been learned can be unlearned, codifies this.

Behaviorists give to social conditions an overt normative weight that few other cultures of care approach. Behaviorists make no bones about the need, in their view, to help patients adjust to society. That is as it should be, given their views. There is no such thing as the "true" self, and there are no such things as innate temperaments and needs and instincts. The way a person comes to be who he is at all—and the whole meaning of life—rests with the positive or negative experiences one receives from the environment. Thus, it follows, as night follows day, that the social environment is the effective point of reference for well-being. There is nothing else available to serve as such a reference.

Whereas psychoanalysis generally considers socialization to be a precarious process, more likely to result in a "false self" or neurotic problems than to promote health, behaviorism sees socialization as the principle source of developing "appropriate" behaviors. Perhaps it is no accident that the problems behaviorism has applied itself to most assiduously are matters defined *as* problems by the larger society itself, or characteristics that interfere with fulfilling normal social expectations. Behavioral treatment of children, for instance, focuses on issues such as ill-behaved children (tantrums, eating problems, aggression toward other children and parents, learning problems, unwillingness to attend school, delinquency, and the like). With adults, behaviorism has its greatest use in the treatment of alcoholism, drug use, anti-social behavior, and anxieties that interfere with what we consider "normal" social behavior. Many of us would want to ask in which cases, or under what circumstances, such behaviors "really" indicate the presence of psychopathology, as distinct from situations in which they are called illness simply because our society does not like them. We would want to ask when turning over "treatment" of such problems to "experts" is morally advisable, and we would want to debate what sorts of experts they should be turned over to—ministers, prison wardens, support groups, etc. Behaviorism cannot engage us in debate on these questions. One of the leading attributes of behaviorism, deriving from its insistence on overthrowing the "medical model" of treatment, is that psychopathology—problems which, in the "medical model," are ascribed to underlying disorders—is seen as just various sorts of behavior, to be explained in terms of the same principles of learning as any other behavior, not the result of some disorder. The behavior *is* the disorder, and it is disordered relative to its potentials for positive and negative experiences in the environment. Thus, to ask a behaviorist whether alcohol abuse sometimes indicates pathology, while other times it indicates a moral deficiency, while other times it represents a logical response to despair, is to ask a question that cannot be discussed in behaviorist terms. The behavior is the behavior, and its consequences are problematic or not, for behaviorists.

This is an inescapable implication of asserting that psychology is explicable through learning theory and that all people, patients and otherwise, learn in the same way. For this assertion entails that there is nothing wrong with the internal functioning of the individual organism. Problems result from environments that lead the person to emit behaviors that do not fit well into society. This has a profound implication: Behaviorism cannot, in principle, repudiate social demands for change in behavior. If the behavior does not fit with the environment, it is disordered. We have no logical basis, within behaviorism, for saying, "The individual is in good working order, but the environment is awry."

What an odd paradox—and perhaps unintentional honesty! Behaviorists, unlike psychiatrists, face the stark fact that they take their definitions of what needs to be altered not from hypotheses about internal order and disorder but from what the patient's environment does not meet with positive rewards. Behaviorism resolutely refuses to develop a normative notion of what a healthy person amounts to. Unhealthy people do not fail to meet any norm of health other than the norm of fitting felicitiously into the environment.

This refusal to develop an overt normative notion of the healthy individual is somewhat paradoxical, though. Behaviorism *does* generate its own norms and possess its own values, and these are not necessarily those of the culture at large. The malleability and immersion in immediate experience that behaviorism entails could be used to generate implicit notions of health and pathology; but in the larger society, we do not, universally or in too great a measure, want people to be overly changeable or too heavily determined by the quality of their immediate experience. Furthermore, behaviorist norms run directly counter to a major strand in American culture: the insistence on self-determination through internal resources. The hard fact of the matter is that none of us has a huge amount of control over what our environments want of us; none of us has much control over what is available outside ourselves to encourage or discourage us. Outside of behaviorism, these facts meet with an insistence that we do have substantial internal control over what we *make* of these things, how we meet them, how we let them affect us, and the like. Outside of the culture of behaviorism, we long to believe that we can, by getting our inner lives in order, rise above, fend off, or turn to our own uses what the environment presents. Further, many people want to believe that their inner resources include a capacity for well-being that is not dependent on the environment. When behaviorists speak of self-regulation, self-mastery, and the like, they talk of these as mediational strategies. Behaviorist notions of self-determination *do not* include anything resembling spiritual, moral, or other inner resources that can outweigh the environment in determining well-being. They may be right, but there is nothing unusual or outlandish about the hope that self-regulation and self-mastery mean more than efficient pursuit of self-interest in obtaining environmental resources.

We need to be clear that inner resources, if we have them, need not be involved in the perennial question of free will. The point is not that our inner resources allow us to escape the laws of nature (or the determinism of the present by the past), but that they are *inner*, that they constitute each of us as individuals over and above what may happen to us in the circumstances of life our environments present us. To understand inner resources, we must ask what, if anything, would constitute resources of well-being that could determine the quality of one's life irrespective of one's circumstances.

For psychoanalysts, inner resources comprise the energies inherent in being a body at all. We need not hold, with the psychoanalysts, that these energies consist principally of libidinal and aggressive energies (though it would seem that such energies certainly are among the elements our bodies bequeath us). We have, as well, other energies from being a body at all—all the energies of being bodies with brains, for instance, including our exalted cerebral cortex, our lush limbic endowments and the proprioceptive enjoyment of location and movement in space. We also have the sensuous pleasures of having vocal cords and receptors for touch and texture, the warm ache of muscles slightly overworked, the feeling of a full belly or sated desire. We have, too, the full meanings of memory, the reservoir of experience which funds the present and makes it far less than fully determinative of our lot at the moment. We have the trajectories of hope that buffer us against immersion in the moment's offerings. We have our incredible imaginations that let us reconceive our hopes and reorient our trajectories when circumstance makes what has guided and oriented us no longer tenable. We even have the horrible deliciousness of grief at what we give up when life makes us change—the rending misery that honors what has been and what we have hoped for even as we lay it to rest. Behaviorists do not make much of these.

Behaviorism, like every other culture of healing, involves a particular view on social relations, morals, and obligation. This becomes most clear in their work in assertiveness training and social skills training—and, though we have not looked at it here, in marital therapy as practiced by behaviorists.

Consider assertiveness training. How behavior science could discover when it is and is not appropriate to assert oneself is almost unimaginable—training as a psychologist, so far as I can tell, does not provide any special understanding of the relative rights and obligations of persons toward each other. Assertiveness training involves a deep assumption, not discovered (and probably, as a matter of social and ethical philosophy, not discoverable) through science: that what goes on in a social interaction is legitimately constituted by two or more individuals each asserting themselves (or failing to assert themselves) and negotiating some mutually agreed upon way of interacting. In actuality, it seems to me, the behaviorist teaches the patient that a certain range of behaviors has moral legitimacy because that is agreed by the behaviorist community to be "appropriate assertion." This may be a helpful thing; it seems a bit much to claim that it follows upon analysis of stimulus and response.

Similarly with social skills training. Training patients in social skills would not seem to be a special province of licensed mental health professionals—I am not aware that psychology training gives one any special social grace. Be that as it may, the social skills that behaviorists teach certainly are not essential to being functional humans—obviously, since so many persons get on well without them. The "life of the party," the eminence holding court in the corner, and a host of other sorts of people manage to get through life without carefully attending to the emotional content of other's conversation, calculating what behaviors to emit to elicit desired responses, and the like. A fair number of people, in a fair number of cultures, even think there is such a thing as prescribed social behavior that should be adhered to whether or not it is pleasant—often prescribed on the basis of one's class, status, age, or gender. Living up to such social prescriptions (which might be something like fidelity to one's station and its duties), for most people in each culture, seems to get them along reasonably well in life, whether they give pleasure or otherwise approximate anything like the behaviorists' notions of social skills or not.

When we look more deeply, it becomes clear that behaviorists take an individualistic view of social relations, morality, and obligation—a sort of view that philosophers call "nominalistic," because this view holds that things are good because *we* call (name) them good rather than because they fall under a principle by which things *are* good. Behaviorists teach individuals to control and assert themselves in pursuit of intrinsically pleasing experience—for such experience is what, in the behaviorist world, is named good. Social skills and relations are instrumental to it. Behaviorists recognize that people *do have* values and see themselves as obligated to each other in various ways. They do not countenance the view that values and obligations lie beyond social convention and particular agreements between particular persons. A person's values and sense of obligation, on the behaviorist view, are learned through conditioning, and they may be changed through conditioning. The only questions of how values and obligations *ought to be* viewed, for behaviorists, are questions of what ways of viewing such things result in maximizing positive and minimizing negative experience. Behaviorists treat values as habits that people happen to have; they treat obligations as something that happens to be expected of the patient in his milieu.

One cannot be a behaviorist without taking such a fairly radically utilitarian view of ethics: An experience is to be sought because of its positive experiential qualities. Moreover, it is a very specific sort of utilitarian view: The utility is located in *specific events of experience for individual persons.* A different sort of culture of care might be utilitarian, but locate utility in a system of *social rules or moral principles,* regardless of the specific experiences that leads to for any particular person. A "rule utilitarianism" (rather than an "event utilitarianism") can deem an act or event as good because it fulfills the demands of a rule that is beneficial to follow, even if that event is unpleasant. Alternatively, utility can be located in promoting the well-being of one's group—a more collectivist notion of good than behaviorism has room for—or in adherence to a larger unit of meaning than immediate experience (like one's membership in one's group or one's projects and purposes), or both. Both a rule utilitarianism and a utilitarianism that locates utility beyond individual events of experience are inconsistent with behaviorism. Both give primacy to the ability to *conceive* of rules, group membership, or life projects apart from any stimulus/response experience—no one *experiences* a rule or a group or a life project as an event, for they are conceptual constructs.

The individualistic, experience-bound utilitarianism of behaviorism may be the correct view, but certainly it is neither obvious nor compelling. There are certainly many credible theories of ethics and social justice that are at odds with them. Yet this view is, for behaviorist culture, essential: Experience is the only thing that can be reinforcing, and individuals are the only units for which reinforcement is calculated. Personally, I think there is much to be said for this way of viewing ethics, though I do not ultimately agree with it. I am sure that "discovered by science to be correct" is not one of the things to be said for it, though.

Behaviorism also values, and teaches patients to value, action— and it finds no particular value in passivity or openness to what is beyond one's control. Behaviorism makes action ubiquitous. This may not seem noteworthy, at first glance; but fundamental to social discourse, and to our ordinary ways of thinking about ourselves, is the distinction between what we *do* and what *happens* to us.

Some things that seem like actions, we ordinarily believe, are not—a twitch in one's arm muscle is something that happens, not something one does, even though the physical motion may be identical in a twitch and a gesture. Similarly, some of one's thoughts (and most or all of one's feelings) happen to one, while many thoughts and maybe some feelings are deliberate. An entire subdiscipline of Anglo-American philosophy, called "action theory," and the Continental traditions of existentialism and phenomenology deal with understanding this distinction, especially what it means that some dimensions of who we are *happen to us.*

In psychoanalytic thought, especially in recent decades, careful attention is given to the fact that the patient experiences much of what goes on in himself as happening to him. Some things are simply part of being a person; whether one likes it or not, sexual, aggressive, and other wishes happen to anyone who exists. An important part of psychodynamic therapy is bringing what happens to a person (simply because he is a person) and what happens to a particular person (because of how his history has shaped him) into the smooth functioning of his psyche. Owning the "it"—the realities of life that are not of one's own making, but that, themselves, make one who one is—is central to the psychoanalytic enterprise.

That behaviorism has to turn internal events into "behaviors" makes it well-nigh impossible to investigate what we *do* versus what *happens* within or to us. That may be good. Perhaps the great number of eminent and astute souls who exercise themselves over these issues are chasing figments. To be a behaviorist is to be relieved of the effort to fathom such deep questions, whether they are important or acts of fiction.

Socially, it would not seem incredible to propose—as a great number of people have proposed—that most of one's life is beyond anything one's actions *can* influence or control. Fate and accident would seem to be fairly important determinants of the quality of life; and it would not be preposterous to teach either a sort of quietude or fidelity to one's lot as a healthy response to these apparently ubiquitous realities. Behaviorism, though, teaches patients always to be poised for action and control. That may be good. Clearly, it is not the only way to comport oneself toward fate and accident, nor is it clearly essential to the healthy functioning of a person.

The Scientific Status of Behaviorism

Behavior therapy was never more than loosely based on findings of behavior science, and it was heavily mentalistic from its inception, despite its disclaimers. Furthermore, and curiously enough, behavior therapy arose just as behavior science began a precipitous decline from dominance in psychology to be replaced by cognitive sciences that insist upon the centrality of mind.

Behavior therapy as a distinct field got its start from the work of Joseph Wolpe,[56] who believed that neurotic problems were principally due to conditioned autonomic responses. That is, the autonomic system, which generates anxiety states, remains in a more or less constant state of arousal because of conditioning that occurred in the past. The anxiety—the autonomic response—is appropriate to the original situation, but conditioning brings about a set of conditioned stimuli that do not, in fact, signal appropriate occasions for anxiety. The neurotic becomes anxious inappropriately, by normal standards, because of this fortuitous connection. This was not something anyone had discovered; it was Wolpe's hypothesis, extrapolated with the help of a massive assumption, from his laboratory work with certain very specific anxieties induced artificially in cats. (That the extrapolation was not warranted by Wolpe's scientific base is not disputed by current behaviorists.) Wolpe's methods depended, in part, on the patient's imagining a progressive series of scenarios pertaining to the putative conditioned stimulus, each slightly more anxiety inducing than the next. Imagination is central to the most influential behavioral techniques, though Wolpe ardently denied that anxiety reactions are mediated by cognition. So behavior therapy from the first rested on a shaky scientific base and required mentalistic activities it aimed to deny.

Wolpe's work probably would not have been so persuasive had it not been for the ethos created by B. F. Skinner's elegant laboratory work and brilliant conceptual polemics in favor of behavioral science in the 1950s and 1960s. Skinner did not do a great deal of research on clinical topics or human populations; his was "pure science," mostly with animals, and his dazzling arguments for behaviorism as a general stance were, he insisted, philosophical excursions. His contribution to clinical behaviorism consisted of giving heart to the intrepid adventurers who *believed* that theirs was the right course.

---

56 For a detailed history of behaviorism, see Alan E. Kazdin, *History of Behavior Modification* (1978).

At the point that behavior therapy arose, then, behavioral science had done relatively little controlled work on humans, for very good reasons. Rigorous behavioral research is at odds with the natural conditions of human life. Isolating and controlling stimulus and response requires a high level of artificiality, obtainable only under laboratory conditions. Further, a great many experiments have to be done with animals rather than persons, precisely because we do not know in advance their effect on the subjects and harm is often predicted (or deliberately inflicted). So most behavior *science* rests on studies of animal species under artificial conditions. Behavior *therapy* concerns itself with human life under natural conditions. As has often been argued, applying the results of animal studies to human life begs precisely the central question: whether human minds introduce important variables that, however complex and difficult to research, are crucial to understanding human life.

The fact that most behavioral science relies on animal studies is not, in principle, a sufficient reason to reject behaviorism; it simply makes clear that further steps are necessary to establish behaviorism. What turns out to be true in animal studies must be formulated into a research program ethically applicable to humans, first under controlled and then under natural conditions. However, the reliance on animal studies *does* mean that, insofar as such studies have not been successfully shown to apply to humans under natural conditions, behavior *therapy* does go beyond the scientific basis it claims to have in behavioral science. Almost all behavior science, in the days when behavior therapy was taking form, consisted of animal studies—as a great deal of it still does.[57] The willingness to make the leap from animal studies on a few phenomena to the body of human neuroses is a

---

[57] As behaviorists eventually began to do careful studies of humans, they found that stimuli, in fact, play an infinitely smaller role in determining behavior than the original behaviorists thought. This, while showing the error of the foundations of behavior therapy, is a good instance of why employing a rigorous scientific method is a good thing—it tends to lead to knowing what one might prefer not to know. Whether one is willing to throw over the principles that have been challenged by what has been found is a different matter—we do not like to abandon our cultures.

matter of cultural faith, not a matter of empirical validation or sound reasoning.

Looking back on the claims of the founders of behavior therapy, Last and Hersen tell us that "some of the [behaviorist] assertions of yesteryear most certainly have a comical ring."[58] The claims of contemporary behaviorists tend to be more humble than Wolpe's own. Harry I. Kalish, for instance, says, ". . . the link between learning [i.e., conditioning] and the origin of the behavior disorders involves a great deal of speculation based an extremely small amount of evidence."[59]

The move into behaviorism, then, was a leap of faith. Sociologically and professionally, this leap has borne fruit. Behaviorism did play an important role in giving psychology a clear field of expertise over which psychiatrists could claim no provenance. That may be the largest accomplishment of behaviorism. For scientifically, it has had an odd fate. The therapeutic faith of behaviorism arose even as the ground under behavior science began crumbling away. Fortunately for psychologists, they brought this about on their own, so psychology did not collapse into the psychiatrists' clutches. But there is something strange about a school of care that develops even as its own putative scientific basis erodes.

Behaviorism as therapy, as we have seen, originated in the late 1950s. That was precisely the moment when the cognitive sciences began to lead most psychologists to conclude that the behaviorist program in science simply would not do. Frequently called "the New Look," this movement apparently showed that there simply *is no such thing* as a stimulus, apart from what the stimulus event is *taken to mean* by the human stimulated by it.[60] The internal processes of mind that behaviorism eschewed began

---

[58] Michel Hersen and Cynthia Last, *Behavior Therapy Casebook* (1985).

[59] Harry I. Kalish, *From Behavior Science to Behavior Modification* (1981).

[60] Jerome Bruner, the father of the New Look, includes a lovely, readable account in his intellectual autobiography, *In Search of Mind* (1983). For his original papers, see *Beyond the Information Given* (1973)—which is more technical than the general reader will probably find comfortable. For a retrospective and current formulation, see his *Acts of Meaning* (1990).

their victorious march back to the center of psychological concern. The New Look set out to make *meaning* central to psychology and to change the discipline's research agenda to the study of how and why meaning evolves and how it operates. By the late 1950s, a number of trenchant critiques of behaviorism—among which Noam Chomsky's devastating review of Skinner's book, *Verbal Behavior*, was one of the most important—had rendered its claims incredible. Between the rise of the cognitive sciences and the formulation of new critiques, behaviorism was mortally wounded.

At roughly the same time, it became ever more apparent that, in psychological science, behaviorist theory has difficulty accounting for behaviorist findings. When behavior is studied carefully, it does not fit anything that should be possible in behaviorist terms. As we have already seen, behaviorists discovered, for instance, "stimulus generalization"—the process by which some feature of a stimulus is abstracted from the complete stimulus and itself becomes an independent stimulus (for example, a person conditioned to fear a white rat may come to fear anything white and furry). But *something*—some internal process apparently not directly observable—has to be doing the abstracting and generalizing. Similarly, behaviorists learned that inconsistent reinforcement of behavior exercises greater control over behavior than does consistent reinforcement. So if a rat is rewarded for a behavior only ten out of one hundred times, it will emit the rewarded behavior more consistently than if it were rewarded fifty out of one hundred times—gambling works on the same principle. In behaviorist terms, this should not happen. The ninety unrewarded efforts should teach the rat not to bother. It also became apparent to behaviorists that a neutral stimulus or a contingent reward could only become conditioned if it could be seen to correlate with the unconditioned stimulus or the behavior to be reinforced. Thus, central to both conditioning and reinforcement is the ability to discern correlations, which requires internal processes of appraisal that distinguish random from correlational pairings. Finally, behaviorists began to discover that conditioning itself does not always work on behaviorist principles. Some things, it seems, we are biologically prepared to know, and some things no amount of conditioning will teach us. Behaviorism, in studying behavior carefully, produced results that made obvious, to all but the true believers, the central importance of mind for understanding behavior.

So behavior therapy is a curious school whose attempts to take over care for psychopathology began out of high-minded scientific wishes and hot-headed emotional contempt for its predecessors, only to find its own growth paralleled by the rapid decline of its putative scientific basis.

One more problem intruded itself. To deal with the problems that we usually identify as psychopathology, behaviorists found they had to include all sorts of activities that had not been investigated by the behaviorist researchers—even activities that made no behaviorist sense—to treat their patients at all. A prominent current behaviorist, Neil Jacobson, put it this way (in 1987, after *three decades* of behaviorist research): "Much of the behavior therapy literature has failed to speak to the practicing clinician. . . . There is no literature on how to treat many of the clients confronting clinicians on a day-to-day basis. The long and short of it is that in our quest for internal validity, we have evaluated the efficacy of our efforts on such restrictive client populations that behavior therapy technology has not been extended to cover many of those who sit in our outpatient waiting rooms hoping for our help."[61]

The idea that behavior therapy is scientific, then, makes little critical sense. That many psychologists continue to trumpet behaviorism as a scientifically valid therapy tells us more about the need to maintain the scientific image of therapy than about the scientific status of behavior therapy.

Behavior Therapy and Mentalism

The distance between behavior therapy and good science also shows itself in the heavy reliance of behaviorism on mentalism: To call upon a principle or force that one's theory denies is the

---

[61] Neil S. Jacobson, "Cognitive and Behavioral Therapists in Clinical Practice: An Introduction," in Neil S. Jacobson, ed., *Psychotherapists in Clinical Practice* (1987).

antithesis of good scientific work. Behaviorism's use of mentalism even as it denies it is not hard to show, to any who are not members of its culture. In even the most rigorously behavioral of contemporary treatments—treatments involving direct exposure to feared objects and situations (about which there is plenty of research literature)—patients are taught to pay close attention to "internal cues," that is, their introspective awareness of the first signs of internal distress. Behaviorists generally interpret these as "signs of physiological arousal." They may well be right, but the hard fact of the matter is that they occur to awareness as moments of feeling. This introspective awareness itself is an internal process of the sort behaviorists should not countenance, if the basic behaviorist project were correct. Presumably, every item of psychology is physiological; so to refer to introspective awareness in this way is to do nothing except fool oneself that one is not referring to it. Further, and perhaps foremost, behaviorists have been forced, for clinical reasons, to adopt cognitive methods; and they have had to come to terms with the fact (odd from a behaviorist perspective but obvious from their own research) that the patient's sense of self-control and self-determination is central to therapeutic success. Indeed, a case can be made that contemporary behaviorism is principally *about* learning self-control, including control of one's thoughts. This is odd, from a behaviorist perspective, because it requires postulating a self of some sort, which is unobservable, and because ascribing causal control to this unobservable internal entity violates the behaviorist principal that reinforcement from external events—contingencies—controls all behavior.

As behaviorists have begun to admit to mentalism, they have only grudgingly shoehorned mind into their peculiar conception of reality. Shoehorning mind into a theory based on denying it results in two sorts of problems: some odd ideas about mind and biases in favor of ideas whose only recommendation is that they disturb behaviorist dogma as little as possible, not that they are scientifically known to be the best portrayals of mind.

We can illustrate the odd ideas by considering the extraordinary powers of self-knowledge behaviorists have ended up ascribing to mind. Behaviorists assume the ability of persons to describe themselves and their behavior accurately, as indicated by the central place given to the reports of patients (and research subjects) on their inner states. For behaviorists, in essence, the describing *is* the inner state, so that there can be no question of whether or not it is accurate. Certainly this is more credible if minds are concerned only with discrete events, rather than with existential projects and the meaning of being oneself in one's time, place, and society.

Yet this seems a bit much. Consider the fact that, with "verbal behavior," what people are capable of saying depends on their vocabulary and how they have been taught to use it. It would seem to follow, from the behaviorist position, that persons with larger and more complex vocabularies possess larger and more complex inner states, since they have larger and more complex "self-vocalizations" or "verbal behavior." Yet when we stop to think about this, it seems questionable. We have no real reason to believe that persons with lower IQs or less education have less complex or extensive inner lives than the intelligent or educated. Since that would seem an inevitable consequence of the behaviorist view, we have to doubt that view.

Perhaps more important, there is no reason to assume that everyone possesses a sufficient vocabulary and uses it correctly. That persons possess inner states that they lack the vocabulary and self-reflection to articulate does not seem implausible. Nor is there any good reason to assume that self-reports are especially accurate. For one thing, it does not seem implausible that persons use (and have perhaps been taught to use) the vocabularies they possess to lie. For another, it certainly would seem that persons may be mistaken about their self-descriptions, as we can be mistaken about anything else.

Logically, then, it would seem that verbal behavior may be a poor indicator of inner states. Not so, for behaviorism. We may characterize the behaviorist culture as ascribing an innocence and adequacy to self-reports that make little empirical or logical sense. The culture of contemporary behavior therapy here, as elsewhere, displays the commitments of its history more than the intellectual imperatives of its ontology. To admit the reality of inner states would seem to require admitting that verbal reports about them might be inaccurate, self-deceptive, and certainly inadequate.

Behaviorism ends up granting to self-reports an accuracy that even the most ardent introspectionists would never claim!

We can also see behavior therapy's heavy reliance on mentalistic assumptions by looking at the ways that social skills, assertiveness, and many other behavior changes are taught by behaviorists. Outside of some academic communities, where training groups can be assembled, such skills are taught mostly one-on-one in the therapy room, mostly by talking and imagining various situations and their possible outcomes. The patient may describe a situation, and the therapist asks questions like, "What did you think might happen?" or "How could you do that differently to get a different response?" or "How do you suppose it would affect you if you tried *x* instead?" When the patient and therapist have worked out some alternative scenario, they will usually "rehearse" it, either by going back over it in conversation or by role playing. Such rehearsal is generally said to be essential to effective learning. What is curious here is not only the obvious primacy of mental events that have no overt reinforcement, but the sense in which the patient is having a new experience. Clearly, he is not having the new experience *within* the therapy room—the whole point of rehearsal is to enable him to go out in the world, where the new behavior will actually produce rewards. More important, if the patient is imagining scenarios, presumably (in behaviorism's view) they are based on a recollection and rearrangement of past experiences. If this is so, and if those experiences are, in fact, more felicitous than his current habits and if anticipated experience governs behavior, we have to ask ourselves why the patient is not *already* acting according to the scenario he and the therapist have constructed. Why didn't his reinforcement calculator—his behaviorist mind—come up with this alternative before? Is it, perhaps, that the important thing here is the authority of the therapist? That the patient constructs the scenario because that is what the therapy situation requires? If this is so, we have to ask ourselves how the therapist got this authority. The answer will depend on a host of beliefs that the patient brings with him into treatment, since he has never before experienced therapy or observed a therapy session prior to his own.

Of course, it may be that the therapist's role is important for another reason. Perhaps the patient lacks the mental ability to construct the scenario without the therapist's guidance. In that case, the therapist would seem to provide something quite different from reconditioning, namely, superior mental ability.

In either case, the concrete realities of how behavior treatment gets done requires positing extraordinary powers of mind. Behavior science does not explain these.

If we admit the existence of mental processes, we must also admit that there is no *a priori* reason whey they must be so closely correlated with behavior that they express themselves through it in ways that let us infer their characteristics. Even with so relatively simple a mechanism as a computer, whose internal processes we know to be mechanical and rule-bound, we cannot infer either how it works or how to reprogram it from the study of its behavior alone. Or consider a business's accounting practices. These certainly influence how the business is run, but we cannot, from observing how it collects and disburses money, infer its accounting practices. Behaviorists who admit the reality of mind, yet continue to insist that the proper study of human life must necessarily give center stage to behavior, in effect insist that mental processes and their relation to behavior cannot be as complicated as computers or accounting practices.

Behaviorists do such research into mind as they do by studying discrete events of mentation, identified primarily through subjects' verbal reports, in relation to observable behaviors. They do not do it this way because there is any strong reason to believe it will show us how minds work—that this is an apt way to study mentation is less than obvious. Behaviorists do research in this way because, in the days when they denied the reality or importance of mind, they decided to study discrete events of behavior, and now they have to make mind look accessible to this method.

I suspect that what matters to behaviorists is not that their practices and methods make good scientific sense, but that they be *overt, discrete, and active.* If a technique has these characteristics, it can be researched using their existing methods. Its components are clearly identifiable, and the therapist's activity can clearly be seen to introduce an intervening causal process upon the mechanisms that bring about the distress. What is *done* is clearly identifiable; what it *does* is therefore assumed to be equally available for study. Thus, behaviorists are relatively untroubled by accounts of mentation that characterize it as consisting of discrete, articulate, verbalizable moments of silent speech. Nor are they troubled by clearly articulate moments of verbal interaction between therapist and patient or between patient and others. What would trouble them, and what they adamantly deny or assiduously ignore, is any account of such moments that portrays them as resulting from internal processes that are not so clearly isolated, that describes them as misleading or in principle inaccurate, or that attributes to such moments of conscious clarity an illusory role in the determination of life. This only allows behaviorists to keep their faith that these practices can be studied by their favored methods, when, in fact, they have not been. By observing the form of behaviorist notions about life, they can continue to believe that someday the substance will follow.

Thus, the scientific basis of behavior therapy was always shaky, the hegemony of behavior science faded away, and behaviorism has not developed a research literature addressing most of the problems of patients. Moreover, even rigorously behavioral treatments have had to include ideas of mind whose repudiation was the justification of behaviorist methods in the first place, and a great variety of quite overtly mentalistic treatments have been developed under the rubric of behaviorism. One would think that, under such conditions, behavior therapy would have been short lived—but one would be wrong. For what motivated and sustains behavior therapy has less to do with its actual scientific credentials and theoretical adequacy than with its ethos. What makes a contemporary behavior therapist a behaviorist can be understood more by the history to which he gives allegiance (and to the motivations behind that history) than by any particular doctrine—for most of the doctrines of behaviorism are defunct.

This raises again an important point about cultures which we have already seen with psychoanalysis: They do not die simply because they come to recognize the reality of something that may undermine their founding beliefs. Even where demonstrable facts and necessary practices violate the organizing assumptions of the culture, those assumptions shape what its members are willing to make of these discrepant facts and practices. They try to work them in, somehow, without giving up the assumptions that brought the culture into existence, upon which its claims to legitimacy and authority are based. They refuse to look at them in ways that would allow for the possibility that they will undermine the culture's way of looking at things. Cultures, even defeated cultures, are inherently conservative; they try to take with them into the future as much of the familiar and meaningful as can be accommodated.

Behaviorism's belated alliance with cognitive therapy illustrates this, for it was not born of scientific considerations so much as allegiance to history. We must remember that behaviorism originated in a wish to repudiate psychoanalysis. Indeed, G. Terence Wilson, one of the current and long-time leaders of behaviorism (who now calls himself "cognitive-behavioral") describes all the forms of behaviorism as sharing two features: commitment to science and repudiation of psychodynamic views.[62] By those criteria, most of the social and cognitive sciences would count as behaviorist, which, of course, they are not. Neil Jacobson explains that behaviorists began using cognitive constructs "to conceptualize and attempt to modify internal events without resorting to psychodynamic concepts."[63] The behaviorists are certainly correct that cognitivist notions of mind are radically different from psychodynamic concepts of mind—since psychoanalysts generally see cognition as subject to unconscious bodily imperatives and riddled with self-deception born of pathology. Still, these seem to be tendentious and political criteria for choosing how to conceptualize internal events. The logic seems to be, "We find that we must admit internal processes, but we will not consider psychoanalytic portrayals of those processes. Cognitivists offer an alternative portrayal. So let's make our alliance with the cognitivists."

---

[62] G. Terence Wilson, "Behavior Therapy," in Raymond J. Corsini and Danny Wedding, *Current Psychotherapies* (1989).

[63] Neil S. Jacobson, ed., *Psychotherapists in Clinical Practice* (1987).

Recognizing the reality of mind *should* have undermined the idea that behaviorism is scientifically legitimate. Behaviorists, rather than moving into a scientific investigation of mind, allied themselves with cognitive therapists—who, we shall see in the next chapter, have not done much scientific study of mind, either—to avoid the clutches of that evil beast, psychoanalysis. Recognizing the reality of mind, behaviorists were not about to venture off into the murky world of the unconscious, primary process thinking, and the prepotent importance of the past. That would have violated their deepest wish about life: that it is clearly comprehensible and manageable, in principle if not in current fact. We can make humane sense out of the immense variety of things that behavior therapy encompasses if we interpret it in this light; we cannot make much sense of it at all in terms of behavior science.

Contemporary behaviorists who use ideas of mind sound like theologians who have accepted evolution: Borrowing it without recognizing that it is antithetical to their project, they manage to miss the point. Perhaps even more, they sound like conservative religious groups dealing with sex. They would just as soon deny its importance, but since they cannot, they ring it about with all sorts of limitations, refuse to explore it in its own right, and end up knowing even less about it than ordinary people do. The behaviorist use of mental constructs becomes at best minimalistic and, more often, *ad hoc* and confusing. Sometimes, as in its excessive reliance on self-reports, it just fails to be credible.

The Place of Behavior Therapy

If behaviorism had proved to be an adequate science of human life, the many things it leaves out of its account would have to be seen as myths and fictions. Since it has not, we do not have to give these up at present. Clearly, thinking like behaviorists is a matter of accepting one culture's radical proposals about how to reform our view of ourselves.

Because behaviorism insisted upon careful attention to what is observable, the best of the behaviorists offered something of immense value: an antiseptic to the intellectual sloppiness of psychoanalysis. Though their explanatory theories did not do much to advance our understanding of life, the very care they took to avoid excess theory biased them usefully toward careful, if sometimes tendentious, description. The behaviorist disdain for the cavalier attitude of psychoanalysis toward observation and the behaviorist's careful attention to whether it refers to things that are real gave behaviorism a ham-handed and constricting notion of science; but it made for a great deal of sound observation.

The problem, of course, is that behaviorism always failed to consider so much of what most of us think needs to be observed and thought about. As behaviorists move beyond the original confines of their culture, they take with them an impoverished notion of what needs to be understood to make sense of the world. They add mental constructs only as they are forced to, and they keep their ideas about mind limited to what they think cannot be avoided. The research of post-behavioral cognitivists continues to be limited by the behaviorist narrowness of vision about what humans amount to.

We can illustrate this by referring to the highly influential work of Martin Seligman. Though Seligman was one of the most important researchers in forcing behaviorism to acknowledge the reality and central importance of cognition, he was trained as a behaviorist and for years his experiments were essentially behaviorist in methodology and standards of evaluation. Based on animal research—shocking dogs until they gave up trying to avoid being shocked—Seligman postulated that depressed persons have been reduced to helplessness by a failure of connection between what they do and what happens to them. Here is essentially a behaviorist idea: If my actions do not lead to predictable consequences (that is, if what happens is not connected to my actions), then there is no point in doing anything. In trying to understand the cognitive activities involved in the resulting listlessness (among other deficits induced by uncontrollable consequences), Seligman formulated the view that a depressed person generally explains the failure of her activities to gain desired outcomes in similar terms, along lines that are internal, pervasive, and permanent—"I failed because of something about me that will endure and pervade my further experience, so there is no point in expecting things to get better." Thus persons, like shocked dogs, learn to give up. The theory is called "learned helplessness."

Exploring this intriguing theory is beyond the scope of this book, but notice several things. First, the unit of study is always the relationship between some discrete event and its effects on other discrete events. Within the bounds of ordinary behaviorist concerns, the science itself is extremely interesting and carefully crafted. That is, Seligman's research looks at discrete events and habits of explaining discrete events. It does not look at how life histories accumulate or whether specific explanatory styles are appropriate responses to the lives of the individuals who have them. The issue of *having to get a sense of one's life* is not considered. Conceivably, a sense of the pervasive, permanent, internal factors that give coherence to one's history may be a crucial dimension of mental health. This does not arise as a question in Seligman's sort of research—probably because, coming out of the behaviorist tradition, he does not consider personal history a fundamental determinant of one's mental health.

Second, the focus of attention is always the person's own actions. Is it obvious that one's distress is always so self-referential or action oriented? We will think so, if we have been trained to see the world in the individualistic, activity-pervaded world of behaviorism. If we have not, we might think that one's receptivity to others, one's status in one's family and community, one's position in society, and one's history have something to do with one's sense of well-being and susceptibility to psychopathology.

Consider the fact that a person's embeddedness in a social community never factors into Seligman's attempts to understand what he studies. Indeed, almost all of the test conditions in the learned helplessness experiments unintentionally make reliance on others impossible. Almost always, individuals are tested on individual tasks, without the option of looking to others for help. The only exception is a rather small body of research on whether people can become helpless *as a group* if some collaborative task proves impossible. There are no studies, to my knowledge, on whether an individual's sense of helplessness is augmented, precluded, or unaffected by the presence of persons she has reason to believe she can call on for help with *her* task. Thus, the effects of one's sense of social support could not possibly be examined. Yet think about the meaning of the word "helpless"—that one will not be helped. For Seligman, it means "Nothing can be done," which, in turn, means for him "*I* cannot do anything." Yet those of us who look at life in a less individualistic way do not find these notions synonymous. "Nothing can be done" does not mean the same thing as "I cannot do anything," which does not mean the same thing as "helpless." If *someone other than myself*, who is obligated to me (and can be relied on to fulfill her obligation) or someone who cares about me (who can be counted on to act caringly) can do something, then the fact that *I* cannot do anything does not mean that nothing can be done. Nor am I helpless, if there is help to be had. So those of us who believe basic worldviews or basic stances toward life are important would want to ask about how *confidence in the benign attention of others in the world* (what Erik Eriksen called "basic trust" and what John Bowlby studied under the rubric of "attachment") affect depression. We might see the kind of attitude Seligman defines as healthy to be very dangerous—precisely because it puts too much burden on the individual and does not make basic attachment to reliable, caring others essential to health. Yet Seligman, as one formed by behaviorism, does not address the issue of how one's social relations shape one's mind and thus prevent or promote helplessness, even after having left the behaviorist fold.[64]

Finally, Seligman and kindred spirits have devised a therapeutic strategy called "learned optimism." With an optimistic bias,

---

[64] Seligman does, of course, know the data showing that persons with good social relations are less likely to become depressed than others, but this has not led him to reformulate his notion of how minds work. His theory remains absolutely individualistic. This confirms my point all the more forcefully: The science is constrained by the culture. For a popular presentation of his views, see *Helplessness* (1975) and *Learned Optimism* (1992). Peterson, Maier, and Seligman, *Learned Helplessness* (1993) is a model of systematically clear, candid science writing. Readers will note that the extensive research does not include social attachment variables. In a recent experiment by the primary author, looking to others for help was described as "using others as a crutch" and was taken as an indicator of helplessness. So radically individualistic is this culture that availing oneself of help counts as being helpless!

one presumes that one's failures can usually be attributed to external, temporary, discrete factors, rather than to internal, pervasive, enduring personal characteristics. As Seligman and similar thinkers well know and (Seligman and those closest to him, at least) honestly state, there is little scientific knowledge of how to change persons' explanatory styles. As they well know, it is a long leap from their findings on learned helplessness to the idea that learned optimism (as a general mind set) is the appropriate antidote. For our purposes, though, the important point is that this idea of learned optimism is framed with little considered regard for its ramifications for the many functions of mind. What does it do to one's thinking processes to deliberately cultivate an optimistic bias? From a behaviorist perspective, the important thing is that changing one's thought habits changes one's actions and thus one's experience: Optimistic people allegedly show greater perseverance on tasks, greater sociability, and other attributes that get them positive rewards. Is instigating activities that meet with positive experiences really so centrally the proper function of mind that it should be given such weight? The question that is never asked by these post-behaviorists is the cost, to other mental concerns, of making positive feelings and positive rewards the main goal of thinking.

How does learned optimism affect our abilities to formulate orienting life projects? How does it affect our ability to assess our internal resources and our senses of our characters? How does it affect our ability to relate to others in our society, who generally will explain our failures in quite a different manner? What kinds of disruptions does it introduce into the lives of persons who have shared some large event but find their interests diverging—say, for instance, two persons who have been married to each other then divorced or business partners in a failed venture? Would "learned optimism" lead these persons to explain the failure as the result of matters external, temporary, and limited in scope (like the other partner)? How would that affect their ability to forge some kind of future relationship? Learned optimism theorists do not have to ask such questions for two reasons: Coming out of the behaviorist tradition, it is simply assumed that seeking positive rewards (and consequent positive feelings) defines the nature of humans (and other animals); and the many other possibly important functions of mind (as we have seen) are simply not considered with any weight.

For those of us who have not had our ideas about mind thoroughly sterilized by the behaviorist disinfectant, the questions that post-behaviorists like Seligman do not even ask may seem to be the most important questions. That they vex post-behaviorists so little is a function of the cultural traditions to which these researchers and theorists answer.

Behaviorism developed a number of clinical techniques that obviously have some value, especially in helping people with phobias and anxiety problems. Knowing just what to make of behaviorist clinical successes is difficult, because we do not know how all the factors behaviorists deny (and thus do not consider or control for) play into what happens. Further, clinical behavior therapy goes so far beyond anything confirmed by good research, even in behaviorist terms, that we cannot be sure what accounts for such effectiveness as it can rightfully claim. For instance, presumably the warmth, support, and empathy of the therapeutic relationship—which even behaviorists now acknowledge as critical—play some role in the therapy's success. We cannot explain this simply in conditioning terms; for behaviorist principles would not explain why the effects of therapy would generalize across the extremely dissimilar conditions that exist outside of therapy. In sum, we *know* that the behaviorist account of how human life works is inadequate; to continue to call on that account to explain why behavior therapy works seems to be just one more act of historical reverence for those notions.

If the basic tenets of behavior science were accurate and if behavior therapy followed from behavior science, behavior therapy would be the treatment of choice for whatever we want changed. But behavior science can no longer credibly claim to be the truth about human nature. Thus, behavior therapy, if it is to continue, must be justified on other grounds. We have to understand that behavioral therapy is *not* necessarily dependent on behavioral science for its utility! Conceivably, behaviorism as a general psychology is wrong and behavior therapy as a general approach to psychopathology is wrong. Perhaps behaviorist explanations of why behaviorist treatments work are wrong. Yet behaviorist treatments may, under certain conditions, be the treatment of choice for certain problems. For this requires only that systems of reinforcement, under specifiable conditions, eliminate or sufficiently decrease psychopathology or its troubling ramifications, without deleterious side effects, to make them a useful treatment.

If behavior therapy is effective at instituting changes that we want, without effects that we do not want, and if it is either more effective than alternative ways of doing the same thing or simply the way we want to do it, behaviorism is fine. If, though, we do not relish the views about human nature that behaviorism promulgates, or if we prefer that people not relate to each other as behaviorists recommend, we have a more complicated situation. We could look for other ways to accomplish similar ends, ways that involve giving up fewer non-behaviorist beliefs. Just as there is more than one way to skin a cat, there may be more than one way to bring about psychological change.

Perhaps behaviorist institutions should be seen in analogy to the Securities Exchange Commission, plumbers and electricians, police departments, architects, and financial advisers. That is, all of these are instruments for accomplishing particular purposes. Just as it is important, for reasons of public policy, to have panels, commissions, and police departments, it may be that society needs experts in behavior modification to accomplish such purposes as decreasing alcohol use and increasing social harmony in schools. Just as it is important for some individuals to have architects and financial advisers, behaviorists in private practice may be useful to individuals who need *their* services. It may even be important, in behavior modification as in architecture and electrical engineering, to have laws governing practice so that we can be more likely to get what we need from such professionals.

However, the cultural *authority* that health care professionals claim *does not apply to behaviorists*. Because behaviorists refuse to develop a normative notion of health, they have no coherent claim to cultural authority: They cannot (even in principle) legitimately claim to tell us what is normal versus what is sick, and therefore what needs to be done (whether we like it or not) to achieve normalcy. At best, they can say, "For certain things that trouble you, we have a way of helping." Theirs is at best only the provisional, instrumental, more or less entrepreneurial authority of those who say, "If you want what we sell, we can give it to you better than anyone else." This is not to say that behavior therapy is intrinsically suspect, any more than financial advisers and architects are suspect. Behaviorist therapy's place in society is precisely dependent upon the legitimacy of the uses to which it is put and the costs of using it to those ends.

The culture of behaviorism began as the ultimate imperialism, possessed of unquestioned arrogance about the rightness of its cause, the inevitability of its destiny, and the inferiority of those alien to it. In effect, behaviorism tried to create, by fiat, a closure on what would be studied and thought about. This premature closure resulted in a defiant pretense to understand more than is understood and, consequently, a mind-boggling refusal to acknowledge how much of life is confusing, beyond our current state of knowledge, or intrinsically (so far as we can now tell) tragic or inhospitable. It is one thing to dispel mystery by understanding; it is quite another to pretend that any mystery we cannot dispel by current methods is unreal. Behaviorism seems not yet to understand how poorly it grasps the realities beyond its ethnocentric (so to speak) agenda.

Behavior science has become an instrument in the advancement of mentalistic psychology. Its effort to establish sovereignty over the field of understanding human life has failed. Behavior science and behavior therapy have developed a host of methods and procedures that clearly do *something*, even if we are not sure quite what that is. Behavior science can now offer only the—very important—promise that it will provide important tools for research. Behavior therapies, by the same token, can point to a substantial body of research literature as containing important data; but that data must now be reconceptualized and new research done to incorporate mentalistic constructs. What behaviorists cannot be sure of, though, is that such reconceptualizing will not eviscerate the behavior therapy program.

Behaviorism succeeded in giving psychology an independent voice in mental health care, and it succeeded in providing care with an alternative focus, shifting attention from the weight of an individual's history to the immediacies of her life. This gave to the mental health community and its consumers a more hopeful orientation toward life and its problems. Behaviorism also succeeding in establishing a tradition of serious research, which would eventually prompt psychiatrists to forsake speculation and turn to its own type of basic research. However, it did not succeed in providing a *viable* alternative to psychoanalysis. Neither its hypotheses about human nature nor its range of effectiveness sufficed to create a school of care that would fulfill our society's hopes for a science of psychopathology and healing.

Culture and Temperament

We have seen many differences between psychoanalysis and behaviorism, and we need not recapitulate them. Before we leave these two cultures, however, we should note that the differences between them probably lead to very different sorts of persons being attracted to each, as practitioners and patients.

Certain sorts of practitioners will find psychoanalysis comfortable: Those who take great pleasure in languorous contemplation of complexity and in reflective quietude, who find great meaning in elaborate conceptual and literary constructs, and who are reticent to intrude actively upon the lives of others. Such practitioners probably also enjoy (or suffer) the brooding presence of the past and long for a sense of continuity and coherence in stories of human life. They tend to be impressed that ambivalence, emotional conflict, and the dark underbelly of human motivation are all central to being a person. For such people, behaviorism is simply not an enlightening or comfortable place to live.

Other practitioners want to see themselves as expert in causing change, and they are more inclined toward activity than passive reflection. For them, life in the present is (or should be) free of the legacy of the past, and they take great pleasure in mastering a finely elaborated body of literature on diverse learning conditions and effects. They find sustenance in the conviction that life is capable of being more simple than ambivalent. For such persons, psychoanalysis is a dreadful bore without much that is gratifying.

For patients, a similar set of considerations also apply, except that patients do not become experts in the literature or therapeutic techniques. Patients who do not want to believe in the vast presence of the past, who want to believe that their problems have more to do with the environment than with their underlying personalities, and the like, will be more comfortable seeking behavior treatment. Patients who seek an arena to think at length and in detail about their inner lives, who long to believe that they are ultimately the centers of their destinies, and the like are more likely to enjoy psychoanalysis, in some one of its current forms.

The issue of personal temperament as a determinant of culture will be etched sharply as we move now to the two current leading contenders for hegemony in mental health care. For cognitive therapy and biological psychiatry have their own very distinctive cultural flavors, and these are likely to sit well only with some practitioners or patients. The culture of cognitive therapy, in particular, can appeal only to certain sorts of individuals and leave others without comfort—as we shall see.

Chapter Five

THE MIDDLEBROW LAND OF COGNITIVE THERAPY

THE PSYCHOANALYTIC AND BEHAVIORAL MODELS SKIRT THE COMMON CONCEPTIONS OF WHY A PERSON BECOMES SAD, GLAD, AFRAID, OR ANGRY. THE COGNITIVE APPROACH, HOWEVER, BRINGS THE WHOLE MATTER OF AROUSAL OF EMOTION BACK WITHIN THE RANGE OF COMMON-SENSE OBSERVATION.

—*Aaron Beck*
Cognitive Therapy and the Emotional Disorders

THERE IS A PAIN—SO UTTER—
IT SWALLOWS SUBSTANCE UP—
THEN COVERS THE ABYSS WITH TRANCE—
SO MEMORY CAN STEP
AROUND—ACROSS—UPON IT —
AS ONE WITHIN A SWOON—
GOES SAFELY—WHERE AN OPEN EYE—
WOULD DROP HIM—BONE BY BONE.

—*Emily Dickinson*
The Complete Poems of Emily Dickinson

✻ ✻ ✻ ✻ ✻ ✻ ✻ ✻ ✻ ✻ ✻ ✻ ✻

✻ ALL OF US EXPERIENCE a variety of cognitive states that demonstrably cause us distress or failure. Consider some technological task in which we know there is a clear, rule-bound, absolutely logical, correct way to proceed: programming a VCR. (For those to whom this is no problem, consider the frustrations even computer mavens often have in setting up a new system configuration.) We know what it is to be so confused by this process that we become anxious, irritated, and unable to think straight; perhaps we throw up our hands in defeat, decide we are stupid, and refuse to try ever again.

Consider a different, more ambiguous situation: Someone believes, subjectively, that he clearly understands something—say, for instance, he has an idea why his business partner has been curt and grumpy lately. He interprets her attitude and behavior as results of a recent difference of opinion, after which she ostensibly came to agree with him. He asks, but she says that is not the problem. He still sees evidence that suggests she is not being completely candid, though—off-hand remarks that seem to refer obliquely to the recent conflict, for instance. So, to be conciliatory, he does what *she* had originally wanted. He anticipates that she will be pleased, the air will be cleared, and life around the business will become more pleasant. But when he graciously and gently reveals to her what he has done, she is dumbfounded, then furious; she had, in fact, been convinced by his earlier analysis, and now she finds that he has taken what she agreed was the inferior course. Upon further discussion, it turns out that her behavior actually has to do with a problem in her personal life, unrelated to the business. Her off-hand remarks were just ways of displacing her frustration and blowing off steam. So even though he was able to give a clear account of why he believed as he did, and even though it made plenty of sense, it turned out he was wrong—and now he has committed the business to a course of action that neither partner thinks is a good idea. This could leave the poor fellow bewildered, suffering in his self-esteem, shaken about his judgment, and faced with the deleterious consequences of his ill-advised action.

Given the significant distress we can suffer in such discrete, relatively straightforward matters, is it not reasonable to assume that we may be equally confused (or wrong) about far more comprehensive, more complex situations—like life? This is the basic assumption of the cognitive therapies. Psychopathology results from fundamentally erroneous ways of comprehending life and the situations that constitute it.

Cognitive therapy got started in the late 1950s and early 1960s. Unlike most of the dozens of alternative therapies that developed then, cognitive therapy has managed to transcend its provincial origins and become a major player in the field. Indeed, it is fair to say that, at the moment, cognitive therapy is the "hot" field among the talk therapies; cognitive therapy is to the early 1990s what behaviorism was to the early 1970s and what psychoanalysis was to the early 1950s.

We saw in the last chapter that the 1950s marked a watershed in studies of thinking. The "New Look" in psychology, the rise of the cognitive sciences, and the behaviorist research that showed the need to introduce concepts of mind into learning theory—all of these fomented interest in how thinking works and what roles it plays in our lives. In general, it is fair to say that what unites all study of thinking in recent decades is "constructivism"—the view that our minds play an active role in constructing how we perceive and experience the world. We know, and appreciate now as no generation has before, that "the world" presents itself to us as various forms of physical energy and chemical compounds that impact upon the periphery of the body in manifold ways, and we know that only a small amount of the physical energy available in the world gets registered by human sensory receptors. Yet we experience something different in kind; we experience a refulgent world of objects, events, situations, histories, directions, and meanings. How does the welter of energies and compounds stimulating our sensory apparatus get transformed, for us, into the world as we experience it? Through the constructive activities of mind. Though cognitive scientists differ radically in their hypotheses and discoveries about this process, what unites cognitivists is a conviction that our experience cannot be understood without reference to the active processes of the mind.

Cognitive therapy rests on the notion that something is wrong with the way a person suffering from psychopathology constructs her world. The distress of psychopathology is the result of pathogenic cognitive processes. In principle, science should be able to identify what normal cognitive processes are, how deviation from them causes distress, and how the pathogenic problems can be corrected. Cognitive therapy takes a straightforward tack: Find the cognitive processes or contents that cause distress, then change them. This will allow the patient to construct her experience in a healthy manner, and the distress of psychopathology will end.

"Cognitive," though, is a bit like "light" was on food products a few years back: the trendy label to advertise. Cognition has become the *zeitgeist* of the age in the social and allied sciences since the late 1950s. Consequently, all sorts of therapeutic cultures have taken up the study, or at least the label, of cognition.

Cognition does not refer unambiguously to some obvious set of events, entities, or processes. "Cognition" means "thinking," and people who label themselves cognitivists differ substantially in what they believe thinking is, how it fits into life, what kinds of cognitive problems cause pathology, and so forth. Therapists who use the term to refer to themselves range across a vast terrain of competing camps and incompatible cultures. In the *Comprehensive Handbook of Cognitive Therapy*, for instance, we find persons from behaviorist, gestalt, psychodynamic, and a host of other backgrounds characterizing cognition in different ways. Larry E. Beutler and Paul D. Guest tell us that even "[a] cursory review of the literature will reveal at least two dozen different approaches ... that, at one time or another, have been identified with cognitive therapy."[65] When a therapist says she is "cognitive," that tells us that she recognizes the reality of

---

[65] Larry E. Beutler and Paul D. Guest, "The Role of Cognitive Change in Psychotherapy," in Arthur Freeman et al., eds., *Comprehensive Handbook of Cognitive Therapy* (1989).

■ ■ ■

thought, attributes a central role in mental health and illness to active processes of mental construction, and works to modify thought. It does not say much more.

The wide range of therapists and therapies calling themselves cognitive could be taken to mean that there is no particular culture of cognitive therapy. Certainly it means that science has not yet told us what cognitive therapy needs to look like. Interestingly, though, one particular brand of cognitive therapy, which Aaron Beck and his colleagues developed, codified, and enshrined in treatment manuals, has taken the lead within the field. While cognition makes for a variety of hybrid cultures and microcultures—an issue we will address in the closing chapter—Beck's version of cognitive therapy does, we will see, possess a distinct culture.

We will devote our attention in this chapter to this leading school. Whenever we speak of cognitive therapy in the remainder of the book (unless otherwise noted), we will be talking about the large number of therapists who take Beck's work as central to cognitive treatment.

Beck's Cognitive Therapy

The main demonstrable accomplishment of cognitive therapy is in the treatment of depression—all the other applications of cognitive therapy are modeled on this. Since our comments on cognitive therapy will have a fairly sharp critical thrust, it is best to concentrate on its strongest suit. In so doing, we will also get an accurate sense of the field, since this work constitutes the paradigmatic achievement of cognitive therapy.[66]

Psychopathology, in the culture of cognitive therapy, results from defective cognitive processes. Thus, like psychoanalysts and—as we shall see—neurologically oriented therapists, and

---

[66] Beck's major works include the following: *Cognitive Therapy and the Emotional Disorders* (1976); (with A. John Rush, Brian F. Shaw, and Gary Emery) *Cognitive Therapy of Depression* (1979); and (with Gary Emery) *Anxiety Disorders and Phobias: A Cognitive Perspective* (1985).

unlike behaviorists, cognitive therapists believe that psychopathology constitutes *something wrong* with the patient, relative to healthy mental functioning. They believe something is amiss in the ways that persons afflicted with psychopathology parse their lives and the situations that constitute them. The minds of the afflicted work differently from healthy minds, and these deviances constitute pathology of cognition.

One of the striking phenomena in the clinical setting is that patients' ways of thinking are frequently quite congruent with their problems. Thus, depressed persons think negatively, anxious persons think in terms of imminent danger, and the like. Moreover, the clinician, who is not in the throes of a particular patient's problem, sees all sorts of data to which the patient seems, to the therapist, not to give due weight. It *looks as if* the patient is somehow failing to think straight; either some belief or some reasoning deficit causes him systematically to misperceive his situation. Cognitive therapists are much impressed by this commonplace of clinical practice; they think it reveals ways that persons with psychopathology differ from other people. They think that persons with psychopathology suffer some set of beliefs and habits of thought that impede their ability to *correctly* understand their situations in life.

In the case of depression, Beck and allied cognitive therapists give what looks, at first blush, like a straightforward and very coherent description of the cognitive problems. A depressive person is deeply sad, discouraged, demoralized, and hopeless. Accordingly, his basic organizing ideas must be ideas of loss, defeat, inadequacy, and a bleak future. Beck says these cognitive attributes form the "cognitive triad": the person holds negative beliefs about himself, his future, and his world. Whatever data come within his purview are interpreted to fit into this negative scheme. Data that others would consider positive are ignored or discounted.

Both this negative ideation in general and the specific forms it takes are determined by the patient's "cognitive schemata." A cognitive schema ("schemata" is the plural of "schema") is basically a mental model of reality or some dimension of it, sort of a blueprint or outline into which various stimuli are taken, by

■ ■ ■

which they are interpreted; on the basis of the cognitive schema, a person predicts what is likely to happen and what, if anything, she can do to influence what eventuates. According to cognitive therapy theory, a person's mind comprises a hierarchy of cognitive schemata, ranging from very general notions about the world down to ideas about specific kinds of concrete situation. The cognitive triad represents the most general set of schemata. These, in turn, influence the subsidiary schemata, biasing them in a negative direction. The effects of the cognitive triad lead the depressed person to interpret particular events as being negative. The specific kind of negativity that colors each interpretation is but the content that concrete situations take on under the influence of her larger picture of hopelessness. This is what makes cognitive therapy, in theory at least, more than merely a descriptive account of the kind of thoughts that occur to depressives. Everybody has always known that depressives have a gloomy outlook and complain a great deal. Cognitive therapy makes an explanatory claim: that these thoughts are the results of cognitive schemata.

According to Beck, the cognitive triad and subsidiary cognitive schemata cause psychopathology because they are "cognitive distortions" that lead to further cognitive distortions. Reality is consistently misinterpreted to be more negative than it is. The patient interprets herself as less capable than she is, unable to bring about any positive outcome. She thus loses the motivation to do anything at all. She interprets events as inadequate to ward off impending doom, and so takes no joy from them. Since she cannot herself bring about positive outcomes, and since the environment will not provide them for her, the future looks valueless. At the extreme, she sees no point to living at all.

With this negative point of view, and under the influence of her "faulty" general schemata, the depressed person exhibits flawed logic. She begins to employ the following illogical principles:

1. *Arbitrary inference:* she draws negative conclusions from evidence that does not dictate those conclusions; the same evidence would be equally consistent with a positive or neutral interpretation.

2. *Selective abstraction:* she notices only such elements of situations as fit her negative cognitive set, ignoring what look to others like equally salient dimensions of the situation. Beck *et al.* say that she takes details "out of context."

3. *Overgeneralization:* from a limited set of experiences, the person draws a general conclusion that most situations will be the same.

4. *Magnification and minimization:* these are errors in evaluating the significance or magnitude of an event that are so gross as to constitute distortion.

5. *Personalization:* she interprets events as having particular significance for her when there is no basis for this interpretation.

6. *Absolutistic, dichotomous thinking:* events are classed according to polar, black-and-white categories.

Because the depressed person draws inferences in service to her negative cognitive set, her cognitive activities ensure that she will structure her experience in dire terms. Whatever happens becomes further evidence of the hopelessness of her situation.

What has to happen, then, is cognitive change at a deep level. The patient must be led to correct his cognitive distortions and make inferences that are logically valid, based on realistic cognitive schemata. The way to do this is to identify one's dysfunctional cognitions, formulate them as empirical hypotheses that can be tested and disconfirmed, and then formulate new hypotheses that, when confirmed by experience, become the basis for new, realistic schemata. Beck says this constitutes thinking like a "practical scientist." The realistic schemata that emerge from the process will enable the patient to see that his negativity is erroneous. As such changes are effected, the patient will structure the world differently, and he will therefore feel and act differently.

How do cognitive therapists go about effecting cognitive change? The basic structure of cognitive therapy is rather thoroughly standardized; *Cognitive Therapy of Depression* is the manual that governs treatment of depression and serves as the model for all other forms of cognitive therapy. Learning this *structure* is no great feat; the expertise of the cognitive therapist consists in her exquisite sensitivity to the idiosyncracies of particular patients and her ability to turn these idiosyncracies toward the standardized routine, so that the patient experiences himself as understood and guided in a way congruent with his own process of thinking. The communicative abilities of cognitive therapists in service to this end—turning idiosyncracy toward the standard routine—are quite finely honed, and acquiring them takes significant training.

Essential to cognitive change is close attention to emotion. Cognitive therapists *do not* discount patients' emotions; this is a mistaken assumption often made by persons who do not understand the intimate connection between cognition and emotion in the culture of cognitive therapy. The only cognitions relevant in cognitive therapy are the ones that cause the problematic feelings; since those cognitions cause those feelings, one cannot deal with the cognitions without, perforce, dealing with the feelings. One might as well try to deal with fire without dealing with smoke! In Beck's version of cognitive therapy, therapists are exquisitely sensitive to the presence of emotions. They recognize that emotions are both the inevitable concomitants of cognition and the only reason to bother attending to cognition. Further, emotions are good indicators of cognitions that need to be identified and addressed; if you want to find a fire, follow the smoke. Good cognitive therapists will not focus on ideas that patients *say* they believe unless they are accompanied by emotion; they will, instead, teach patients to be intricately aware of emotion, precisely so that authentic cognitions—those actually extant and effective in the patient's emotional life—come under scrutiny.

At the same time, we must remember that cognitive therapists believe that negative emotions are based on distortions that have to be corrected. Cognitive therapists do not believe that "getting out" emotion has any intrinsically curative force or that awareness of one's emotions is, in itself, a helpful thing. The value of emotion in cognitive therapy lies in its potency to let the therapist understand empathically how the patient experiences the world and to let the patient give full expression to that experience in consort with an empathic guide to remediation. The point of emotion in therapy is to facilitate understanding and alteration of the cognitions that cause emotion. By definition, "getting out" emotion *should not* accomplish anything by itself, for cognitivists; unless the cognitions that cause them are changed, the therapy will not accomplish anything.

In Beck's version of cognitive therapy, cognition is assumed to be coterminous with consciousness; in recent years, Beck and his colleagues have admitted the reality of unconscious information processing, but this has not led to any significant change in the therapy process. Rather, they have simply stipulated that unconscious cognitive processes are readily accessible to consciousness. Beck believes that consciousness itself contains all the relevant cognitions (or at least those that are direct causal consequences of the problematic schemata), but he believes that patients have to be trained to pay attention to the full range of consciousness. Of especial importance are what he calls "automatic thoughts." Beck believes that persons with psychopathology—and everyone, at some time or another—suffer from a divided consciousness, in which a running commentary accompanies perception. Thus, a depressed person whose friend does not compliment him on his appearance will have both the perception of no compliment and an automatic thought such as "She thinks I look like an idiot." These automatic thoughts are one of the ways that general cognitive schemata reveal themselves in consciousness.

Thus, a principal task of cognitive therapy is "training"—this is Beck's word—the patient to "pay attention" to automatic thoughts. Once he identifies them, he is asked to look at them logically, applying basic rules of evidence. He is asked to identify the evidence for his automatic thoughts and to evaluate whether this evidence might not be consistent with some alternative schema. Where the evidence seems to confirm the negative ideation, the patient is asked to test it further, along with alternative positive hypotheses consistent with the same data.

These are the basic strategies of cognitive therapy: Identify problematic thoughts, consider the evidence, formulate hypotheses, and test them empirically. The therapy process itself aims to help patients do these things and, equally important, to teach them the skills that will enable them to continue to think properly once they are out of therapy.

Cognitive therapy is a short-term therapy, usually around six months in duration—sometimes less, sometimes more. The process is highly structured, and the therapist has custody over making the process go according to structure and timetable. In the first session, and usually also in the second, the therapist "explains" the cognitive perspective: that one's ways of thinking determine one's feelings and that, by careful attention to conscious experience, one can discover the sequences of thoughts that lead to distress. The patient is told that in therapy he will learn to identify and correct his mistaken cognitions and thus to alleviate or eliminate his distress. "Target" feelings are agreed to; the therapist and patient agree to study these feelings in order to determine the cognitions behind them and assess their reasonableness, considering alternatives and subjecting both the cognitions and the alternatives to logical and empirical tests.

Thereafter, each session and the time between sessions are highly structured. The therapist and patient agree on homework assignments that will help the patient to identify and assess "dysfunctional" cognitions, then they focus on those cognitions and the tests to which the patient has put them. Presumably, the patient will not suddenly begin to think rationally and realistically. The therapist must empathically understand how the patient has thought about and undertaken the homework assignments and how he is processing information in the sessions. She must adroitly communicate to the patient where these efforts are infected with dysfunctional cognitions and help the patient formulate better cognitions. As a result, the patient learns to examine the contents of consciousness, identify and assess patterns of cognition and emotion, formulate alternatives, and—most important—therefore control emotion through reason.

Cognitive therapists have developed a variety of tools to help in this process, including forms for recording dysfunctional thoughts at specified times each day and "clickers" worn on the wrist—golf-score counters, actually—that the patient is instructed to click each time he recognizes a dysfunctional automatic thought. These tools are intended to make clear not only the nature of the patient's automatic thoughts but also how thoroughly they pervade and influence her.

As cognitive therapists see it, dysfunctional cognitions occur at several very different levels of generality. Specific dysfunctional thoughts are caused by pathogenic schemata of greater generality, ultimately by the patient's negative view of himself, his world, and his future. Cognitive therapy aims to change the schemata themselves. Otherwise, the patient remains always vulnerable to the recrudescence of the depression whenever the underlying assumptions are reactivated. These underlying assumptions, cognitive therapists claim, warp cognition (and therefore emotion) into perpetual negativity. They are the root of the psychopathology.

The Taming of Mind

The culture of cognitive therapy is very lovely: calm, deliberate, sufficiently careful to avoid great catastrophes, cautiously optimistic, not given to grand terrors and deep *angst*. Cognition is reason, reason is subject to conscious control, and conscious control is deliberate and methodical. Problematic ideas and inferences make themselves easily available for identification and tests are simple to come by. Changing one's life is as easy as changing one's mind, and changing one's mind is as easy as thinking empirically and logically. A healthy mind lets us clearly grasp our environment and carefully calibrate our wishes to what is possible. Appropriate feelings and actions follow. Minds unafflicted by psychopathology do not draw dire conclusions from ambiguous data or hold themselves to standards not readily attainable. Healthy minds are quite well adapted to furthering well-being. The world from which we construct our experience is not terrifying or demoralizing; profoundly negative ideas can safely be assumed to be false, the result of cognitive distortion.

So genial, so thoughtful a way of therapy seems on its face only laudable. Who could argue against patients learning to think more carefully, to test their ideas against their experience, to modulate their emotions according to disciplined reason? Who would even want to criticize therapy that urges patients to avoid

leaping to grand and debilitating conclusions, excoriating themselves needlessly, and seeing the world as less promising than
need be?

Unfortunately, when we think carefully about cognitive culture, we will see that it possesses a very peculiar notion of mind
and a very peculiar notion of the world within which minds work.

Consider the idea of "cognitive distortion." Cognitive therapy
rests upon a constructivist notion of mind, as we have seen: It
is because of the claim that mind actively constructs experience
that mind is given a central role in determining the quality of
experience. Constructivism, in turn, rests on the recognition that
how information presents itself to humans is not sufficient to
determine how humans experience the world. Constructivism has
taken as a central body of data the immensely varied ways people can structure experience. Reality (if by this we mean the
world considered apart from the way it is experienced) leaves an
extraordinary amount of room for reasonable persons to differ.
Because many different ways of parsing reality truly are possible,
terms like "misperception" and "unrealistic" become highly
problematic once we accept constructivism. Constructivists do
not claim that we can or should get along without assuming that
reality exists independently of what we think about it; nor do
they deny that our views have to match up with it sufficiently,
whatever that may mean. But since there is no one right way to
construct experience out of reality's impingements upon our
nervous systems, the fact that one person's views differ from
another's—or that one person's views differ at different times—
does not imply that one of them is wrong. What counts as a true
perception or belief, then, becomes a highly vexed matter.[67] Yet

---

[67] Persons who do not understand constructivism very well sometimes make two erroneous
assumptions about it: that it means "any view is okay" and that it entails a regressive relativism.
Actually, within a given construction, conditions for specifying truth are quite possible, and constructions can be compared for their adequacy on various counts. Further, constructivism is
about constructing *experience*. It does not follow from this that we cannot use scientific methods
to generate an *explanation* of experience. Such an explanation would include the general laws
that minds follow in constructing experience—though these laws themselves would not be
matters of experience. A science of mind will not consist in describing particular mental constructions—though those will be its data—but in discerning the laws, principles, and operations
by which construction takes place.

in the culture of cognitive therapy, patients are taught that, in very straightforward ways, they can identify distortions; they start making lists of these distortions from the first session. How can that be? What are they being taught? They are being taught that undistorted ideas are those that follow elementary principles of empirical investigation and logic. This seems a strange sort of constructivism. If there is no such thing as the right way to construct one's experience, how can there be a simple set of rules that allows people to begin identifying distortions—"wrong" constructions of experience—after less than an hour of instruction? In effect, cognitive therapy teaches patients that simple methods of logical, empirical investigation possess amazing power— namely, the power to dissolve the perplexities of constructivism, to identify distortions, and to discover truths about oneself, one's world, and one's future.

Leaving aside the complexities of constructivism, think about how difficult it *seems* to be to learn important truths about oneself, one's world, and one's future. People go to school for years simply to master the methods needed to arrive at reliable beliefs about these things. Yet, according to cognitive therapy, simple empirical tests suffice. Form a hypothesis, test it in only a few instances, and one discovers something capable of falsifying fundamental beliefs. Consider, though, how difficult testing a hypothesis *really* is—as illustrated by how many different schools of psychology exist, for instance, or how many different ways there are of conceiving of how cognition works. Consider how many different views of one's personality are held by people in one's social and work lives (or by oneself at different times). For any discrete body of evidence, we can usually formulate a great number of hypotheses consistent with it. In cognitive culture, people somehow manage to avoid this messy fact. Consider next how very hard it is to calculate probabilities—most psychology students dread their courses in statistical methods precisely for that reason. Yet somehow, cognitive therapy patients have a special talent for calculating probabilities that enables them to use a handful of uncontrolled observations to revise their view of the future. If distortion is so easy to identify and truth so easy to find, why is education so demanding and why is there so little agreement among psychologists (and others)?

■ ■ ■

Cognitive culture permits itself a corollary assumption: That reality is quite transparent to reason. Somehow, from early in therapy, patients can get at the truth about themselves, their worlds, and their future. A fair number of people, not to mention the extraordinarily complicated and controversial histories of science and the liberal arts, would testify to the contrary: that reality is maddeningly recalcitrant to reason. In cognitive culture, though, everyone has the mental ability to identify "dysfunctional" assumptions and make "realistic" corrections of those "errors."

Cognitive therapy practitioners and patients also get to ignore a fairly substantial logical distinction between learning about reality and assessing possibility. Most of the sorts of beliefs that Beck deems pathogenic—especially those concerning one's future—could not *possibly* be judged as to their "realistic" or "unrealistic" status, because they are not even, on their face, *about* reality; they are about the patient's sense of *possibility*. To assess the adequacy of one's sense of possibility is a very different thing from assessing descriptions of reality. (Philosophers call the logic of possibility "modal logic" and the logic of reality "propositional logic.") Cognitive therapists and their patients get to ignore this crucial distinction. Somehow, in the culture of cognitive therapy, possibility is the same sort of thing as reality.

Cognitive therapists and their patients also have a peculiar take on words and utterances (including the things one says to oneself). They regard all sorts of verbal actions as if they were transcripts of mental actions, and they treat all mental activities as if they were perceptions, beliefs, or inferences. It would seem, though, that we do all sorts of things with words other than report our cognitive activity, and we do all sorts of things within our minds other than perceive, believe, and infer. What we say can be a social act, not a report on an inner state, and we can cajole, punish, exhort, manipulate, pose, and fantasize, among other things, in our minds. If someone says, "I went off my diet yesterday; I have absolutely no will power—getting to the weight I want is hopeless," the cognitive therapist would treat this as a report of one simple event leading to a series of inferences: I went off my diet, therefore I have no will power, therefore I have no hope of success at weight loss. The patient is taught to treat this as "globalization" or "excessive inference." Yet this is obviously not the only way to think of these mental activities.

Saying these words may reflect a series of inferences—though not be an instance of globalization or excessive inference—but the verbalization may be something else altogether. Yesterday's event may simply be one more instance in a huge body of data from which one has logically concluded that one's will is powerless over food. This entire series of sentences may be an expression of the inference, I have a long history of such experiences and this is one more instance of my lack of control over my eating. The verbal account may be a way of communicating something to the therapist. "I have no will power" may be a way of expressing antagonism toward the therapist: "Don't even expect me to comply with this treatment regimen." Similarly, the patient's hopelessness may be an expression of opposition to treatment, or it may be a form of posturing to provoke sympathy, attention, or reassurance.[68]

The mental activities underlying this speech act may not be inferences or beliefs at all. "I have no will power" may be self-punishment or an exhortation akin to those coaches use when they insult team members with remarks like "You're a bunch of no-talent wimps." This works, in some situations: We do not like the image of ourselves we are presented with, so we try to do the opposite.

In cognitive culture, then, patients learn to think of speech acts as reports on inner activities, and they learn to think of inner activities as perceptions, inferences, and beliefs. Minds concern themselves mainly with assertions about the world, and the assertions of healthy minds meet the standards of simple empirical logic, which possesses a power beyond that of the most

---

[68] It also seems to be the case, outside of cognitive culture, that emotions themselves may be actions—we may induce anger, self-pity, or other emotions for a variety of reasons. Perhaps more important, emotions are social acts—we become angry or sad or listless or filled with longing in order to affect others or make them act in certain ways. Cognitive culture pays little or no attention to the intentionality or purposiveness of emotions as actions. They are, in this culture, always primarily internal affects.

sophisticated methods of investigation known to psychologists and others. Very peculiar.[69]

Unhealthy minds, of course, fail to follow such methods— through "distortions" and illogical thinking. But on reflection we realize that illogical thinking is neither abnormal nor pathogenic, and false beliefs are not particularly pathogenic. A person can, and most people quite often do, draw true conclusions by illogical thinking. As philosophers have known for several centuries, how a conclusion is reached does not determine its truth or falsity. Since illogic does not even imply falsity, it cannot imply distortion—or pathogenicity. Furthermore, a conclusion drawn by thoroughly rational means can be false. This can be due to a false premise, limitations of the data sample, or the presence of factors that one does not have any reason to suspect need to be taken into account. Hardly any of us is so omniscient that we always take account of all the data we need to consider. Presumably, we frequently draw false conclusions through altogether logical processes. Surely the cognitive therapists cannot be saying that a false belief, so long as it is reached by logical means, cannot cause acute distress. Thus, it would seem that whether or not a belief is logically reached cannot determine whether it is distorted or accurate.

A serious problem, for cognitive therapy, is the finding from social psychology that *in fact, the ordinary mental processes of most people are irrational.* A host of social psychologists, studying cognitive processes, have validated the robust phenomenon that the rules of reasoning used by most people most of the time are quite at odds with basic standards of logic and evidence.[70] Furthermore,

---

[69] Some of the case illustrations offered by Beck do not even fit elementary principles of logic. He offers an example of a woman who feared she was a bad mother but decided that, in fact, she was just "not a morning person." Logically, the latter does nothing to falsify the former. There is nothing logical about inferring from "I am not a morning person" to "I am not a bad mother." Indeed, it would seem quite possible that not being a morning person could have deleterious consequences if one's children have to awaken themselves, find their own clothes, and go off to school unfed, and if one becomes inattentive to the anxieties children face as they approach their daily tasks. See Aaron T. Beck et al., *Cognitive Theory of Depression* (1979).

[70] R. E. Nisbett and L. Ross present an excellent account of this work in *Human Inference: Strategies and Shortcomings of Social Judgment* (1980).

we know that only about thirty percent of adults are able to function fully at the level of formal reasoning; fifteen percent are incapable of abstract thought of the sort required to question one's beliefs, consider alternative views, and weigh the evidence for each. Most people are not cognitively capable of what the cognitive therapists characterize as healthy thought.[71] Philip Johnson-Laird, certainly one of the leading cognitive scientists in the world, has argued that ordinary thinking does not even proceed by the use of logical rules and evidentiary considerations at all, but by the construction of imagistic models and intuitive comparisons between models and events.[72] The cognitivists seem simply to be wrong that health has any correlation with sound logic and sound evidence. Normal thinking is not rational thinking. Thus, irrational thinking cannot be the source of psychopathology.

Worse, it is not at all clear that the thinking of depressives is either illogical or false! In the last fifteen years, a substantial body of data has accumulated showing that depressives are actually much more accurate than nondepressed persons in their appraisal of themselves and their circumstances. Most people's characteristic ways of understanding themselves are, in fact, inaccurate and overly positive.[73] What is most powerful about this data is that much of it comes from situations that are unambiguous. We are not talking about people giving themselves the benefit of the doubt. We are talking about outright lying to oneself—

---

[71] D. Kuhn, J. Langer, L. Kohlberg, and N.S. Haan "The Development of Formal Operations in Logical and Moral Judgment," in *Genetic Psychology Monographs* 95 (1977).

[72] Philip Johnson-Laird, *Mental Models* (1983).

[73] See, for instance, S.E. Taylor, *Positive Illusions* (1989). Christopher Peterson, Steven F. Maier, and Martin E.P. Seligman also include an excellent account of this work in *Learned Helplessness* (1993). What this body of data means is far from clear. It raises a host of questions about the essential functions of cognition and about the relationship between mind's "natural" functions and its *desirable* functions. We can accurately say that one major value of "civilized" culture is to maximize truth—to learn to discipline one's thinking toward what is true. If "natural" functions of mind are at odds with that, do we tend to make people "sick" by insisting on higher epistemic standards? Should we enshrine positive illusions as benchmarks of health? This body of data also raises serious questions about what makes minds "adaptive." If adaptivity requires illusion, we have a lot of rethinking to do about how minds evolved, what they naturally do, and what sorts of changes in these natural functions we can socialize people into, in the interest of our society's values, without rendering minds maladaptive.

misremembering in a self-favoring direction one's grade on a test, for example. In one interesting study involving parents and children over several years, parents consistently misremembered their earlier parenting techniques so that they were in accord with whatever was currently considered good parenting. This is especially interesting because the parents knew that the techniques they used earlier were on record from earlier interviews![74]

Curiously enough, the data showing that depressed people think more clearly than others probably shed light on why cognitive therapy helps people get undepressed. By becoming a member of this culture, one gets to believe an overly simple, inaccurate, optimistic notion of how minds work and what simple methods of empirical logic can accomplish. How oddly paradoxical that cognitive therapy teaches people to have inaccurate, excessively positive beliefs about thinking! Cognitive therapy lends the authority of the therapy industry to positive illusions, and it bolsters these illusions by calling them sound thinking. That may be the cleverest form of self-deception yet invented.

An even more peculiar idea of the culture of cognitive therapy is that one cannot rationally hold sweeping negative beliefs about oneself, one's world, and one's future. The justification for this seems to be the fact that the therapist can usually find some way to see the data presented by the patient in a less negative light. Yet what it is reasonable for one person to think, given the evidence available to her, is a different matter from what it is reasonable for someone else to think, given the same evidence and additional data to add to the mix. The cognitive therapist assumes, without doing any empirical investigation, that she has a more accurate grasp on the patient's life than the patient does— even though the patient always has more data about his life than the therapist has. The therapist assumes the patient's view to be both false and irrational and proceeds to try to "correct" the illogic and distortions that are simply assumed to be present.

---

[74] Ulric Neisser, *Memory Observed* (1982).

There is no need for the therapist to investigate the realities of the patient's life before deciding that the patient suffers from cognitive errors, for in this culture, a patient cannot rationally have reached a true, negative appraisal of her lot.

Many depressives have long histories of failure at love and work, often beginning with a failure to be loved and to meet the expectations of their families or communities of origin. In my experience, many of them can detail with perfect accuracy all the reasons they ought to be able to expect good things out of life—their talents, abilities, and so forth. But they face the hard fact that, in spite of their abilities and best efforts, they have failed to get what they want. There is nothing irrational about concluding from a long history of failures that this is one's lot in life. When the same sort of thing happens many times, in different circumstances, it is fully rational to consider that the factor present in all those circumstances—oneself—may be the problem. The characteristics that cause the problems may be resistant to change. Whether or not this is true in any particular case, considering it is certainly rational. Ruling it out *a priori* is not.

Moreover, it seems obvious that a great many talented, able people come to bad ends—most of us have known such people. There is nothing irrational about considering carefully the possibility that one will suffer such a fate oneself. Indeed, while it may be "healthy" to avoid dwelling too long on such possibilities, a fully rational appraisal of one's situation demands that one consider them. A fully rational appraisal, after all, requires that one consider all legitimate hypotheses, and this *is* one of the things we know humans to be prey to. Simply assuming it cannot happen to oneself may have its uses, but it is not a sign of rationality. I do not recommend resting in the belief that one is doomed. I am sure, though, that arriving at such a belief is not necessarily a matter of irrationality, and getting past it is not merely a matter of sound empirical investigation and logical thinking.

One way that cognitive therapy avoids facing the fact that many persons have sound reasons to be distressed is by ignoring the individual's history. The immense amount of evidence one has gathered about oneself and one's world, the years and years of turning that evidence into an understanding of oneself and one's life—these are not trivial sources of information. Yet, in cognitive culture, one is supposed to put one's history aside in the name of current investigations. In asking patients to change their beliefs based on the flimsy evidence of cognitive therapy's procedures, cognitive therapists are asking patients to ignore huge bodies of data. This seems a peculiar concept of sound cognitive process.

Consider this possibility. Someone correctly recognizes something about himself that substantially diminishes his prospects—or stops dead some project that he has invested many years in pursuing. He suddenly faces serious limitations on what his life is likely to amount to. He sees that achieving what he thought he was capable of is now quite unlikely or impossible. He is faced with the fact that he cannot have as good a life as he had hoped. He has to come to terms with a change in his projected history (that is, his sense of the future) that, by all rational measures, will cost him a great deal. Moreover, his past has been conducted, at least in part, in pursuit of his projected history; events have been evaluated in terms of their fit with this now defunct projected history. He faces a past that no longer can mean what it meant when he went through it. He may become despondent, even depressed, as a result. This does not seem an unreasonable possibility, does it?

The person facing such despair has to come to terms with *a reality he already understands quite clearly*. Precisely the most cold-eyed appraisal of the facts has caused his depression. In my own experience, this kind of situation is rampant in clinical situations; a great many patients are troubled by the facts they face. Yet in cognitive culture, such people do not exist. Patients who see themselves in this way are taught to think of themselves as suffering instead from cognitive errors.[75]

---

[75] Cognitive therapists claim that even under such conditions they can help the patient "see the positive" in his or her situation. Perhaps that is the case. However, it seems clear that this is a matter of imposing on the patient a certain task—coming to a positive view—not a matter of correcting cognitive errors or making the patient more rational. This task imposes a gross bias that is anything but rational: One must consider only such evidence and ways of thinking as will lead to a positive view. The fact is, a fully rational appraisal of one's situation, considering both good and bad dimensions, may lead one rationally to a negative view.

Those of us who believe that such a situation does not reflect cognitive errors can be reasonably sure that the patient *will* have to undergo cognitive change—envisioning a new future, creating new ways to understand his world and his place in it, re-evaluating the meaning of his history to date. This seems unlikely to amount to correcting some misperception or remedying logical fallacies. Nor does it seem likely that cognitive change is all that is involved in coming to terms with the recognition that one's life is not going to be as one wished, that one's talents or character is not as one hoped, or that the world does not work the way one always believed. Courage, endurance, and the acquisition of humility may have something to do with making the needful changes.

Here we approach what is perhaps most odd about cognitive culture: its extraordinarily constricted image of cognition and emotion.

Cognitive therapy's ideas about how minds work leave out an immense range of mental activities that—though we do not understand them scientifically—seem fairly obviously real. In a situation like the one we have just sketched, the patient will probably have to come up with a substantially new way of looking at himself, his world, and his future. That seems reasonable enough. Yet are we to think that straightforward empirical, logical methods will enable him to do this? Generating such a new conception is not rule-bound, so far as we have yet discovered; we do not possess methods for inducing creative thought. As Lewis Wolpert puts it, " . . . it is no use for anyone to pretend that there is, at present, any real understanding of the creative process in any human activity."[76] Original thought, by its nature, escapes the sorts of rules we know about so far; originality breaks past extant ways of conceiving of things. Whenever a patient has to come up with something significantly new, we can be reasonably sure this will require powers of mind that cognitive therapy does not teach.

---

[76] Lewis Wolpert, *The Unnatural Nature of Science* (1993).

Rationality, under such conditions, seems a richer, more complex, more difficult process than cognitive therapy describes, and it seems to require much patience and even moral fortitude. Even when we can call upon empirical and logical methods in the course of deep change, they take place within very complicated, messy, disorderly processes of imagining—and feeling—our way through our perplexities. We create—no one knows how—ideas of new possibilities. We think them through, envisioning how they fit (or fail to fit) with our other beliefs and wishes and commitments. We see whether we can imagine their working out in ways we can tolerate. We rest with or flee from the ways these scenarios ramify through our complicated and convoluted systems of meaning and feeling. We find ourselves, quite often, *believing what we cannot help believing.* Some new way of seeing works its way through our considerations to present itself as the solution that cannot be denied, no matter how little we may understand how we reached it.[77]

Deep change seems rarely to be under control of consciousness and will. At best, one wills to put oneself in a position of pondering possibilities, struggling with ideas and information, and making one's self open to change. One attends to one's processes of thought for clues and considers new ideas that present themselves to consciousness. At best, one makes one's self faithful to the dialectic process. How that process develops, when it ripens, and what it makes of itself is not fully subject to one's timetables and conscious decisions. How difficult it is to have the patience and perseverance to stay with a process of thought, through its distressing confusions and bafflements, long enough to bring it (or let it bring us) to a conclusion that makes sense. This bears no resemblance to cognitive change as cognitive culture describes it.

---

[77] The complexity and lack of inherently orderly procedures in rationality has begun to be not only appreciated but formalized by some scholars and scientists of cognition in recent years, especially under the influence of research into artificial intelligence. Most of this is highly technical and difficult to follow. Chapter three of Robert Nozick's *The Nature of Rationality* (1993) includes a reasonably readable (though very dense) presentation of some of the issues and possibilities involved. (The two equations in the chapter—and the pages explaining them—can be skipped over, if need be.)

Equally important, in cognitive culture, passion plays no great role in the process of change. Cognitivists do know that "affective arousal" is intrinsic to change, and this makes sense from their perspective: If cognition causes emotion, working with the cognitions that actually inform a person's life will arouse emotion. The ideology of cognitive culture has it that emotion is caused by cognition, and the goal in cognitive culture is always for reason to control emotion. When we have an emotion, there must already be a cognition that has caused it—we need only identify it and test it. Doesn't it seem, though, that we are sometimes given to passions larger than we can understand or articulate—passions that surpass our cognition? The experience of trying to articulate that by which one feels taken and possessed, prior to and in oblivion to one's ability to give voice to it—the sort of thing that makes for genius and for culture-shaking art when it occurs to people of large talent—this is not something to which cognitive culture would have its members aspire.

Further, the ethos of cognitive therapy (to provide quick improvement of mood) overlooks the fact that significant change is very painful. A vast literature (in the liberal arts, religion, and autobiography) testifies that engaging in serious reflection and enduring the confusion of remaining faithful to a process of significant thought make one feel substantially worse long before they make one feel better. Thus, substantial change requires substantial courage; deep cognitive change is terrifying. In the cognitive view of mind, terror can have no plausible role. No courage is required to realize that one has simply been mistaken in one's negative expectations; that would in fact be only an immense relief. For most of us, though, it seems more likely that coming to terms with the facts of our lives and facing the uncertainty inherent in changing basic beliefs about ourselves, our world, and our future is often a sobering experience, to which despair is not always alien. Cognitive culture elides such experience from its concept of emotion and cognition.

At least one other crucial feature of cognition and emotion seems to be omitted from cognitive therapists' notion of mind. We might think that well-being depends substantially on the fabric of faith and trust—in others, ourselves, and our world—

■ ■ ■

that constitutes social life and personal relationships. How much of what we believe about ourselves, our loved ones, our friends, our community, and even our business networks depends on empirical and logical thought? How much, instead, depends on images that we construct and vest our faith in? How much do social relationships require an implicit contract that we will live up to our images of each other? Doesn't it seem that the ability of mind to construct images beyond anything we know, and our ability to invest these with trust and hope, are central to social life?

Keeping faith with those who rely on us does not seem to be simply a matter of bearing out some sound empirical prediction they have made about our behavior. When someone lives up to our image of them, we do not react as we would if they had simply verified a prediction. Rather, we feel gratitude and appreciation. These do not seem to be feelings appropriate to someone's doing what, given the empirical realities of the situation, we had been able to predict they would do. When someone disappoints us or violates our trust, we do not react simply as if we had made an erroneous prediction. Rather, we feel let down or betrayed. These do not seem to be feelings appropriate to recognizing we had been mistaken. By cognitive therapy's own logic (that cognitions cause emotions), the cognitions involved in faith and trust must be different from the cognitions involved in making logical assessments of empirical reality.

Conceivably, a fair amount of depression is precipitated by others betraying our trust, irreparably rending the fabric of our lives. Some depression may be precipitated when others tire of our failure to keep faith and remove us from their circle of friends, intimates, or trusted employees. Conceivably, much—maybe most—optimism relies on our vesting our trust in images of others that *they* cherish *and aspire to* precisely because of their feelings about us: They do not want to let us down, so they become what we see them as being. Such processes seem quite central to how we live and grow.

In cognitive culture, the ways in which mind and feeling operate in social and personal life to construct such vital relationships receive no attention. Neither does the vexing question of regaining faith that has been destroyed. Cognitive therapists would have us think that we can have reliable social relations simply through common-sense empiricism; keeping one's faith, then, would be no more than making a good investigation—like having faith in one's calculations of how much food will be needed for dinner. Our ability to construct a life by creating images of what we will be together and for each other, then keeping faith with those constructions, does not seem to me to be that sort of thing.

Mind is probably much more than cognition and cognition is certainly more than reason. Rationality, logic, evidence—these are subsets of cognition, and just what they are good for needs to be seriously thought about. A poet exercises cognition, but this is rather different from the cognitive processes of which cognitive therapy speaks. The poet Rilke, for instance, engaged in cognition as he moved through a career in which he first possessed a sense of the Holy in nature, then moved to a sense of the deep inwardness of meaning and the nothingness of everydayness. These cognitions constitute, for those to whom they speak, ways of grasping what it is to have one's life. Evaluating them is not a matter of logic and evidence, any more than Rilke's evolving vision was a matter of scholarly or scientific investigation.

The issue of possibility needs to be thought about in this light. One's sense of possibility depends very much on ways of grasping the world that cannot be determined either by common sense or by rational inquiry. Indeed, to confine one's sense of possibility within such bounds is to ensure that one will never create anything new, will never find novel ways of putting together a life, and will always be constrained by received opinion about what is possible. One of the more intriguing functions of cognition is how imagining creates new possibilities. Creating new possibilities requires an inventiveness that does not primarily derive from what already exists—from what can be found through empirical investigations or logical elaborations of extant conceptual schemes. Furthermore, one would think that pursuing new possibilities defies the odds—and requires a courageous heart.

Coming to see cognition and its place in one's life as cognitive therapists do is to eviscerate cognition and diminish some of thinking's most magnificent capabilities—those involved in radically reconceiving ourselves and the contents of our lives and in pursuing passion and mystery that originate beyond reason. Such passions and mysteries may surpass our best efforts to understand, but insofar as they can be parsed by cognition or respected in their unsayable strangeness, they open us to life in ways that reason, as cognitive therapy understands it, cannot possibly do. Because cognitive therapy enjoins us to depart from its favored ways of thinking on pain of psychopathology, it militates against the powers of mind that offer most for lives of rich meaning. Cognitive therapy makes of cognition something far thinner, less exciting, less powerful, and less dangerous than cognition probably is. That seems to me a surpassingly peculiar concept of mental health.

The Values of Cognitive Culture

The values of common-sense reasonableness and optimism obviously pervade cognitive culture. We need to notice that these values rest on a normative belief that life is not tragic. For the last 2500 years or so, a fair number of fairly intelligent people, from Euripides to William Faulkner (and beyond) have thought that the reality of who a particular person is, coupled with the reality of her time and place, inevitably entails the loss or destruction of what is most important to the person, in at least some cases. This tragic sense of life must be seen, in cognitive culture, as cognitive distortion. Since no one can accurately believe that she is doomed, they believe, it follows that tragedy cannot possibly be an apt portrayal of reality. Writers of tragedy and those to whom their works speak suffer negative schemata, which need to be given up through common-sense reasonableness.

We are in a position now to see that the fundamental value of cognitive culture is *approval of and conformity to the conceptual and social status quo.* The assumption that profoundly negative beliefs cannot be true points us in this direction: "The way things are is not so bad; who I am, how the world works, and the reality of my situation allows for a good life," is the essential message of that assumption. More important, one *cannot* think as cognitive therapy teaches patients to think without accepting the status quo as benign and as the basis of one's thinking. One cannot, otherwise, come to the kinds of conclusions, or even engage in the kinds of therapeutic exercises, prescribed by cognitive therapy.

To make this point requires some rather complicated and perhaps subtle reflection. First, we need to look at three things that cognitive therapists often say and how radically at odds with reality these elements of their ideology really are. We will weave together these three strands of our considerations and look at the conditions under which the ideas in question can *seem* true— namely, when the status quo is approvingly conformed to. Then we will bolster this conclusion by seeing how some other characteristics of the culture make sense in its light.

The first strand of thought pertains to when and how empirical, logical reason works. Beck frequently explains cognitive therapy by reference to Thomas Kuhn's notion of paradigms and paradigm shifts. Beck says that a patient's old paradigm is dysfunctional and a paradigm shift has to take place. Yet Kuhn developed these ideas as part of a radical critique of the common idea that science is rational and empirical. He argued that this image of science is only true during periods of settled beliefs, when the scientific community is working within a given paradigm that its work does not call into question. His main point was that significant discoveries are *not* fundamentally rational or capable of being generated (and decided) by empirical tests. Contrary to the received interpretation of science, its empirical and logical work is always constrained within a given paradigm, which defines the terms of empirical inquiries and the sorts of inferences that are acceptable. Change from one paradigm to another, and the choice of what to move to, throws those definitions into question. When a new paradigm has emerged, it will define new terms of inquiry and reason. The need to give up an existing paradigm, the interregnum between paradigms, and the choice of which way of looking at things will emerge as the new paradigm—all of these have to do with emotional and aesthetic preferences, philosophic musings, politics, and a variety of other considerations. Choice of belief, and especially choice of when to change beliefs, is *not* fully the result of empirical or rational procedures.

For Beck and his allies to make use of Kuhn's ideas, while claiming that the patient's old worldview is "mistaken" and must be "corrected" (and teaching the patient that this change and "correction" will take place by the patient's learning to think like a "practical scientist") is palpably odd. What Beck seems not to understand is that paradigms are not given up because they are "wrong," nor are they replaced by new views chosen because they are correct. Nor does he seem to understand that empirical and logical work, by definition, must proceed in terms of the *existing* paradigm; for that is the paradigm that structures experience. Paradigm change cannot be determined through empirical and logical tests, precisely because a paradigm shift requires developing a new set of categories and a new conceptual order within which to approach the world.

Since the methods of cognitive therapy are solely those that can be used within a settled paradigm, it seems safe to bet that cognitive therapy cannot bring about paradigm shift.

The second strand in our argument that cognitive therapy fundamentally values benign adherence to the status quo has to do with what cognitive therapists say about values and valuing. Cognitive therapists spend a great deal of time "helping" patients come to "realistic values"—opposing the "tyranny of shoulds," in Karen Horney's pithy phrase, which cognitive therapists often quote. They see getting "realistic values" as a cognitive process.

There are two serious problems with this. Outside of cognitive therapy, valuing is not generally held to be either a cognitive process or a process that can be "realistic" in any straightforward sense.

The idea that valuing is a rational process has suffered immense assault in this century. Beginning in the late nineteenth century, social scientists and philosophers began to argue that values are largely determined by one's culture and emotions, not by reason. In twentieth-century intellectual culture we tend to assume that valuing makes essential reference to "values" that are matters of neither rational principle nor logical or evidentiary discovery. Indeed, the idea that reason can mediate value disputes has generally been discredited, replaced by the idea that reason can mediate such disputes only where there is substantial agreement on some range of values held in common by the disputants. As Herbert Simon (surely one of the most important cognitive scientists in the world) puts it: "Reason is wholly instrumental. It cannot tell us where to go; at best it can tell us how to get there. It is a gun for hire that can be employed in the service of any goals we have, good or bad."[78]

Indeed, what can it mean to speak of "realistic values"? Values and facts seem to be different things. At least, we use different words to refer to them, and getting people to agree on values seems to involve different processes than getting them to agree on facts. No matter how much one uncovers about reality, one cannot infer from what is real to its value. As a simple logical point, even an infinity of statements about how things are cannot imply how they ought to be: You cannot derive "ought" from "is," anymore than you can derive "run" from "observe," "talk" from "purchase," or any other predicate from sentences that make no reference to it. Describing reality and assessing value seem to be different sorts of processes.

Here is what it can mean to talk of "realistic" values: Where we already have a set of stable values, we can, indeed, use reason in their service. We can ascertain what conditions exist, and we can envision what possibilities are congruent with those conditions. We can apply our values both to the conditions and to the possibilities, and reason to that extent can help us see which of the things we value are most likely to be attainable. When we know what things are worth, as it were, and how much money we have, we can use reason to allocate our resources. Where worth has not been established, we cannot. Think of shopping in a store where there are no price tags, with a pocketful of foreign currency with which you are unfamiliar, and you will understand what it would be like to try to think rationally about values in the absence of established habits of valuing.

---

[78] Quoted in Robert Nozick, *The Nature of Rationality* (1993).

The kinds of evaluative processes that cognitive therapists undertake with patients seem very similar to what we can do once we have an established set of values. Where we have a set of established values, we can, indeed, deploy empirical and logical means to determine the probability of various alternatives and what we have to do to achieve them. We can do a "cost/benefit analysis" to determine what the benefits and relative costs of the various alternatives mean to us. In the same way, we can probably use the methods of cognitive therapy to determine "realistic" values only where we are putting reason to work in service of prior values.

We can put the first two strands of our present critique together with a third. This third line of thought pertains to the cognitive therapists' perpetual use of "adaptive" and related terms—they claim to help people get "more adaptive" ways of thinking. "Adaptive," though, is neither a cognitive concept nor one applicable to individual beliefs. In its legitimate scientific use, "adaptive" is a term drawn from evolutionary biology and related disciplines, and it refers to traits that confer reproductive advantage on individuals who possess it. An adaptive trait is genetically determined or at least genetically enabled.[79] A trait that is adaptive exists because of something that can be passed on to offspring through genetic material. What cannot be genetically conferred is irrelevant to natural selection. Furthermore, adaptive traits are those that members of a species possess because natural selection, operating through the reproductive activities of members of the species, selects them. *That* is the point of the term: to enable us to understand how a *species* comes to have certain traits and not others.

"Adaptive," in its legitimate scientific use, is useless as a criterion for determining beliefs, except for beliefs that are both

---

[79] Christopher Wills, in *The Runaway Brain: The Evolution of Human Uniqueness* (1993), makes the ingenious argument that environmental conditions may lead to a new utility for genetic traits that had previously been of no adaptive relevance. The genetic capacity may be present but not put to use prior to the environmental conditions that make it adaptive. Thus, the genes do not "cause" the emergence of the trait, but they enable its emergence under needful environmental conditions.

genetically determined and sufficiently advantageous for reproductive success that they have become characteristic of a species.
When we consider adaptivity and cognition, the question is how
evolution has shaped our basic neurological wiring—not those
beliefs which are up to individual choice and empirical consideration. Adaptive beliefs probably do not require much individual
choice, since by definition they are genetically determined traits
of members of the species. We do not have to sit around asking,
"Is this one of those beliefs I am supposed to hold because
natural selection has given me genes that make me believe it?"
Adaptive traits come naturally to members of a biologically
successful species.

There probably are beliefs that we are hard-wired to accept, by
the way—such as the beliefs that snakes are dangerous and cliffs
should be avoided. Interestingly enough, one way we can identify
such cognitive traits of our species is precisely their failure to fit
the criteria that Beck and company identify with good mental
health. They are beliefs people hold even when they have little
or no reason to hold them. Fear of snakes, for instance, is widespread even among people who have little or no experience with
snakes or reason to fear snakes—we even find this fear where
there *are no* poisonous snakes! Infants show an instinctive fear of
cliffs, even though they have no evidence that these are dangerous and certainly have not undertaken careful deliberations on
the harm contingent on venturing near a cliff. There is also some
suggestion, from twin studies, that some persons are genetically
inclined toward religious belief. Presumably there is something
adaptive about religious beliefs, even though—so far as I know—
no one comes to religious belief by logically considering evidence
for religious doctrine.

Of course, if Beck had in fact identified a group of people for
whom natural beliefs did not come naturally, or if he had discovered that depressives are lacking some cognitive wiring necessary
for reproductive success, his would be extremely important discoveries. Indeed, they would fit the basic idea of psychopathology: failure of essential human traits. I think we clearly do not
know yet what beliefs are essential expressions of our genotypes,
but we can note two facts: Most mental health patients do not
show reproductive incapacity, and very few, if any, come for help

on problems that have anything to do with adaptive fitness. Most patients are adults, well past the age of puberty. Indeed, Beck's cognitive therapy more or less has to be restricted to biological adults, since the capacity for formal reasoning does not develop until puberty. Almost all of them, since they can afford treatment, are able to work and secure food and shelter. So far as natural selection is concerned, most psychotherapy patients are fine. Adaptivity is an irrelevant issue.

To be fair, Beck and company are not alone in this misleading use of the term "adaptive." The term has gained currency throughout the mental health disciplines, probably to try to give the cachet of the biological disciplines to various dubious doctrines. Of course, the evolutionary disciplines do not have a copyright on the term, and psychologists could give an account of what makes a belief "adaptive," in some other sense, if they chose. That would probably only promote confusion, though. When mental health professionals are not talking about evolutionary advantage, they should come up with a different term rather than using the same word with a different meaning. But the fact is, Beck and his colleagues (like most mental health professionals) have not bothered to define the term differently. They use it *as if* they were talking about the same thing other scientists mean, but they are not. For the usual meaning of the term has nothing to do with correcting the cognitive errors of individual patients who do not fail to show reproductive eligibility.[80]

In fact, most of the cognitions Beck talks about have nothing to do with reproductive success at all. Patients who think "negatively" about themselves, their futures, and their worlds are usually not preoccupied with acquiring food, shelter, and children. They are concerned with whether or not they are good, what

---

[80] An interesting issue in the biology of mind is why we evolved with the emotional repertoire we come wired with. Emotions presumably serve adaptive purposes in their own right—a presumption that is bolstered by recognizing that animals share many of our emotions, though they do not share significant parts of our range of cognition. If Beck were really serious about understanding adaptivity, he would have to give emotions a more significant role in providing information and guiding action. This, of course, is the point of the Emily Dickinson poem at the head of this chapter: Emotion may serve profound purposes that cognition cannot—that, indeed, emotion may save us where "an open eye would drop us, bone by bone."

accomplishments or failures will define their lives, how they measure up to their obligations and the values of their peers, and the like. To understand the kind of negativity that afflicts the patients described in cognitive therapy case material we do not need to think in terms of adaptivity. We need to think in terms of the existential and cultural meanings that make the lives of patients worth having or not.

Hence it seems that cognitive therapy cannot institute paradigm shifts, that valuing can be seen as a cognitive exercise only when reason is put to use in service of existing values, and that adaptation is not a criterion for choosing beliefs. Both the methods of determining "realistic" values and changing one's beliefs can work only within established modes of thinking and valuing. We have to conclude, I think, that what cognitive therapy does is help—or at least attempt to help—people think and live within the status quo in a way that makes them feel positive. There is, in fact, a term with a long history in mental health care that *does* seem to describe this: social adjustment. *That*, I think, is what Beck is talking about when he uses terms like "adaptive."

We can bolster this conclusion by considering three facts. One is that Beck frequently says that the problem with "dysfunctional" cognitions is that they are "idiosyncratic." Now, what logical justification can be given for considering idiosyncracy a *prima facie* reason for dysfunctionality? I would suggest that none can be given at all. That an idea is peculiar to an individual does not mean it is false, distorted, or problematic. That Beck says this so often, without even bothering to explain why idiosyncracy should be considered pathogenic, seems to presuppose that healthy minds are those that conform to the consensual version of reality embedded in the status quo.

The second fact is that cognitive therapy aims to be short-term, though it claims to bring about major cognitive change. If change that can take place in short-term work is major, then the measure of needed or possible change must be a short yardstick. If we believe that the status quo is basically fine, and that patients only need to be changed so that their thoughts and values are approximately the same as those of others who get on well within the status quo, we might imagine that short-term work could accomplish this. All that has to be done is indoctrinate the patient into the views we already expect him to come to. We can be reasonably sure that most patients already possess the necessary categories of mind to conform to the status quo, simply because those are the categories of mind that society has given them. Where therapy is just a matter of getting people to deploy their existing repertoire in a way we already believe fits nicely into the status quo, it can probably be done quickly. For the patient possesses the means and the therapist already has an idea of what is "reasonable." However, if we believe that major change involves substantial creativity and originality, we are not likely to consider what can be done quickly to be very major.

The third fact to bolster our conclusion is this: As we have seen, cognitive culture elides from its concept of mind imagination, passion beyond reason, and the radical dialectic of creative thought. If the basic value is submitting approvingly to the status quo, it makes sense to devalue these dimensions of mind, for they are precisely the ones that tend to take us beyond received forms of thinking, valuing, and living. We can therefore understand why cognitive culture does not pay much attention to these crucial elements of mind.

This is why I characterize the culture of cognitive therapy as middlebrow. It certainly gives reverence to mind, but it resides within an already existing conceptual and empirical world and does not partake of any significant creativity or existential courage. Cognitive therapy's version of the life of reason is analogous to the musical life of a certain sort of seasonal subscriber to symphonic concerts. Such people go to the symphony because that is what cultured people do. For their benefit (and continued patronage) symphony programs always include (as their latter half) some popular warhorse of the repertoire that everyone will recognize. These people listen to music at home for distraction or comfort but not for instruction or guidance; they show little evidence of ever being deeply disturbed or challenged by music. Such folk are appreciative, at a distance, but not too deeply moved by the passions that created the very thing to which reverence is paid, not too open to the breaking up of our basic emotional and intellectual vocabulary by new ways of parsing experience.

The basic norm of cognitive therapy is this: Except for how the patient thinks, everything is okay. Reality is not pathogenic. Just think straight and life can be good enough. A person should think of herself in terms consistent with how most people in her society think of someone like her. She should pursue values congruent with the social milieu she occupies. She should convince herself of a generally optimistic view of how life works in this time and place—and confine her imagination to possibilities consistent with this. She should quell passions that would put her at odds with the status quo. She should not let her mind drift off into thoughts about life that might make her conclude that she (being who she is, living in the time and place fate has bequeathed her) is unlikely to find fulfillment. If she feels profoundly negative about herself, her world, or her future, she should refuse to consider that such emotions may be highly instructive. She should not even consider that such disquiet may be pointing toward important truths, and instead should find ways to negate such feelings. If she does all of this, she will have a life meaningful and satisfying enough to banish depression.

That may well be good advice, and perhaps people who can take it would be foolish to do otherwise. Yet it raises serious questions. What about those who cannot—or *choose* not to? Are they doomed to mental illness? Or has cognitive culture drawn its diagnostic categories too broadly, including in the psychopathology of "depression" a variety of distressing but humanly authentic and important emotional states? Haven't the members of this culture decreed that, by definition, one cannot face profoundly negative truths without becoming ill? What would a society that enshrined such values in the name of mental health be like?

Consider, to start with, the experience of persons who are officially ostracized or oppressed by our society. Such persons may have characteristics that are not pathological but make it highly unlikely that their lives will go well. To a great extent today, and almost completely not long ago, an African-American of intellectual and artistic bent could be reasonably sure his life would frustrate his deepest values and abilities. Is the "mentally healthy" thing for him to see his intellectual and artistic concerns as "unrealistic" values and to realize optimistically that he can, so long as he knows his place, have a less distressing life? In most of America today, and in almost all of it a few decades ago, a gay male would be wildly irrational to assume that his life is not going to be quite difficult. How is he to banish pessimism? Consider next the distinct possibility that many people have other characteristics that do not fit well into our society, even if they are not objects of overt ostracism—Adrienne Rich's wonderful book, *What Is Found There: Essays on Poetry and Politics*, presents a compelling argument against America's disdain of poetry and a moving lamentation on the lot of poets (and others). Some people are objects of overt ostracism; others just do not fit into the society that determines their opportunities. I think there is very much room for many sorts of people, coolly and rationally appraising the evidence, to conclude that ours is a society that does not value their most important attributes. They are not wildly irrational to decide that their lives are not likely to go well unless they abrogate what they value most about themselves. How would cognitive therapy have such people understand themselves? Are they to change what they value about themselves, in the name of "realistic" values? Are they mentally ill to be perpetually distressed that what they find most important about themselves is negatively valued by their society?

These are not questions Beck addresses, and we should not be surprised by that. For the orientation and values of cognitive culture assume that how things are is okay. People can fit, if they just think straight. It would follow, then, that persons who think they do not fit in, who think the status quo is seriously lacking, who are troubled by what is required to embrace some positive vision of life within the status quo—such people are just guilty of cognitive error.

Recognizing that cognitive therapy enshrines the status quo gives us a possible explanation of a consistent, puzzling research finding: that cognitive therapy produces no "specific effect." That is, while its patients (like the patients of all the mainstream therapies) get better, they do not show any cognitive patterns different from those of persons treated by other methods. Though cognitive therapy claims to induce specific changes in patterns of thinking, many studies have shown that the cognitive changes shown in patients of other methods are indiscernible from the effects of cognitive therapy. One way to understand this is that cognitive therapy does not actually change anyone's way of thinking. That seems plausible, since its portrayal of mind seems rather unrealistic. Yet we might understand it differently: The work of cognitive therapy may be to convince patients to think like people in our society generally do.

The Scientific Status of Cognitive Therapy

No great effort would be required to show that the relationship Beck asserts between cognition and pathological emotion is not a matter of scientific discovery. All we would have to do is show the radical disparities between various scientists on emotion and cognition. The fact of the matter is that fairly little research has been done on such issues until recently. In 1985, Izard, Kagan, and Zajonc wrote (in a masterful compendium of state-of-the-art papers, *Emotions, Cognition, and Behavior*), "For most of the past two decades learning theory and cognitive psychology in general, as well as social-psychological and personality theory, was largely devoid of emotion concepts. . . . [N]one of these areas produced empirical research dealing with emotion concepts." They also said (now that research into emotions has begun), "What is surprising is that the theoretical sophistication reached by cognitive science, the new technological and methodological developments in mental chronometry and story analysis, have not yet been formally absorbed into the study of emotion."[81] Research on the relationship between cognition and emotion is extremely new, and little unanimity has been reached.

Research within the cognitive therapy community has been less than stunning.[82] Beutler and Guest (who are sympathetic

---

[81] Carroll E. Izard, Jerome Kagan, and Robert B. Zajonc, *Emotions, Cognition, and Behavior* (1984).

[82] Several essays in Arthur Freeman et al., eds., *Comprehensive Handbook of Cognitive Therapy* (1989), present the state-of-the-art in cognitive therapy research. See especially Goldberg and Shaw, "The Measurement of Cognition in Psychopathology;" Beckham and Watkins, "Process and Outcome in Cognitive Therapy;" Beutler and Guest, "The Role of Cognitive Change in Psychotherapy;" and Coyne, "Thinking Postcognitively about Depression."

to cognitive therapy) say that cognitive therapy's theory would entail that

> (1) disturbed cognitive patterns or distortions will occur more frequently in pathological groups than in normals; (2) disturbed cognitive content will predict the nature of psychopathology that will appear in times of stress; (3) cognitive therapies that are designed to impact these cognitive contents and dysfunctional processes will do so at a faster rate than therapies that are not so designed; and (4) changes in cognitive patterns will coincide with changes in symptoms and signs of emotional disturbance.

Their assessment is straightforward: "None of the[se] . . . hypotheses is strongly supported by current research."[83]

The quality of the research has not generally been admired, outside of the circle of true believers. James Coyne (who has written some of the more careful reviews of the cognitive therapy research literature) says that ". . . in the large body of research it has generated, the measurements that have been made have typically been crude, confounded, and incapable of supporting precise distinctions between possible cognitive concepts."[84] The research is consistent with a wide variety of hypotheses other than those of Beck's cognitive therapy.[85]

---

[83] Larry E. Beutler and Paul D. Guest, "The Role of Cognitive Change in Psychotherapy," in Arthur Freeman et al., eds., *Comprehensive Handbook of Cognitive Therapy* (1989).

[84] James Coyne, "Thinking Postcognitively about Depression," in Arthur Freeman et al., eds., *Comprehensive Handbook of Cognitive Therapy* (1989).

[85] One of the immense problems of cognitive therapy research is that Beck and company have not been able to establish the causal relationship between cognition and psychopathology that is central to their views. In recent years, Beck and other cognitive therapists will sometimes say that they are *not* claiming a causal role for these cognitions; yet they continue frequently to make direct causal claims. Further, their language and activities make obvious that they do believe that these cognitions are pathogenic. They say that the problems "are derived from," "stem inevitably from," "result from" the cognitions; they say the cognitions "lead to" the problems. They say that how one structures the world "determines" how one feels and acts. (See, for instance, Beck and Marjorie Weishaar, "Cognitive Therapy," in Arthur Freeman et al., eds., *Comprehensive Handbook of Cognitive Therapy* [1989]). What they tell patients, according to their published case materials, is quite straightforward. *They tell patients that their thoughts cause their feelings.* Certainly if cognitive therapists claim to provide an explanation of depression (and other psychopathology), they cannot avoid causal claims.

To illustrate the kind of problem Coyne identifies, consider that the fact that depressed persons say negative things more often (or more quickly) than nondepressed persons does not tell us anything about cognitive schemata or about any causal relationship between cognition and emotion. Negativity is perfectly consistent with having basically the same sort of schematic repertoire as anyone else but *accessing* the negative categories more often than others when depressed. Depressed persons could be accessing negative categories more frequently for any number of reasons. They could simply be "primed" for negative categories because of recent unpleasant experiences—which is a normal process. A person with a perfectly ordinary mental apparatus can, under stress or negative conditions, become highly attuned to negative possibilities, prone to negative perceptions and judgments, and more apt to infer from available information that negative outcomes are more probable than others.

The most common sort of cognitive therapy research has patients fill out a pencil-and-paper questionnaire that contains statements they can agree or disagree with along a scale of possibilities—say, 1 means "strongly agree" and 7 means "strongly disagree." This kind of research has several problems. At best, it tells us what kind of thinking the subjects are doing, but it does not tell us why. Nor does it tell us whether they are thinking such things with or without good reason. However, this kind of research does not even clearly tell us what subjects are thinking. Subjects can answer based on how they want to be seen, how they feel about taking the test, or some general behavioral stance that has little to do with whether the statements actually reflect their thinking. They can endorse a statement because it expresses something similar to how they feel, even if they have rarely thought such a thing. Finally, as we have seen in the previous chapter, self-reports cannot be assumed to be accurate, unless we impute to subjects omniscient introspective powers and flawless honesty.

Another sort of research is to have a depressed person, who believes she cannot succeed at anything, succeed at some trivial laboratory task—like sorting cards. Lo and behold, this tends to brighten her mood and decrease her complaints. Beck interprets this as showing that the person's cognitive schema has been falsified. But this cannot be a reasonable interpretation. A cognitive schema about oneself is, by definition, highly general. If it were susceptible to change under such trivial and specific conditions, we would have to see the schema as very unstable. A person whose basic orienting schemata were so fickle would exhibit a degree of instability in excess of even the most dire psychopathologies. Even borderline personality disorders show more stability than this, and the thought disorders of schizophrenics are remarkably resistant to change. The most reasonable interpretation of this kind of work, in fact, is that the person's basic schemata include positive dimensions that are activated by positive experiences. The flip side of this interpretation is that her prevailing negativity, too, is due to the kinds of experiences she has been having.

We should note in passing that, as both a conceptual and an empirical matter, it is not obviously true (or generally agreed within the mental health community) that all depressed persons exhibit the thoughts that Beck ascribes causal status to, much less that they show the pattern he claims to find among them. Conceptually, the DSM-III-R diagnostic criteria include, in addition to the dysphoric mood characteristic of depression, eight symptoms, only any four of which need be present for a diagnosis of major depressive episode. The kinds of thoughts Beck talks about constitute only two of the eight symptoms. Unless a clinician decides, on her own, to require such symptoms for a diagnosis of depression, all sorts of persons without the thoughts Beck describes will merit the diagnosis.

For clinicians who do not make these thoughts definitive, it is certainly the case that a great many people whom everyone would describe as depressed do not obviously exhibit the cognitive pattern Beck describes. It is not unusual to find persons with deep dysphoric mood, appetite and sleep problems, loss of interest in normally pleasurable activities, agitation or retardation in motor activities, difficulties in concentration, and the like, who have become compulsively, slavishly enmeshed in work—or religiously involved in twelve-step programs or other self-help groups—because they believe that they can push through the depression by dint of their own efforts. They believe they can bring about a state of affairs in which they no longer feel bad. Thus, they are, quite literally, actively invested in the belief that they are capable of producing a better future. This directly contradicts the "cognitive triad" hypothesis.

More interesting than the indecisive quality of cognitive therapy research is the significant disparity between Beck's concept of mind and the views of mind developed in the sciences that study cognition directly.

If we look at the work of Jerome Bruner, the father of the New Look, we do not see a concept of mind anything like Beck's. Indeed, it is possible to make a case that Bruner's work on cognition enables us to understand the depressive's cognitive processes as normal cognition functioning in negative circumstances. Curiously enough, most of what Beck calls pathogenic is, by Bruner's lights, normal.

In general, we can say that Bruner insisted that cognition is always embedded in the life of the person and cannot be understood solely by reference to logical and evidentiary considerations. Bruner argued that cognition in general cannot be understood apart from the purposes it serves in fulfilling needs, situating persons in their social milieus, and the like. That is, thinking has multiple purposes *not* determined by principles of logic and evidence but by a variety of noncognitive motivations. He also showed that specific acts of cognition serve specific tasks within a general orientation. Bruner was extremely interested in the social processes that determine cognition—one's need to affiliate oneself with a group, to externalize one's internal values, and the like. Beck consistently warns cognitive therapists against seeing motivation as an issue, and he consistently argues that studying deviation from logical and evidentiary principles suffices. Beck and colleagues do not even ask what their patients are trying to accomplish by their existing cognitive habits. Beck never even considers how crucial to cognition social purposes are.

Further, Bruner argued that the purpose of mind, by its very nature, is to generalize beyond the available evidence, to derive hypotheses and rules that can be deployed in other situations.

Moreover, attention by its nature is selective; information is often (and normally) purposely distorted in accord with values. For cognition to accomplish its tasks, it has to overgeneralize, apply rules to situations about which it has not yet collected evidence, and direct attention selectively. Since it serves specific purposes, it "distorts" information according to the values behind those purposes. Beck consistently argues that generalizing beyond the evidence, selective attention, and distortion are pathological.

Bruner thought that adult minds possess a conceptual repertoire that transcends particular instances, in two senses. First, one's cognitive repertoire is the result of generalization across an immense body of concerns and experiences over one's history. Second, a cognitive repertoire is fairly resistant to being changed by particular instances because its function is to give rules that cover large categories and to relate those categories in theory-like ways. The highly general, theory-like schemata of adult thinking generally take precedence over particular items of information. Contrary information is more likely to be discounted than to cause a change in one's cognitive repertoire. The kinds of procedures that Beck says suffice to change one's schemata should have very little effect on one's conceptual repertoire, if they work as Bruner says they do. Very substantial challenges (not a few exercises) are necessary, from Bruner's perspective, before one's orienting habits of thought will change.[86]

When we look at contemporary work on cognition, the discrepancy between cognitive therapy and what seems to be true of minds is amazing. We have already noted robust findings that depressives are more accurate than nondepressed people in their perceptions of themselves and their world. We have also noted

---

[86] Bruner and other scientists of mind try to do what, as we noted in note 67, scientists of mind have to do: find the laws, principles, and operations by which experience is constructed. *If* a clinical researcher could show that these principles of construction are violated in psychopathology, he or she would have shown something important. Beck, as we have seen, has shown no such thing. A comparison of his view with Bruner's seems to show, instead, that his account suggests that the minds of the psychopathological are functioning in accord with the principles that animate mind. He has thus completely failed to show pathological reasoning behind psychopathology.

the demonstrable distortion in a self-serving direction that is common in normal thought. We have seen that the principles of inference most people use are radically illogical. We will look very briefly at three other areas of contemporary work: "split brain" research, a variety of fields studying "parallel distributed processing," and social psychology on how ideas get determined. We will tie these together by considering emerging ideas about consciousness, since Beck imputes immense powers of self-knowledge to conscious awareness.

Split-brain research is a fortuitous benefit of a horrible condition. Some epileptics suffer massive seizures that cannot be controlled by medication. To reduce the seizures, the tract that connects the left and right hemispheres of the brain is severed. This enables scientists to study the respective functions of the hemispheres. For our purposes, two phenomena are especially interesting. First, we now know fairly conclusively that when information that is fed to the right hemisphere causes an emotional reaction, the left brain produces an explanation in terms of information that has been fed to *it*, and this is what the subjects are conscious of. The information used in the explanation is, in fact, irrelevant to the emotions being felt. Yet the person doing the feeling and explaining finds her explanation to be obviously correct and congruent with the emotion.

Most of us, of course, do not have split brains, so the relevance of this research may not be immediately obvious. What it shows is that we inveterately explain ourselves to ourselves and believe our explanations, even when the explanation is quite irrelevant to what caused our mood. When we have a feeling, the information we use in explaining it to ourselves may have nothing to do with what actually caused the feeling. One very well-known phenomenon is that the expressions of self-deprecation that are common among depressed Americans (and other Westerners) are not usually associated with depression in Eastern countries. That suggests that we use culturally induced ways of explaining misfortune—a moralistic orientation derived from Western religions, for instance—to explain bad feelings. It also suggests we are probably mistaken in these ubiquitous explanations. "Identifying" a cognition that "causes" an emotion is not a very reliable process.

The second interesting thing about the split-brain research is the support it lends to a "modular" theory of mind. Minds (assuming that mind is a function of the brain) are not inherently unified, but consist of many modules that need not work in synchrony with each other. The modules controlling one's emotional state at a given time may have little to do with the modules processing other information and feeding ideas to consciousness.

That leads us to the issue of "parallel distributed processing." One of the curious things about the human nervous system is that it conducts electrical activity extremely slowly. The least powerful home computer moves information around faster than any part of the brain could possibly do. So how is it that the brain is so powerful? The answer seems to be that, for any task at any moment, a great number of different parts of the brain process information at the same time. Rather than having one central processor to process a million instructions per second, the brain can distribute the work among, say, two thousand processors working at the rate of five hundred instructions per second.

Parallel processing fits very well with the fact, discovered by neuroanatomists and psychologists, that brains are modular. Visual processing, for example, does not take place in just one part of the brain but in (at least) a couple of dozen. This characteristic of brains has been repeatedly verified—there are, for instance, many different "spatial maps" in different parts of the brain, not one central map for processing spatial information.

What these considerations have to do with cognitive therapy is this: It follows from them that consciousness cannot possibly be a very complete or accurate reporter of what is going on in the brain. No one knows yet just what consciousness does and does not do; but we are sure that it does not provide a mirror into how we think.[87] For instance, visual consciousness is always serial—

---

[87] For a beautifully written popular account of a leading current contender among theories of consciousness, see William H. Calvin, *The Cerebral Symphony: Seashore Reflections on the Structure of Consciousness* (1990). For a well-written and intellectually more challenging work, see the wonderful book by the philosopher Daniel C. Dennett, *Consciousness Explained* (1991).

that is, we experience one set of images, followed by another set of images, followed by another set, *seriatim*. Yet we know that in the brain, huge numbers of visual processes go on in parallel. What appears in consciousness does not tell us about those parallel processes or how they create unitary images in consciousness. It only makes sense to assume that the same is true for our conscious awareness of ideas and emotions—especially since we know what we know from split brain research.

The idea that consciousness is not a good indicator of what goes on inside our minds is bolstered by social psychology research on cognition. Over and over again, social psychologists have shown that the ways we make decisions are determined by cognitive processes we cannot explain accurately. Put differently, our explanations of how we reach conclusions are frequently at odds with what we have actually done. Take two groups of people and "prime" them differently—give one group something predominantly negative to read and give the other something predominantly positive. Then have the two groups read an identical story about someone who is ambiguously described. Have the two groups describe the protagonist of the story. The first group will evaluate him negatively, the second group positively, and both will think they reached their conclusions through a careful reading of the story. In fact, each group has been influenced by categories of thought activated by the "pretest" reading, though no one is likely to say, "I saw the character as negative [or positive] because I read that negative [or positive] stuff before." This is but one example of the immense distance between how we think and how we *think* we think.[88]

The central role of consciousness in cognitive therapy is just not consonant with anything scientists have discovered about minds. Knowledge of our operative beliefs about ourselves, our world, and our future is not a simple matter of being trained to pay attention to what goes on in consciousness. Most likely, our ideas about ourselves—including our ideas about what is

[88] R. E. Nisbett and L. Ross, *Human Inference* (1980), contains a rich lode of examples. See also the fourth chapter of Eliot Aronson's *The Social Animal*, 6th ed. (1992).

going on cognitively—are like all our ideas: active constructs. Probably what we really do is formulate theories about ourselves and interpret ourselves accordingly. Owen Flanagan has said, "Accurate self-understanding requires understanding and internalization of the best available scientific theories about the kinds of creatures we are, as well as collective cultural wisdom about human nature and human history."[89] Cognitive therapy teaches patients to formulate theories of a specific sort: Theories about cognitions causing emotions, as well as theories about distortion, illogicality, and dysfunctional beliefs being easily identifiable, pathogenic, and correctable by the techniques of cognitive therapy. As we have seen, these are not likely to be very accurate theories.

Beck and his allied cognitive therapists, in my view, are to cognitive science somewhat like the nerve doctors of the nineteenth century were to the emerging science of neurology: They draw an aura of authority from an emerging science that actually has yet to shed much light on psychopathology or its alleviation. When Helmholtz showed that the nervous system involves electrical charges, it created an atmosphere in which George Beard and others could make up myths about nerve force and convince people to submit to being shocked. As cognitive science began to show the importance of cognition in how we experience the world, the atmosphere was right for Beck and his allies to promulgate their own myths about thinking.

The Appeal of Cognitive Therapy

Why have Beck's myths been so persuasive? Why has cognitive therapy been so appealing to so many people when, as we have seen, its ideas do not bear scrutiny? I think that cognitive therapy appeals to beliefs that the mental health community and our society already held long before cognitive therapy came

---

[89] Owen Flanagan, *The Science of the Mind*, 2d ed. (1991).

into existence. It seems to offer a culture based on those ideas without some of the problems entailed by psychoanalysis and behaviorism.

The first of these ideas is the belief that the individual's normal inner functioning is sufficient to guarantee freedom from pathological distress. We have already encountered this idea in psychoanalytic culture. We can understand Beck's views as psychoanalysis stripped of bodily imperatives, the unconscious, and the presence of the past. Stripping psychoanalysis of those central elements leaves an emaciated structure, of course. But Beck's notion of normal cognitive processes is just the psychoanalytic notion of secondary process thinking, and his ideas of distortion and reality testing fit any psychoanalytic textbook from the 1950s. His emphatic insistence that the problem is within the patient, and his blithe assumption that reality cannot be the cause of pathology, are both central psychoanalytic notions, as we saw in chapter three. We can understand part of the appeal of Beck's work in these terms. He spoke to mental health workers who had been primed by psychoanalysis, but who (for whatever reason) did not want to consider internal bodily imperatives, the dynamic unconscious, and the presence of the past as essential to psychic functioning. Beck allows us to sustain the myth that avoiding pathological distress is a matter of straightening out one's inner life, but he lets us believe that this is a much more straightforward task than the psychoanalysts would have us think.

The second idea that was held long before Beck, which prepared for finding his work appealing, is the belief that the problems of life are easily manageable. Beck's notions that the environment is basically congenial, that problems are clearly and discretely definable, and that fairly simple operations suffice to institute major changes all resemble behaviorist culture. His minimalist concept of mind offers disillusioned behaviorists a way to maintain their optimistic philosophy while making reference to cognitive processes. We can be reasonably sure that chastened behaviorists would not want to hear about the dimensions of cognition that Beck leaves out of his account, and he obliges their wish to ignore such mysterious matters.

The most important reason that Beck has been persuasive, though, probably has less to do with concerns of the mental health community than with one of the grand myths of Western culture. This is the belief that reason can shape the emotions, so that a rational life is a good life. Consider that, from Plato to Aquinas to Freud, the Western tradition of moral rationalism has held that passions and emotions come before reason, operating in their own sphere but capable of being directed and subdued by reason. At first blush, it seems that cognitive therapists turn this upside down: Cognition plays a central role in causing emotion, not just in taming it. In the grand tradition, as we may call it, the effort to make reason ascendant is an arduous moral task. Reason comes to hold sway over the passions only after a long process of education and cultivation, and a life of equanimity and well-being constitutes a Herculean triumph. Cognitive therapists have it differently: Reason by its very nature determines what we feel and do, and a life of distress represents a failure of ordinary reason.

On closer inspection, we can see that cognitive therapy has found a way to deliver an everyday version of this Western tradition to consumers. To achieve the attitude prescribed by cognitive therapy is, indeed, to achieve something *resembling* the triumph of reason that moral rationalism recommends. Normal, healthy minds, for cognitive therapists, think logically and with circumspect care, modulating actions and emotions by well-balanced consideration. One's life is good because one's mind is clear. As the neurological theories of the eighteenth and early nineteenth centuries dressed up classical metaphysics in the language of the sciences of the day, so does cognitive therapy incarnate a specific moral philosophy in the language of psychology.

The philosophy of moral rationalism has much to recommend it; I think it constitutes a virtuous and effective way to conduct one's life, if circumstances allow. Whether cognitive therapy actually helps people to achieve the life of moral rationalism seems doubtful, but I think it undeniably allows people to *believe* they are achieving the triumph of reason over emotion that our culture has revered for millennia. Most of us like believing that we can achieve the supreme values of our culture. A therapy that promises to help us do that simply through common sense offers immense reassurance.

Evaluating Cognitive Therapy

Whenever we can resolve our difficulties with minimal reconstruction of our basic beliefs and minimal disjunction from our community, it is probably wise to do so. For persons whose educations have not provided them with the habits of mind that enable such an adjustment, the personal attention of a therapist devoted specifically to imparting those habits should, we can imagine, usually be a good thing. If cognitive therapy actually helps people think in the ways it claims to, it probably improves the acculturation of those who have not been successfully inducted into society's consensual notions of reality. For people whose talents, temperaments, and proclivities have a valued place within that social reality, cognitive therapy should be a good thing, helping them to find their place. Even those who generally show excellent acculturation and deployment of their beliefs can sometimes get so bollixed up in distress that someone has to help them see the simple way out of the maze they are in. To the extent that cognitive therapists help them recover perspective, it should help.

For others, the social adjustment offered by cognitive therapy may be less helpful. This social adjustment is very different from recognizing, as all of us must, that we have to *come to terms with* the status quo. Cognitive therapy requires that we learn to think and value *in accord with* the status quo. That is not the same thing as recognizing what the status quo is and finding a way to live with it. The status quo obviously provides the milieu of every person's life. Individuals or groups can recognize that and still believe that the values of our society are warped, that traditional ways of thinking are infected with skewed and constricting notions. They can recognize that received forms of thinking and valuing are not well suited to their temperaments, talents, and proclivities. They have to find substantially different ways of thinking and valuing, ways that let them find a viable life within the interstices of society or in opposition to its values and ways of thought.

How many people need more effective acculturation into their society, and how many would not find that adequate? No one knows. Certainly a great many depressives feel like misfits, and it is not inconceivable that their sense of themselves is accurate. Conceivably, some significant number of depressives (among others) are trapped within, or suffering from the collapse of, ways of life that suit them poorly. For such people, effective change probably requires a great deal of creative, imaginative work. Perhaps for them the cognitive component of depression is a failure of imagination, and what they need is help in putting imaginative courage in service to their passions. Perhaps such persons must come to possess the courage and fortitude to live at odds with accepted social values. They may have to come to terms with the fact that conventional ways of making a living, having friendships, achieving status in the community, and fulfilling their needs are not open to them—or will not work very well if they are made available. Thus, they have to come to terms with the fact that life will probably be harder for them than for people more suited to the mainstream. I think such persons would be poorly served by cognitive therapy.

Whether or not cognitive therapy actually changes how patients think, it does provide a rhetoric that enshrines certain ways of thinking. Thus, it supplies the larger society with a set of rationalizations for endorsing some ways of thinking and devaluing others. Our evaluation of cognitive therapy as a player in society will depend largely on how we value the forms of thinking and valuing that it puts its weight behind. For persons—conservative or liberal—who are basically happy with the status quo, these probably will not seem problematic. So long as one believes that our existing forms of living, valuing, and thinking are adequate for meeting the problems of life, shoring up the claims of optimistic common sense and elementary logic will not seem threatening. If we believe that our existing forms of discourse and modes of life are significantly inadequate for a substantial number of people, we are less likely to be happy with cognitive therapy as a social institution.

Persons who believe that truth is important should be troubled by cognitive therapy's ruling unacceptable, in the name of mental health, a whole class of beliefs—namely, profoundly negative views and the sense of life (or individual lives) as inherently tragic. The equation of optimism and mental health in effect declares a host of possible, if difficult or dismal, truths out of bounds, regardless of their intellectual merit. Both the great geniuses of our culture who have embodied tragic visions in art or essay and those to whom their works speak bear witness to important dimensions of experience, for which the culture of cognitive therapy seems to have little room. In the world of cognitive therapy, such negativity calls not for moral courage but for correction by logical thinking that adapts one to the world as currently conceived. Ruling out a whole host of possible truths in the name of sound cognition, without bothering to consider the evidence, seems to me quite frankly a travesty.

Many critics have claimed that mental health care is just a way of making people conform to the values of the dominant culture. Cognitive therapy effectively (if unconsciously) exemplifies what such critics are complaining about. The irony seems quite rich: institutionalizing conformity in the name of intellectual rigor.

This amounts to biting the hand that feeds you, however. For cognitive therapy is parasitic upon the existence of intellectual traditions that could not exist if cognitive therapy's views about mind were true. Living a life of reason, tempering one's emotions through careful thought, are cultural achievements, not a natural state of affairs. Our understanding of the rules of logic and evidence depends upon centuries of work by great geniuses, embodied in our cultural traditions and passed down through our educational institutions. What a society counts as "reality" is equally a cultural phenomenon, as constructivists insist.[90] All of us, most of the time, dwell in ways of worldmaking—ways of seeing the world and construing information—that we acquire from the culture that spawns us. That culture has been constructed over generations, as the exotic and immense originality of the most imaginative among us has wended through everyday life, amended and qualified by the million smaller originalities

---

[90] Richard Schweder, *Thinking through Cultures* (1991).

and creative deformations of the more ordinary among our forebears. The creative ways of thinking that make culture possible are left out of cognitive therapy's account of mind.

The culture of cognitive therapy devalues those attributes of mind most likely both to create culture and to take us beyond the status quo—imagination, passion, and the courageous, painful process of bringing new ways of thinking and living to birth. It amounts to an endorsement of middlebrow life under the authority of "good mental health." *That* does not seem a good thing at all. Roberto Mangabeira Unger has expressed well the consequence of allegiance to received forms:

> Our membership in historically given and flawed communities provides us with the only standards of sense and value we have. These standards form the unavoidable basis of communication and self-reflection. But unless we constantly push our experiments in self-reflection and in practical collaboration or passionate attachment beyond what established society or available discourse can countenance we incur a double loss. Not only do we fail to make many discoveries about the world and to find more successful ways to reconcile the conflicting conditions of self-assertion, but we may find ourselves increasingly reduced to an unconscious servitude. We may begin to act and to think as if all our thoughts and actions could indeed be governed by a lawlike structure we were powerless to escape or revise.[91]

When we enshrine the "standards of sense and value that we have" as the conditions of good mental health, we make the way things are *now* look like laws of nature—and to the extent that we discourage imaginative, passionate disruption of our current sense of reality, we make the discovery of new ways of living less likely.[92]

---

[91] Roberto Mangabeira Unger, *Passion: An Essay on Personality* (1984).

[92] The issue here is not rationality, but the way that cognitive therapy's version of rationality confines us within received forms of thinking. Rationality itself can include passion, imagination, and the generation of new ways of thinking. See Robert Nozick, *The Nature of Rationality* (1993), as well as Roberto Unger, *Passion* (1984).

Cognitive Therapy and Cultural Criticism

Beck's cognitive therapy seems to me a case of a good idea, but bad execution. Looking at the role of cognition in health and illness was probably a good idea, as it remains. Identifying mental health with rationalism was probably a mistake. Beck's view of how rationality works is probably badly mistaken.

That Beck and his allies were able to establish themselves as authorities on thinking and mental health illustrates the problem of the undeserved status of the mental health professions. Cognitive culture offers perspectives that stand at odds with important elements of our culture and important scientific findings. If cognitive culture draws on the prestige of moral rationalism, alternative traditions of Romanticism, existentialism, and transcendentalism offer perspectives from which to critique it. Both humanistic and scientific studies of cognition offer substantially different ways of understanding mind. If a philosopher, cognitive scientist, poet, or social theorist had presented Beck's view of mind as a serious intellectual hypothesis, she probably would have been hooted out of serious consideration—Beck's views are that blithely oblivious to the major issues of reason, knowledge, and value that have animated Western culture in the last century. That this view was delivered as a discovery about mental health allowed it to become the animating ideology of significant institutions. As we have seen repeatedly, an idea does not need much of an intellectual pedigree to become the basis for clinical work. All that is required is some initial plausibility together with a set of clinical practices, and clinicians will put the idea to work to deal with the problems of patients. Because of this, we possess institutions of cognitive therapy that have to be radically altered or displaced before better ways of understanding cognition and health can gain control of the field.

Rightly or not, hardly anyone doubts that changing how people think can change the quality of their lives. We can well imagine, as the opening paragraphs of this chapter illustrated, that some persons are sufficiently confused about life, or think about it in such cockeyed ways, that they are miserable from running their lives on such misdirected bases. Cognition may turn out to have a significant role in a significant number of psychopathologies; there is no reason to rule out this possibility. Nonetheless, whether thoughts can induce psychopathology, rather than ordinary misery, has yet to be shown.

As various sciences create a rich lode of information on cognition, emotion, action, and the relations among them, we can expect this information to generate more sophisticated notions of how cognition can be understood (and addressed) in therapy. We thus have the perfect opportunity—and obligation—for precisely the kind of discourse on mental health and therapy that I am recommending. Work on learned helplessness and learned optimism, on positive illusions, and on social cognition pose substantial questions about our concepts of the healthy mind. This work, as sound as it is scientifically, addresses only small slices of mental functioning. At the same time, we possess in our cultural heritage a rich and diverse body of serious thought about thinking—and a few centuries of experience with shaping how people think (in educational institutions, for example). These should not simply be dismissed in deference to scientific fragments. All intelligent, educated thinkers need to give serious thought to what will be made of those scientific findings and how we will think about what it is to think healthily.

We need such critical thought about thinking simply because thinking is important—whether or not it causes psychopathology. Establishing a role (or many roles) for thinking in mental illness and health requires us to think about another question, though: whether psychopathology may have less to do with psychology than with biological malfunctions in the machinery of mind. To that issue we now turn our attention.

Chapter Six

BIOLOGICAL PSYCHIATRY'S CONFUSION OF TONGUES

. . . MAKING CORRELATIONS BETWEEN SPECIFIC NEURAL SUBSTRATES AND SPECIFIC BEHAVIORS IS ONE OF THE MOST DIFFICULT CHALLENGES IN ALL OF BIOLOGY, AND THE HISTORY OF ENDEAVORS IN THIS AREA IS A RECORD OF MANY DECEPTIONS AND DISCOURAGEMENTS. THUS, ANY APPARENT CORRELATION OR CLAIM MUST BE REGARDED WITH HEALTHY SKEPTICISM.

—*Gordon M. Shepherd*
Neurobiology

IN CLINICAL PHARMACOLOGY, CONTEMPORARY TECHNOLOGY PLAYS A DOMINANT ROLE IN SHAPING IDEOLOGY. WHAT WE LOOK FOR IN PATIENTS DEPENDS TO A GREAT DEGREE ON THE AVAILABLE MEDICATIONS.

—*Peter D. Kramer*
Listening to Prozac

✖ ✖ ✖ ✖ ✖ ✖ ✖ ✖ ✖ ✖ ✖ ✖ ✖

✖ WHILE COGNITIVE THERAPY is the hot form of talk therapy these days, the hottest topic in the field of mental health care is, in effect, to what extent talk therapy is legitimate at all. The alternative is that mental and emotional problems are due to problems with biological functions, requiring biochemical interventions—drugs.[93]

Not all psychiatrists are biological psychiatrists; not even all psychiatrists who prescribe drugs regularly share this perspective. Biological psychiatry is a distinct perspective claiming that psychopathology is a matter of biological malfunctions. Talk therapy, in this view, is only an adjunct to necessary chemicals. As Paul Wender and Donald Klein, two of the most important figures in the renascence of biological psychiatry put it, ". . . the biopsychiatric approach does not hold that psychotherapy is always a waste of time but that *by itself* it is useless for disorders in which constitutional deviations and physiological abnormalities are the basis of malfunction."[94] Since biological abnormality is, in this culture, the defining characteristic of mental illness, drugs are essential to all treatment of mental illness.

Notice that (at least) two questions are conflated here: whether psychopathology is biological illness and whether psychopathology requires biochemical intervention. The answer to one does

---

[93] An excellent account of what is and is not known about the biology of psychopathology and the use of drugs is Marvin E. Lickey and Barbara Gordon's highly readable textbook, *Medicine and Mental Illness*. The best expression of the general biological psychiatry position that I know of remains Paul H. Wender and Donald F. Klein, *Mind, Mood, and Medicine*. While they are strong advocates of biological psychiatry, they are generally good at identifying where their beliefs go beyond the evidence. Nancy Andreasen's *The Broken Brain* is a highly popular and widely available presentation of the biological perspective. Ronald R. Fieve's *Moodswing* exemplifies the faith of the true believer.

[94] Paul H. Wender and Donald F. Klein, *Mind, Mood, and Medicine* (1981).

not logically dictate the other, as we will see. Biological illness might be caused and cured by psychological (or social) factors, and drugs may be useful in treating pathologies of a psychosocial nature. In this culture, though, the two become one for a simple reason: Drugs are the driving force of the culture. The "biological illness" hypothesis seems to justify pharmacology as the treatment of choice, while drug effectiveness seems to support the biological illness hypothesis. The conflation of these two issues is not necessary scientifically or logically, but we will come to understand the cultural forces that make it imperative within biological psychiatry and the larger society.

Biological psychiatry is not new, of course. As we saw in chapter two, since the nineteenth century attempts to explain both insanity and neurotic problems biologically have been common. Biological psychiatry fell from favor earlier in the century for two major reasons. It did not manage to come up with many effective treatments, and the physical deficits that biological psychiatrists hypothesized could not be found. Two things have changed. The first is that, since the 1950s, many effective treatments have been found. The second is that the neurosciences and related scientific disciplines have made astounding gains in their understanding of the brain. A corollary, probably consequent, change is that the secularization of society since midcentury has made acceptable to most people the idea that humans are material organisms, not dualistic organisms comprising a material brain and an immaterial spirit. The ideas that the person is the body and the mind is the brain have become almost common opinion, so that antipathy to biological explanations is much less ingrained.

These new developments have made biological psychiatry more credible than ever before. Yet it is a stretch of the imagination to say, for most psychopathology, that the neurosciences (and related biological disciplines) have found biological abnormalities in mental patients. The culture of biological psychiatry exemplifies the thesis of this book most clearly of all. For the science is excellent—but it has not yet shown what biological psychiatrists believe it will show someday. Rather, the culture's commitments shape the science itself: The intent to discover biological bases for mental illness leads its members to do certain kinds of research and not others. More important, they interpret their research (and the research of others) in a manner consistent with the "biological illness" hypothesis, though most of the research to date is consistent with other explanations of much psychopathology. The concept of disease is reshaped, as well, to fit the current state of research and practice. As in behaviorism, clinical care is shaped by assumptions exceeding the research.

When biological psychiatrists marshal evidence and interpret it to support their contentions, they may be doing nothing more than justifying their agenda. They can show that research into the biology of the mind has come of age and that pursuing their culture's agenda can, with good reason, be seen as promising. Honestly done, this is unobjectionable, for a culture pursuing an agenda that would amount to a revolution. Significant research works that way: Revolutionary assumptions generate hypotheses that guide research, and both the assumptions and the hypotheses necessarily transcend what is already known—otherwise, they could not guide further research. Since the research necessary to pursue the agenda is expensive and time-consuming, and since it requires an arduous acquisition of extensive knowledge and research skills, justifying the agenda is essential to its ever being fully carried out.

Biological psychiatrists may be doing something else, though. The debate over whether to regard psychopathology as biological pathology is, at the current state of knowledge, fundamentally a cultural debate about *how to think about* psychopathology. Shall we think about it in the terms of biological systems, or shall we think about it in psychosocial terms (or some as-yet unspecified combination)? When biological psychiatrists claim to have *shown* that psychopathology is biological pathology, they are simply getting ahead of themselves (and the rest of us), trying to short-circuit the debate.

So long as the devotees of biological psychiatry acknowledge the difference between their hypotheses and the results of their work, we can only wish them well (or ill, as may be our wont). What is objectionable is the attempt to persuade patients, the public, and clinicians (especially psychiatrists) outside the

■ ■ ■

research community that the scientific work has already shown the culture's agenda to be correct, capable of fulfillment, and significantly fulfilled.

How Biological Psychiatry Rallied

By the 1950s, as we have seen, care for all but the actively psychotic had come to be dominated by psychodynamically oriented therapies. Yet, in the 1950s, biological psychiatry began a rally that would, over a period of about twenty-five years, bring it back to a place of power. During that decade, several serendipitous discoveries coalesced. Several drugs developed for other uses were found to have what seemed to be desirable effects on psychological distress.[95] Techniques for studying neurotransmitters had by then developed to the point where the effects of psychoactive drugs on neurotransmission could be investigated.[96] (Neurotransmitters are the chemicals that transmit messages within and beyond the nervous system. The study of neurotransmission had begun about three decades earlier, when Otto Loewi proved that the nervous system exercises chemical rather than electrical control over the heart.) Though almost all these drugs had a variety of effects other than psychoactivity, by the end of the decade physicians and drug companies could rightly claim to have found biochemical ways to modulate mania, depression, anxiety, and schizophrenia. Clearly, these drugs acted on biological processes, and they produced some clear and apparently desirable effects. Further, studying the effects of these drugs on neuro-

---

[95] Richard Restak's *Receptors* (1994) presents a highly readable, entertaining history of drug discoveries. Samuel Barondes' *Molecules and Mental Illness* (1993) is equally good and also gives more detail on what is known about how drugs work in the brain. It has the advantage of beauty, with four-color photographs and blowups of microscopic photos of molecular phenomena and very well done charts and schemata to explain the relevant neurology. Both books accurately convey the serendipity and accident that characterize the history of psychoactive drugs.

[96] Solomon H. Snyder's *Drugs and the Brain* (1986) includes some description of techniques for studying neurotransmission. This book, like Barondes' *Molecules and Mental Illness*, contains excellent graphics. Peter Kramer's *Listening to Prozac* includes descriptions of techniques of discovery, as well.

transmission had led to a number of reasonable conjectures about the brain activity involved in some psychopathology.

The first effective drug treatment for psychopathology came in the late 1940s (though it did not become widely accepted until the 1950s), when John Cade, an Australian psychiatrist, discovered that lithium could control mania—the euphoric, grandiose, agitated, psychotic dimension of manic-depression. The discovery, in a significant way, made no sense. Cade had no general theory of mind or mania that would have predicted lithium's beneficial effects; to this day, no one understands why it works.

Cade was conducting very crude experiments to find a "toxin" that he hypothesized caused mania. He injected the urine of manic patients into rats, and sure enough, they showed serious impairments that did not occur in rats injected with normal urine. He tried to figure out which chemical agent in the urine caused the problem and settled on urea. He then wanted to experiment with urea itself rather than urine. Uric acid seemed to increase the toxicity of urea, and he wanted to study this interaction. Fortunately for thousands of manic-depressives, uric acid does not dissolve well, so to make a useable experimental solution, Cade turned to lithium urate, which is highly soluble. To his surprise, lithium did not increase the deleterious effects of urea. Instead, it protected the rats against those effects. Cade was appropriately startled, and he decided to investigate lithium itself. He used lithium carbonate (a safer form of lithium), and found that it not only protected rats but made them placid while still fully alert. In due course, he tried it on manic patients, and it worked. To this day, lithium remains the treatment of choice for most patients with manic-depression (now called "bipolar illness"), and it is one of the most consistently effective psychoactive medications.

Cade never found any toxins causing mania, and he could not find any reason to explain the effects of lithium. Mania is clearly not caused by a lithium deficiency in the body, any more than headaches are caused by aspirin deficiency. What he did, though, by paying careful attention to fortuitous events, was to make the lives of manic-depressives infinitely better.

The next major development came in the management of schizophrenia and—even more than Cade's discovery—it was more accidental than planned. Henri-Marie Laborit, a French surgeon, was using antihistamine drugs to try to prevent surgical shock. He stumbled across chlorpromazine—what we know as Thorazine—and found what he wanted. Chlorpromazine induced a deep calm and sense of detachment, without substantially impairing consciousness. Laborit suggested that psychiatrists try it on agitated psychotics. Though Thorazine has come to have a fairly negative public image, it immediately changed the face of care for psychotics, clearly for the better. Psychotic symptoms lessen (though they frequently do not disappear), and the ones that remain trouble and agitate the patient far less; the patient may continue to hallucinate, but he finds the hallucinations less disturbing. Many persons who would have been condemned to a life on the back wards were able to return to their families (if they had them) and function passably in the community. Again, though, no one knew how chlopromazine worked its wonders. (We now know that it decreases the activity of dopamine, which is now generally assumed to be involved in schizophrenia. Just how and why it is involved is not known.)

The third major discovery came in the treatment of depression. Isoniazid, a drug developed for tuberculosis, produced a general excitement, vitality, and happiness in the TB patients to whom it was given. The obvious conjecture was that it might, by having a similar effect, counteract depression—and it did. No one knew why, but isoniazid fit an emerging hypothesis. When a neurotransmitter is released from a neuron, it crosses a gap—called a synapse—to the next neuron. The neurotransmitter left in the synaptic cleft after transmission is either reabsorbed into the first neuron for later reuse or metabolized (broken down). One class of neurotransmitters, the monoamines (which include norepinephrine, serotonin, and dopamine), are broken down by monoamine oxidase (MAO). Isoniazid (in addition to whatever else it did) inhibited the action of MAO. That means it causes the monoamine neurotransmitters to remain in the synaptic cleft. A theory arose that depression arises from a deficiency of one or more monoamines, and efforts to find more chemicals that would inhibit the metabolic action of MAOs led to a variety of antidepressants.

Meanwhile, an attempt to find a more effective antipsychotic than Thorazine had led to the development of imipramine. Imipramine proved useless as an antipsychotic, but it turned out to be effective against both depression and panic attacks. To this day, no more effective treatment for depression is known; in controlled tests, today's wonder drug, Prozac, is no more effective (though it has fewer obvious noxious side effects and is, for that reason, more desirable). A derivative of imipramine, chlormipramine, was accidentally discovered to be effective for obsessive-compulsive disorder; it, too, remains as effective as any other known medication. Imipramine and chlormipramine both work differently from the MAO inhibitors. Instead of preventing the breakdown of monoamines, they block the routes by which monoamines are reabsorbed into the neuron from which they originated. Thus, they remain in the synapse, to be augmented by the next burst released from the neuron.

The first breakthrough in the general treatment of anxiety, Miltown, was discovered accidentally in the course of a search for antibiotics. Miltown was widely prescribed and praised, until it proved to be highly addictive and to cause liver damage. Its successor in popularity was Librium. By the late 1950s, drug companies had noted the immense market for psychoactive drugs and had begun funding massive research. Hoffman-La Roche hired Leo Sternbach to synthesize chemicals and try them out on laboratory animals. One class of chemicals that he synthesized yielded no promising results in the animal trials, despite over forty different derivatives, and Sternbach gave up on it before testing the last of his derivatives. Over a year later, an assistant came upon the untested substance while cleaning up the lab. He suggested testing it, and it turned out to be what we now know as Librium. Librium opened up an entire new class of chemicals, the benzodiazepines. Though only a tiny fraction of benzodiazepines turned out to have useful psychoactivity, Serax, Valium, Atavan, Xanax, and many other anxiolytics have emerged from this fortuitous discovery. (Recent research suggests that these work by augmenting the activities of GABA, an inhibitory neurotransmitter.)

With these discoveries, two very different sorts of developments were set in motion. One was the use of these drugs as tools (called "drug probes") in neurobiological investigation. By comparing various drug actions, scientists could begin to ferret out just what biological processes were being altered to produce their effects. When it became clear, for instance, that the antidepressant imipramine made the neurotransmitters norepinephrine and serotonin more plentiful, while reserpine (a drug used to decrease high blood pressure) decreased norepinephrine levels and brought about depression, it became reasonable to hypothesize that norepinephrine was somehow involved in at least some depression. (The idea that norepinephrine is the principal neurotransmitter involved in depression has been the dominant source of hypotheses about depression for most of the last four decades. The serotonin hypothesis has become more widely known because of the popularity of Prozac.) The use of chemicals as research tools has been, and no doubt will continue to be, an important avenue into understanding how the brain works.

The other development was the rapid rise of an entire culture of clinical care and research, funded in large part by pharmaceutical companies, to deliver biochemical treatments for the real-life complaints of patients.

Distinguishing these two developments is important, though they have fed into each other and can rightly be considered part of the same general trend in the science of understanding human life. Neurobiology, which aims to understand the biology of the nervous system, is a very different science from psychopharmacology, which aims to develop drug treatments for brain disorders. The two rest on (and seem to require) very different rationales. Using chemicals to do neurobiological research into how brains work does not require the assumption that what the chemicals are working on is biologically aberrant. If we discover that serotonin transmission is somehow involved in depression, we need not (as neurobiologists) assume that serotonin's role in depression represents a malfunction of the serotonin system. (The serotonin system conceivably may be responding appropriately to information from other parts of the brain, including the perceptual, memory, or anticipatory systems.) In psychopharmacology (and in the clinical use of biological psychiatry), the general ideology holds that what the drugs act on is in some way abnormal. If changing the serotonin system ameliorates depression, then something must have been wrong with the serotonin system to cause the depression. This assumption is a function of the traditional idea that mental health care remedies deficits. Without the rationale of correcting biological abnormalities, clinical psychopharmacology has difficulty defending itself against the charge that it provides boutique drugs for the respectable classes—the psychic equivalent of steroids. Making people feel better with drugs that do not correct a deficit generally falls outside our traditional notions of what it means to restore health.

Research into clinical psychopharmacology has been a rather different matter than basic neurobiological research using drug probes. In the latter, knowing the specific functions of specific chemicals is crucial; a chemical with attributes that are not known is at best crude as a drug probe, if not disastrously misleading. In the former, what matters is simply that the drug have a desirable effect, however little we may know about why. Until recently, psychopharmacological research followed a fairly standard routine: Synthesize drugs (more or less at random), try them out on laboratory animals, and see what kinds of behavioral effects they have. If their behavioral effects seem analogous to something we might like to see in humans, try them on humans. If those tests show that they do have the effects we want, market them.

Of late, the process has been somewhat improved. Neurobiology has helped clinical psychopharmacology synthesize drugs more intelligently and target parts of the brain where concentrations of neurons using specific neurotransmitters are found. (Most neurotransmitters are found in many parts of the brain, as well as in other parts of the body. One mode of designing drugs is to try to create molecular configurations that will bind with neurons at some locations and not others.) These drugs are said to be "cleaner," since their effects tend to modulate more limited brain systems. Even here, the process ultimately involves trial and error. Drugs are synthesized to fit hypotheses about what will make them more specific, then variants on that drug are tried to see whether, in fact, they bind with greater specificity.

Then they are tried out for clinical effectiveness, in the usual trial-and-error way.

Understanding just why some drugs work and some do not is generally beyond the current capabilities of science. Even understanding how the ones that clearly work manage to accomplish their tasks is beyond current knowledge. Most of the original hypotheses about neurotransmitter deficiencies or excesses have not stood up especially well to testing; even where we do understand the effects on synaptic transmission, no one understands why that should translate into changes at the level of thought, feeling, and action. In the sixth edition of their highly esteemed text on neuropharmacology, Cooper, Bloom, and Roth say that, ". . . at the molecular level, an explanation of the action of a drug is often possible; at the cellular level, an explanation is sometimes possible; but at a behavioral level, our ignorance is abysmal."[97] For clinical uses, that is not a crucial failure; so long as we know what conditions the drug helps, we can use it.

Neurobiology and psychopharmacology interact fruitfully; advances in one raise new issues and open new possibilities for the other. Yet, the old saw that the more we know the more we realize how much we don't know applies to this collaborative effort in spades. For each of the psychopathologies that biological psychiatry can medicate, a host of different hypotheses exist, and further research keeps turning up counterevidence for each (as well as data that simply do not fit). At least sixty neurotransmitters have now been identified, and recently an entire new class of gaseous neurotransmitters was discovered. Only half a dozen neurotransmitters have been investigated for their effects on psychopathology, and no one knows what effects the many others may have on psychiatric issues. Neuroanatomy—the study of the structures and organization of the brain—has undergone a vast upheaval, and how that will affect hypotheses about psychopathology has yet to be sorted out. Such developments lead to further questions, more elaborately framed hypotheses, and

---

[97] Jack R. Cooper, Robert H. Bloom, and Floyd E. Roth, The *Biochemical Basis of Neuropharmacology*, 6th ed. (1991).

new hypotheses. The multiple hypotheses about drugs working mainly at the synaptic level, for instance, now face rival hypotheses about neurotransmitters functioning more globally—about the presence of monoamines having a more diffuse effect throughout the brain (and body). Ideas that monoamine systems are the source of pathology contend with hypotheses that the problems originate elsewhere—in hormones from the endocrine system, for instance.

The immense ferment in the neurosciences is all well and good. However, it makes ever clearer the fragmentary nature of our understanding of the biological bases of even those psychopathologies that are well researched.

The point of all of this is that drugs drive biological psychiatry, in two ways. First, the fortuitous discovery of certain drugs enables the development of research tools. The refinement of our knowledge of these drugs through their use as research tools, and the development of further research tools, create a body of chemical agents that can then be used clinically. Second, the discovery of drugs with clinically desired effects, even before their biological action is understood, creates a body of practice that has to be rationalized and justified.

It is altogether conceivable, as we shall see, that biological pathology does not entail the need for drug interventions. Indeed, biological psychopathology, like many known physical illnesses, could yield to various regimens of therapy that do not involve drugs. No one has discovered that drugs are more effective at changing biology than other conceivable regimens for changing biology. Indeed, the question has not even been studied; research into how other regimens affect biology is hardly a research priority in this culture, probably at least partly because drug companies have no interest in paying for it. One need not be a scientist to understand that drug companies do not want to discover that the changes brought about by talk therapy include the stabilization of neurotransmitter regulatory systems.

To understand the culture of biological psychiatry, we have to understand the central place of drugs both as research tools in basic science and as clinical agents whose actions drive the rationales and habits of mind of clinicians. It is most decidedly *not* the case that biological abnormalities have been discovered and drugs then developed to treat them. Drugs have been found that do things that are valued within the culture of biological psychiatry, and the value placed upon these drug actions drives the development of the culture. The culture of biological psychiatry is largely devoted to making sense of drug effects, along lines dictated by a certain conception of illness.

Even though research has yet to lead to a coherent understanding of most psychopathology, effective drugs and a powerful research industry make biological psychiatry a strong and credible presence in mental health care—and in how our society thinks about mental illness and help. No responsible thinker can refuse to take seriously the possibility that at least some psychopathology is biological illness—whatever that means.

Biological Psychiatry's Concept of Mental Illness

What are biological psychiatrists claiming when they tell us that psychopathology is biological? Presumably they are saying something significant—something that tells us how care should be delivered and how disease should be conceptualized. Yet the statement that psychopathology is biological is fairly vague. To understand what biological psychiatry says about mental illness, we need to distinguish between two very different assertions: that psychopathology is biological and that it is biologically pathological.

The distinction is crucial. The former is simply the idea that dualism is false—mental phenomena are biological phenomena, and psychopathology no less than mental health is biological. Biological psychiatrists sometimes seem to be saying nothing more than this when they say things like, "Defenders of the medical model assert simply that dualism is wrong. The brain is, beyond doubt, the machinery of the mind."[98] Hardly anyone in

---

[98] Marvin E. Lickey and Barbara Gordon, *Medicine and Mental Illness* (1991).

the mental health community would bother to argue against this. No major contemporary culture of healing believes in matter/ spirit dualism, and all of them are consistent with materialism. More important, simply to say that dualism is false, and that psychopathology is therefore biological, leads to what philosophers call a distinction without a difference, or an empty distinction: To say that dualism is false, so that the mind is the brain, does not tell us anything about the nature of psychopathology, since mental health is also biological. The argument over dualism versus materialism is a metaphysical argument that cannot shed light on the difference between mental health and mental illness. Thus, if biological psychiatrists are only saying that dualism is false, they are not telling us anything about what distinguishes psychopathology from mental health and how to conceptualize and treat it.

If, though, biological psychiatrists are saying that psychopathology is biological *illness*, then they are saying something more relevant. They are saying that the biological machinery is not working as it should. In this case, we have a meaningful distinction, for in mental health, the machinery is presumably working as it should. Biological psychiatrists frequently sound as if this is, in fact, what they are saying.

Most biological psychiatrists have been fairly clear that only problems involving biological pathology should be considered mental illness. Generally, biological psychiatrists do not deny that many problems of many patients result from difficult circumstances and personal histories. They generally do not deny that talking to a mental health professional may help one get a clearer view of what, if anything, can be changed to make one happier. They just do not consider such problems to be illness. Wender and Klein, after an interesting and insightful discussion of how reality factors and one's history of learned behavior can cause misery, say, "Having taken a look at the possible contributions of reality and mislearning to unhappiness, we return to our primary concern—mental illness. In our view . . . mental illnesses consist of poorly functioning brain regulatory mechanisms . . . ." Psychosocial difficulties do not count as mental illness, in this culture.

It seems fair, then, to assume that biological psychiatrists are saying that psychopathology is a matter of biological abnormality or malfunction, even though they sometimes seem to say less than that. It seems fair to assume that they are saying something that is meaningful, not empty, especially since the idea of biological pathology is used in this culture to distinguish between those who have mental health problems and those who suffer problems with living that are not illnesses.

Why bother to point this out? At the present state of our knowledge of the brain, we cannot say whether (or which) biological processes involved in psychopathology are normal or not. Neurobiologists do not understand enough about the normal processes of the brain or the processes that are involved in psychopathology to say whether the biology of psychopathology involves biological abnormality. The ways in which biological psychiatrists go beyond the current state of knowledge to ostensibly prove that biological abnormality underlies psychopathology constitute major elements of their culture, and play a central role in how they conceptualize mental illness. Like the other cultures of healing, they claim scientific validity for ideas science has not validated.

The culture of biological psychiatry justifies its belief in the biological pathology of psychopathology on the basis of several premises. First, since some psychopathologies sometimes respond to some extent to drug treatment, they must be biological. Second, some evidence indicates a genetic component of some illnesses. Finally, some evidence shows that some of the brain functions involved in psychopathology are different from the functions of persons who do not suffer from psychopathology. The curiosity here is that each of these lines of evidence lends weight to the argument against dualism, but none is a strong premise from which to infer biological illness. Biological psychiatrists are confused as to which idea their evidence strongly supports. They have provided strong evidence for an idea that no one in the mental health community would bother to argue with—an idea perfectly consistent with the other cultures of healing. Yet, they have derived from this a concept of illness that a great many people argue with vociferously.

These premises are certainly consistent with the idea of psychopathology as biological pathology, but they do not entail it. Their persuasiveness is a function of the culture: Persons wanting to believe that psychopathology is biological pathology overestimate their weight. Perhaps more important, the notion of biological pathology that rests on these premises is not even necessarily the only one possible. Psychopathology may be biological pathology, but not of the sort that plays the critical role in this culture.

We will take these premises in reverse order. When neurobiologists or psychiatrists discover some process or part of the brain involved in psychopathology, biological psychiatrists take this as evidence that psychopathology "is" biological pathology. Yet, to identify the brain process involved in a phenomenon is simply to say, "This is where this particular process takes place." Knowing whether the process is biologically pathological requires that we know something else: whether it is a malfunction of that part of the brain, or whether it is precisely what that part of the brain is supposed to be doing, under the conditions in which it is working. Thus, simply to show that serotonin or dopamine or the raphe nuclei or the inferior surface of the left frontal lobe is involved in psychopathology does not tell us anything about the biological normality or pathology of the process.

A similar illusion is the heavy reliance on showing that something about the brains of persons suffering from pathological states differs from those of persons who do not. But once we recognize that *all* mental events are biological, we cannot say that "something different" about the biology of a psychopathology shows that the psychopathology is a biological pathology. *Of course* the biology of a pathological state will be different from the biology of a state in which that pathology does not exist, because every state *is* different from the state in which it is absent. That is nothing more than the simple logical law of identity: Everything is itself and not something other than itself. At present, biological psychiatrists seem to think they have established something when they show that depression is biologically different from nondepression or that obsessive thinking is biologically different from thinking that is not obsessional. They haven't quite established so much by that. Once we accept the falsity of dualism, this kind of difference follows as a purely logical necessity. It is consistent with every non-dualistic view.

To the question, "Is depression, or anxiety, or a narcissistic personality, or whatever, biological," the answer (assuming that dualism is false) is, "Of course. Everything is biological." To ask, "Is each psychopathological state biologically different from each healthy state," the obvious answer is, again, "Of course. Each sort of state is biologically different from each other sort of state." To prove that depression, say, has a different biology than non-depressive affect is to prove nothing that we did not already know. It is like saying, "Since spaghetti has a different chemistry than ice cream, we know that spaghetti is not ice cream." But we knew that before we did the chemical assay of the spaghetti and of the ice cream. Discovering the precise biology of each state of an organism is truly a great thing; but that sort of discovery does not amount to a discovery of whether such states are to be understood as biological malfunctions.

The culture of psychopathology tends to be preoccupied with genetic studies as a way of establishing biological pathology. Wender and Klein, for instance, say, "Our belief that mental illnesses arise frequently and sometimes exclusively from biological functioning of the brain stems in large part from studies of genetic patterns of mental illness."[99] Consistently, biological psychiatrists tell us that psychopathology "has a genetic component." This is a fairly vague statement—as well it should be, for genetic studies to date have yielded only very vague results.

Genetic studies of psychopathology have focused mostly on schizophrenia, manic-depression, and major depression. Some studies have been done on anxiety disorders, eating disorders, and a few others. Each of these shows a substantial genetic influence. The degree of genetic influence on most of these conditions is roughly the same as the genetic influence on a variety of personality traits—like leadership, caution, aggression, traditionalism,

---

[99] Paul H. Wender and Donald F. Klein, *Mind, Mood, and Medicine* (1981).

vocational interest, and adult criminality. The degree of heritability for all these traits is roughly in the forty to sixty-five percent range (manic-depression is a bit higher, at seventy-five percent), meaning that genetics accounts for forty to sixty-five percent of the trait's existence. Put differently, for two persons with identical genes, the probability of sharing the trait is forty to sixty-five percent. Another trait that falls into the high end of this range, surprisingly, is alcohol consumption by nonalcoholics.

Most genetic studies on psychological or behavioral matters are done not on genes but on populations. This is not a bad thing, but it is crucial to understanding the significance of the heritability figures. Statistical methods of great sophistication are used to calculate the effect of genetics (versus environment) on traits shared by members of the population (or on differences in traits, if that is the focus of the study). When biological psychiatrists say that psychopathology has a genetic component, they are almost never saying that the genes involved have been located. They are saying that careful statistical analyses of populations entail heritability.

The reason this is important is that we can know that a trait is substantially heritable without knowing just what the genes involved actually determine. Genes do not cause traits. They cause the body's various systems to develop in specific ways, and a great many genes work together to determine most systems. What these systems amount to, in terms of personality traits, is also a function of the environmental conditions under which they function, including social conditions. There is, for instance, probably no leadership gene, intelligence gene, alcoholism gene, and so forth. There are probably a great many genes that act together to produce personal potentials that, under average social and environmental conditions, bring about leadership, intelligence, and so forth. To understand what genes determine, we have to know what systems they generate and the conditions under which those systems function. Conceivably the heritability of much psychopathology will turn out to be a function of some relationship with perfectly innocuous, nonpathological traits. Indeed, it is quite conceivable that at least some psychopathology may correlate with highly desirable personality traits; psychopathology may be the price we pay for some highly desirable kinds of neural wiring. The psychopathology may be a matter of such wiring functioning exactly as it should under certain conditions—exquisite sensitivity to environmental stimuli may be a good thing, for instance, but cause great pain under certain conditions. Similarly, a ruminative temperament may be a valuable trait, but when the reality of one's situation is very difficult it may make "positive illusions" impossible.

Consider an analogy. Fair-skinned people are more susceptible to sunburn than persons with oilier complexions. The fairness of skin is genetically determined. There is nothing pathological about having fair skin. In no sense can it reasonably be said either that the genetically determined mechanisms that make one susceptible to sunburn are deficiencies or that sunburn is genetically determined. That complexion is genetically determined informs us of nothing about how to avoid and treat sunburn. If we were as ignorant about the causes and treatment of sunburn as we are about psychopathology, it would be easy to do genetic studies and conclude that sunburn has a substantial genetic component. Similarly, we do not know whether (or when) a genetic propensity to psychopathology represents a biological pathology or a biologically well-integrated (though not universal) set of systems that, under specifiable conditions, result in distress.

Thus, to show a correlation between genetic endowment and psychopathology does not tell us much, *unless* we know the biological systems that the genes shape (which mediate or cause the susceptibility to psychopathology), the role of those systems in the mind, and the role of environmental conditions. Until we identify and understand the biological systems that the genetics of each psychopathology correlate with, we cannot know whether those systems are malfunctioning when psychopathology occurs.

Biological psychiatry's infatuation with genetics is precisely an attempt to leapfrog the question of what biological systems are involved in psychopathology and whether they are abnormal. It enables biological psychiatrists to say, "We have no idea what the biology of psychopathology is, but since psychopathology is genetically determined, we can be sure that there *is* a biological pathology." Yet, as we have seen, the logic here is just plain wrong. The fact that psychopathology has a genetic component certainly does mean that biological systems are involved—as we would expect, since so much of human life (normal or not) rests on genetically determined biological systems. It does not mean those systems are abnormal.

Genetic studies are, in principle, extremely important. As they become more sophisticated and are correlated with more sophisticated knowledge about brains, and as that is correlated with more sophisticated studies of child and personality development, genetic studies will begin to provide extremely important knowledge as to where in the brain, or in the experiences that shape the brain's makeup or functions, we should look to understand psychopathology. For now, though, biological psychiatrists claim for them a probity that they do not yet have.[100]

The strong suit in biological psychiatry's hand is effective drugs. Biological psychiatrists frequently make the argument that, since specific drugs alleviate specific psychopathologies, they must be addressing specific disorders. Imipramine relieves depression but makes nondepressed persons feel awful. Miltown stabilizes emotion in nervous people but has no discernible effect on calm people. Imipramine, but not the benzodiazepines, has been found to be effective in curbing panic disorder. Such specificity is assumed to mean that the drugs affect a specific biological process and that, since that hypothetical process causes psychopathology, it is biologically pathological. A significant amount of research uses differential responsiveness to variant forms of chemicals (different forms of an antidepressant, for instance) to try to distinguish between types of biological illness. Since it is

---

[100] As an example of the kind of illogicality the culture of biological psychiatry exhibits around genetics, consider this statement from Solomon Snyder, certainly one of the most astute and logical of scientists, in his book *Drugs and the Brain:* "It is quite possible, however, that there also exists a subclass of individuals in whom pronounced anxiety is genetically determined and *should therefore* be regarded as a disease unto itself. . . ." [italics added] Dr. Snyder would probably call this a slip of the pen, a casual statement whose need for qualification he well understands; but that such a sentence should so casually slip out reflects how common this type of thinking is.

generally assumed that depression and anxiety are both names for an indeterminate number of different underlying processes, such drug probes aim to delineate how many different kinds of depression or anxiety disorders there are.

To infer from the specificity of a drug's effect that the state affected is pathological, though, is illogical. At best, specificity of drug action proves that a specific chemical is acting on a specific brain process to cause a specific state change. It does not prove that the state changed was pathological. There is nothing in the specificity argument that is inconsistent with a "steroids for the brain" argument. A well-crafted drug may simply induce certain psychological states or make certain states impossible—altering specific processes so that some things cannot happen.

Conceivably, antidepressants, for instance, may in effect put a "floor" under negative moods, setting a level of negativity below which mood cannot go. Suppose someone was thinking about the fact that one's spouse wants a divorce. This might activate memories, plans, and ideas about the meaning and worth of the person's life. The unmedicated limbic system (the parts of the brain most involved in emotional evaluation) might assess the emotional meaning of this information to produce profound "ordinary" (that is, nonpathological) depression. The combination of the cognitive information and the depressed mood might then lead to further imaginings of a very hopeless future, and the limbic evaluation of that might be something like clinical depression. Suppose, though, that such an emotional evaluation involves a pattern of neurotransmission that cannot take place when certain levels of serotonin are present. Serotonin levels increased by drugs, then, would prevent that emotional information from being formulated. Maintaining a constant level of serotonin in the brain's synaptic clefts might be analogous to masking certain sounds by generating a constant level of another sound.

Additionally, specificity is in the eye of the beholder; it is the way the culture of biological psychiatry shapes the perceptions of its adherents that lets them see specificity where the rest of us might see something far more vague. Consider the fact that all drugs have "side effects." What makes an effect a "side" effect rather than a principal effect or just an effect? One thing, and one thing only: that the effect is not the one *we want* the drug to have. Biologically, all the effects are effects, period. As the eminent neurobiologist Steven Rose has put it, "Introducing an exogenous chemical like a drug into the body has a multitude of biological consequences, some anticipated, others unexpected—but never 'side-effects.' The phrase is a misnomer, concealing the reality that such consequences are inevitable, even though they are ones that the researcher or the clinician doesn't want or hadn't thought about."[101]

The fact that all drugs have side effects means that no drug does specifically what we want it to do. For instance, increased serotonin levels cause sexual dysfunction in rats, and most anti-depressants cause sexual dysfunction in some patients—either impaired ability to reach orgasm or, in some men, decreased potency. Depressed persons, we may assume, are not generally in search of sexual dysfunction, but the effects of the drug include this.[102] Similarly, the antischizophrenic drugs, which alter dopamine functions, result in an irreversible condition called tardive dyskinesia, in which various disabilities of movement occur. Presumably persons who want relief from schizophrenia are not in search of involuntary movement disorders.

Side effects are not necessarily an issue of the drugs being "dirty"—affecting multiple neurotransmitters—for they are present in the cleanest of the antidepressants and neuroleptics (antipsychotic drugs). To say such drugs are specific for certain diseases, then, is rather misleading. Side effects actually provide a strong argument against specificity: Since drugs affect many more things than the pathology they are aimed at, it seems fairly clear

---

[101] Steven Rose, *The Making of Memory* (1992).

[102] Interestingly, psychoanalysts could easily make the rhetorical point that this allows for a hypothetical psychoanalytic explanation of the effectiveness of antidepressants. Since it seems fairly clear that antidepressants specific for serotonin decrease sex drive, or the potential for sexual arousal beyond a certain point, any neurosis that is driven by sexual conflict loses its force. No drive, no neurosis. Decrease the sex drive, and the amount of sexual energy available may be within the bounds that the defenses can easily handle. Whether this might be true is not known, but it seems logical enough as a possibility.

that they are inducing changes at a more general level than the processes involved in the psychopathology. This would not seem to provide much support for the idea that the specific processes addressed by the drugs are pathological.

Since a great deal about what drugs do in the brain is beyond our current knowledge, claims of specificity are, in fact, culture bound. Of all psychoactive drugs it would be accurate to say: "We see certain of the things we have looked for occurring. Other things we had not thought about have intruded themselves too obviously to escape notice. We do not know enough to determine what else may be going on."

The idea of specific effects also makes less sense in reality than in the laboratory. In reality, psychiatrists rarely know just what drug to prescribe to what patient. They listen carefully and try to find similarities between a particular patient and others who have responded well to specific drugs. Even so, finding an effective drug (and dosage) for each patient is largely a matter of trial and error, and the extent to which each patient responds is highly individual. More important, psychiatrists generally do not know who will and who will not respond to drugs at all. Biological psychiatrists are generally quite honest that allegedly biologically based psychopathologies frequently cannot be distinguished from other miseries prior to trying drugs and seeing whether they work. The specific effect is inferred from the effect itself, which is obviously a case of begging the question.

Specificity also makes less sense when we realize that drugs tend to have a wide range of applicability, even when they are carefully crafted to affect a circumscribed brain system. As drugs with fewer obvious noxious side effects (like Prozac) are developed, psychiatrists can try them on people who in the past would not have been considered candidates for medication at all. It certainly seems that these drugs help persons who do not meet the diagnostic criteria of the illnesses for which the drugs are supposedly specific. (Until recently, the side effects of most drugs were sufficiently unpleasant that patients felt they had a negative effect on their quality of life even when they worked. As a result, they tended to be used only where necessary. The idea that drugs like imipramine, for instance, decrease pathology but make normal people miserable may be a function of nondepressed persons finding the side effects completely unacceptable, whereas depressed persons tolerate them to get some relief.) Biological psychiatrists interpret the drugs' wide-ranging effectiveness as evidence that some undetected pathology underlies many disorders. That may be so, but we do not know that. As a line of argument it is clearly circular, designed to preserve the idea of specific effect.

Specificity is also partly an artifact. When a drug is accidentally found that relieves distress, drug companies try to develop new drugs by synthesizing chemicals that have the same sort of chemical effects. The fact that subsequent drugs for a given disorder act in a similar manner is a function of the style of research. In reality, clinically effective drugs often have very different modes of action—there are effective antidepressants that do not block serotonin or norepinephrine reuptake (or inhibit MAOs), for instance. Antipsychotic drugs in low doses are not infrequently used to treat anxiety, though their effects do not seem principally to result from augmenting GABA efficacy. The fact that a great many chemicals addressing specific systems have been marketed tells us as much about the economics of the pharmaceutical industry as about brains. If, as seems clear, drugs acting on very different brain systems can have similar effects, we cannot infer from drug efficacy that a specific brain system is the site of psychopathology. We therefore also cannot infer that the site of a drug's action is biologically abnormal.

None of this is to say that the search for more specific drugs is a bad thing, or that delineating specific responses is anything other than crucial in research into the particular brain systems involved in psychopathology. Obviously, this is critical to finding out how the brain works and whether the processes addressed by drugs are abnormal. The specificity of drugs effects, though, is less impressive than those already devoted to biological psychiatry would have us believe, and it tells us less than they claim. Such specificity as drugs have does not necessarily amount to more than the elementary principle that specific chemicals acting under specific conditions have specific effects. This does not mean that the processes affected are biologically aberrant.

These three ways of justifying the biological illness hypothesis, together with an unpleasant fact about medication, shape how this culture conceives of psychopathology. The unpleasant fact is this: Psychoactive drugs do not cure anything. Withdrawing psychoactive medications results in an extremely high level of relapse. This fact, combined with the idea that the processes affected by drugs are pathological, that they are genetically determined, and that drugs are the appropriate type of intervention, shape how this culture conceives of psychopathology. To biological psychiatrists, psychopathology is a chronic constitutional problem inherent in one's makeup, that can be managed but not cured. It is likened to rheumatoid arthritis, diabetes, and other chronic illnesses. The difference is that this way of looking at psychopathology is not a discovery but an article of ideology. The role of drugs as a premise, not a conclusion, of discovery once more becomes evident: The nature of drug effects defines how disease is conceptualized.

This view of mental illness is not necessary to seeing psychopathology as biological pathology. Most biological diseases are not chronic, constitutional, and genetically determined. Psychopathology could be biological but analogous to a bad back that develops out of years of misuse and lack of exercise. It could be analogous to a muscle tear or a sprained ankle—or bound feet. It could be like malnutrition. It could be unique. Nor does the idea that psychopathology is a biological abnormality entail that drugs are the treatment of choice. Once we accept the falsity of dualism, we have to accept that everything is physical—and that includes talk therapy, new experiences, and changes in one's habits of life. All of these have biological effects. There is no *a priori* reason to think that the biological changes needed to treat psychopathology cannot be effected by non-pharmacological regimens. Anyone who has fallen in love (or felt betrayed by a lover) knows that psychosocial factors have biological effects. Lickey and Gordon recognize this: "Psychotherapy produces biological effects just as a drug or electroconvulsive shock does. Through talking and personal interaction, psychotherapy changes the state of the brain."[103] The culture of biological psychiatry holds a view

---

[103] Marvin E. Lickey and Barbara Gordon, *Medicine and Mental Illness* (1991).

of biological pathology that is both insufficiently evidenced and conceptually unnecessary.

Disproving this concept of disease is not easy, even though other cultures claim to have lower relapse rates. For many psychopathologies, whether they are even chronic is highly debatable. Some recent evidence (from epidemiological studies) suggests that many people suffer an occasional isolated episode of mental illness rather than a chronic disease requiring medication. A fair number of psychopathologies tend to improve in middle age. (Even in schizophrenia and manic-depression, which do tend to be chronic—and are the best candidates for biological pathology—some patients have only one or a few episodes fairly early in life, then stabilize.) Whether or not this concept of disease eventually proves correct, this is what biological psychiatrists teach their patients. This is how one learns to view one's problems.

The biological psychiatrist's view may be true for some mental illnesses, and it may someday be discovered to be generally true, but for now it seems a large and dire view to take as one's definition of mental illness. As Wender and Klein understand, "The biological assertion is far more frightening [than psychoanalysis], implying that cogitate as one will, analyze as one will . . . still one may be unable to manage it." Nonetheless, they say, one need not be so gloomy, because ". . . certain medications may markedly help even organic conditions. Further, recognition of the persuasiveness of the biological evidence can lead to a more realistic restructuring of life in accordance with any limitations that may be indicated."[104] In other words, Yes, this is very scary, but as long as one takes one's medication and alters one's life to fit the biological psychiatrist's ideas about one's chronic vulnerabilities, one's illness may be manageable.

The Clinical Practice of Biological Psychiatry

If biological psychiatrists confined themselves to treating schizophrenia and manic-depression, hardly anyone would quarrel with

---

[104] Paul H. Wender and Donald F. Klein, *Mind, Mood, and Medicine* (1981).

them—nor would we be talking about them in this book. Intuitively, their concept of illness seems applicable to these syndromes. If biological psychiatry held to its neat and plausible distinction between mental illness, which involves biological abnormality, and other problems that bring people to mental health professionals, we might want to argue with them, but they could reasonably claim that this distinction is important and in principle susceptible to scientific investigation. Biological psychiatrists do not confine themselves to psychoses, though, and the distinction they make between illness and health is, at the present time, almost entirely speculative and incapable of being applied to patients. Thus, the ideology is used to interpret the problems that patients bring for treatment and, as in all the other cultures of healing, exercises an influence over how people think of themselves that derives from the culture rather than science.

In the laboratory, biological psychiatrists and neurobiologists work with animals or carefully chosen study groups of patients, and they work with carefully delineated goals of changing target signs and symptoms. In clinical practice, the situation is extremely different. People who come for care are not so neatly packaged as the assiduously homogenized study group populations, and the patients' ideas about what needs changing and what will count as adequate improvement is not governed by research definitions.

An important fact of clinical practice is that *in no case whatsoever* is diagnosis made on biological grounds. Despite immense efforts to create biological tests for psychopathology, none has been found that satisfies minimum criteria of reliability. *All* the diagnostic indicators are behavioral, emotional, or psychological. Thus, the neat distinction between mental illness with a biological base and problems of living becomes a subjective matter of clinical judgment. As we would expect, the psychiatrists' judgments of which psychological and behavioral matters are signs of underlying biological illness differ radically from the judgments of ministers of other cultures looking at the same data.

Peter D. Kramer's *Listening to Prozac* displays with extraordinary self-awareness and reflective appraisal how thinking happens in the culture of biological psychiatry. The effects of Prozac that Kramer reports vastly exceed anything that has been scientifically verified; but that does not affect the excellence of the book as an account of how biological psychiatrists think. As Kramer makes very clear, once psychiatrists have a drug and a clinical sense of the conditions it can change, they begin listening to what patients say for signs of these conditions. As psychoanalysis converts patients' manifest reports into signs of unconscious process, biological psychiatry turns them into signs of pathological physiological processes. As psychoanalysis converts the realities of one's life into derivatives of unconscious infantile conflicts, biological psychiatry converts them into derivatives of constitutional pathologies. "Listening" to a drug—the point of Kramer's title—means that one takes drugs as the guide to what one looks for and how one assesses its meaning.[105]

Biological psychiatry has, at present, drugs to medicate only four classes of complaint: depression, anxiety, schizophrenia, and manic-depression. Effectively, most problems of most patients have to be seen as manifestations of depression or anxiety, if they are to be amenable to drug treatment—or they are interpreted as *having been* sequelae of depression or anxiety *if* they prove amenable to medication. Since all extant antianxiety drugs (called anxiolytics) are addictive and capable of being abused, whereas many antidepressants are not, antidepressants tend to be prescribed wherever possible. This means that clinical syndromes get interpreted as sequelae of previously undetected chronic depression wherever possible.

In the culture of biological psychiatry, the problems of living associated with psychopathology are understood to be consequences of the underlying biological problem. They may be efforts to cope with the pathology or psychosocial expressions—

---

[105] I have been surprised how many of the reviews of Kramer's book that I have read and how many of the people I have talked to have missed the point, which is so clearly indicated by the title. Kramer's point is that our conceptions of life and illness are reshaped by listening to drugs and their effects—by drawing inferences about life and pathology from drug effects. Put differently, Kramer's point is precisely congruent with mine: that what we believe is not a function of science but of the culture.

consequences—of the biological abnormality. Here is one example:

> The dilemma of someone with a chronic undetected depression of probably biological origin—whose major manifestation is an insatiable need for the love and support of others—sometimes leads to other psychological strategies to allay the unquenchable needs, usually without the person's awareness. In order not to drive others off, such an individual may try to anticipate their expressed and unexpressed wishes, keeping his own wishes in abeyance. Thus, he may be predisposed to become passive and compliant. Being assertive, giving vent to his own wishes, is seen as a risky business because of the possibility of antagonizing others or provoking their withdrawal. Furthermore, since it is painful to want something and not act on it, the individual is likely to suppress or repress his self-assertive and selfish desires, unconsciously pushing them out of awareness.[106]

This way of looking at patients allows biological psychiatrists to agree with other kinds of therapists on the psychosocial patterns that patients' complaints involve, while insisting that the explanations offered by other cultures are backwards. Where a psychologically minded therapist, of whatever culture, ascribes causal status to the psychosocial factors (and can see the biological dimensions as effects of these), the biological psychiatrist denies explanatory force to the psychosocial data. The hypothetical biological abnormality explains the observable psychosocial characteristics of patients.

Explanations of this sort are at present entirely speculative, as theoretical as psychoanalytic ideas. They carry weight by virtue of their association with the aura of scientific validity attaching to medications. The evidence for these explanations derives from the fact that some patients who receive medication and who

---

[106] This example is from Paul H. Wender and Donald F. Klein, *Mind, Mood, and Medicine* (1981), which contains many others. Peter D. Kramer, *Listening to Prozac* (1993) also contains many good examples of this sort of explanation.

are enculturated to believe these stories about their problems of living do, in fact, change in the ways psychiatrists enculturate them to. The "psychological strategies" do not change automatically upon ingestion of the drugs; the psychiatrist has to (in Wender and Klein's terms) "reeducate" patients and "explain" that the psychological patterns are the malfunctional sequelae of the depression. The patients take the medicine, feel better, then buy the story and presumably live differently. The power of the medication to make them feel better greatly enhances the psychiatrist's power to indoctrinate patients into her view of which psychosocial patterns are "strategies" resulting from the depression and how they need to change. Anyone who has ever given someone a gift or done a favor knows that making people feel better greatly enhances their receptivity to one's message.

These hypotheses hold immense fascination, and they are susceptible to scientific study—in principle. How can we know whether they are true, at present? We cannot. In this culture, though, a positive response to medication and adjunctive therapy is assumed to be evidence of the truth of these conjectures—as every culture assumes its effectiveness is evidence of its truth. The presumption is that problematic traits that yield to medication reveal illness, even though at present we cannot distinguish problematic traits biologically. This presumption has an intuitive appeal, but it is not very sound. Once biological psychiatrists admit (as most do) that persons with biological illness and persons with psychosocial difficulties (but no illness) cannot be reliably distinguished *prior* to drug response, they must admit that drug response does *not* correlate with a known distinction. The idea that drugs work on biological illness but not on psychosocial difficulties requires that we first be able to distinguish between these two, then that we see which group responds to drugs. If drug response is the method of distinguishing the groups, obviously no correlation is possible—except the tautological one that persons who respond to drugs respond to drugs.

Consider the recently recognized seasonal affective disorder (SAD). There is some controversial evidence that persons suffering from SAD have decreased melatonin levels. (Melatonin is a neurotransmitter manufactured from serotonin in the pituitary gland.) There is also evidence that persons who suffer from SAD but who are allowed to sleep when they want overcome the disease. Characteristically, they stay up later at night and rise later in the morning. This would seem to indicate that the problem is with social expectations—requiring people to show up for work every day at the same time—rather than with a biological system. In these cases, a person may respond well to medication that increases serotonin availability (presumably because it is the precursor of melatonin) and accept the psychiatrist's indoctrination into the idea that he has a brain disorder. What seems equally likely is that the patient has a perfectly healthy brain that, like an overused muscle, becomes malfunctional under the conditions in which he has to live.

In clinical practice, then, there exist no biological tools for distinguishing between biological psychopathology and similar problems that do not involve biological abnormality. The patient's account of her life is mined for indicators that a particular drug may be effective. Speculative theories about how an underlying biological pathology may influence one's life govern interpretation of the patient's problems. If a drug does provide relief, this is taken as evidence of biological abnormality, and the patient is taught to change her psychosocial life in line with the speculative theories. Biological psychiatry, no less than other schools of care, is a culture whose claims far exceed its scientific basis, and it teaches people to think about problems in definite, but scientifically unverified, ways.

Confusion of Categories

Biological psychiatry suffers from and promotes profound confusion, for it has yet to think through the consequences of the collapse of dualism. Though biological psychiatry has to say something more than "dualism is false" to say anything significant, it cannot say less than this. Yet biological psychiatrists say things that make sense only if dualism is true, and they derive from the denial of dualism things that simply do not follow from it. As a result, they say many things that make little sense upon careful reflection. This may seem esoteric, but their confusion distorts understanding—and gives biological psychiatry a specious credibility and drugs a specious aura of significance. Equally important, this confusion is conscripted into service in the turf wars against nonphysicians (and psychologically oriented psychiatrists).

Biological psychiatry makes no sense unless dualism is false; everyone would agree to that. We all recognize that for biological psychiatry to make sense, mind must not be something different from matter; there cannot be not two distinct realms of reality. If mind and matter were different in kind, mental problems should not be amenable to material interventions. Clearly they are, so dualism must (it seems) be mistaken. What follows from this? Almost nothing relevant to mental health care—which biological psychiatrists fail to realize. If everything is material, it does not follow that biology has priority in understanding the mind and its problems. Quite the contrary. It means that psychology (and other sciences) have as much claim to explain material states as biology has to explain psychological ones. We are all talking about the same thing, though we are saying very different things about it. The various sciences (and the activities of all creatures) are all matters of matter. Biological psychiatry's confusions on this issue cause its patients and the public to think about mental health and illness in profoundly confused ways.

Consider the idea that mental illnesses are brain diseases. Nancy Andreasen articulates it in this way: "Psychiatry now recognizes that the serious mental illnesses are *diseases* in the same sense that cancer or high blood pressure are diseases. Mental illnesses are diseases that affect the brain, which is an organ of the body just as the heart or stomach is. People who suffer from mental illness suffer from a *sick or broken brain*, not from weak will, laziness, bad character, or bad upbringing."[107] This statement makes sense only if dualism is true—and also only if it is false. It is therefore quite literally nonsense. Andreasen maintains

---

[107] Nancy C. Andreasen, *The Broken Brain* (1984).

the traditional distinction between matter and spirit when she says, in effect, that because psychopathology is a brain state, it is not a spiritual state. One cannot infer that brain states are not spiritual states unless one maintains dualism. If dualism is false, weakness of will, laziness, bad character, and bad upbringing are, in fact, material states. A weak will may well be like a weak bladder; a broken brain may entail a broken character. If one's brain is one's mind and one's brain is diseased, it follows that one's mind is diseased.

Andreasen, like many biological psychiatrists and their patients, is profoundly confused because she thinks that biological psychiatry should make us less moralistic toward the mentally ill. Certainly we should be more compassionate and tolerant toward the infirm, but for moral reasons, not for reasons having to do with whether or not the mind is the brain. Frankly, it is not at all clear how insisting that brains are diseased helps make compassion and tolerance imperative. We would not decide that someone is a reliable worker or deserves a job simply because his inability to do it is due to a physical illness. Similarly, to explain a person's psychological incapacities or deficiencies as biological disease does not make that person any more capable of socially valued attributes or worthy of a positive evaluation. Quite the contrary. By obliterating any distinction between matter and spirit, the denial of dualism entails that people have no moral character, good or ill, over and above their brain states. Thus, to say that a person is constitutionally, genetically, chronically impaired biologically *is* to say that the person is chronically, constitutionally, genetically impaired as a person. How is that supposed to help increase tolerance of the mentally ill?

Once we accept that the mind is the brain, brain diseases must be seen as *very* different from liver, kidney, or heart diseases. Our kidneys, livers, and hearts are essentially the same as those of other mammals, and they are not generally central to our sense of ourselves—or to our decisions about whom we will love, hate, depend upon, or avoid. The mind is central to our identity and our capacity for all distinctly human functions. Most of us can lose a kidney or have a liver or heart transplant without suffering any deep assault on our sense of who we are. To lose one's mind is the obliteration of oneself. To lose it in part is to suffer the erosion of one's being as a person. Defects of mind modify our capacities as individuals and as participants in relationships and communities. The idea that brain diseases are not substantially different from other diseases only makes sense if they do not affect our distinctly human qualities and capacities. That, however, depends precisely upon maintaining the dualism of brain and mind.

Segregating a person into who she is versus the disease that afflicts her makes some sense when the affliction is *not* a disease of an organ central to being the human one is. Calling mental illness a brain disease does not fit that description. Calling mental illness a brain disease—and a chronic, constitutional brain disease, at that—actually confirms every patient's worst fear: This problem bears witness to something fundamentally wrong with the person I am.

By failing to think through what it means to say that the brain is the mind, biological psychiatry also makes many nonsensical claims about its own status and its relationship to other fields of study. Once we abandon dualism, the distinction between different disciplines becomes a distinction between types of discourse and levels by which reality is organized. All the structures and systems composing reality are made of the same stuff. Thus, to speak of physics versus chemistry is to speak of different modes of discourse addressing different levels of how reality is organized. The same is true of chemistry as distinct from biology or biology as distinct from psychology—or sociology or anthropology. To say that dualism is false says nothing about which sciences are necessary to explain human life (or anything else). To claim some superior or more foundational status for biology simply because the mind is the brain is mistakenly to confuse materialism with one kind of science.

Back in the seventeenth and eighteenth centuries, when physics had first been discovered, theorists smitten with its promise predicted that eventually everything—including human thought—would be explained in terms of physics. We now know that is not true. While (presumably) nothing in the universe can violate the laws of physics, all sorts of things are possible, given physics, that do not exist. Reality reflects only a subset of the possibilities that are consistent with physical laws. (The laws of physics, for instance, are oblivious to the direction of time. They apply just as well if time moves backwards. Reality seems rather more constrained by the direction of time.) Chemistry is presumably consistent with physics, but the laws of physics do not predict the laws of chemistry—chemistry could be other than it is and still be consistent with physics. Similarly, biology has to be consistent with laws of chemistry, but chemistry does not predict biology. Psychology has to be consistent with biology, but we have no reason to think that biology will be able to predict psychology. Yet biological psychiatrists often sound a lot like the eighteenth-century materialists who believed that physics could explain everything.

To think—and to teach patients and the public—that because some things about the mind can be explained in terms of biological sciences, the biological sciences will be able to explain the mind is simply a conceptual mistake. From the fact that something illuminating can be said in biological terms it does not follow that psychological terms are not needed for an adequate explanation. To argue that they are not is exactly like saying that the power of physics makes biology superfluous. Thus, the fact that some important things can be said biologically does not mean that the agenda of biological psychiatry can be fulfilled or that it has any claim to explanatory superiority over other ways of understanding the mind and its problems. We simply do not know yet what matters will require psychological explanation and what will yield to biological explanation.

Psychological information is presumably encoded physically. For most of the problems patients present with, we do not have accounts of the physical encoding or its transformations; that is, biological (or other physical) accounts of most psychological processes do not even exist. Nor do we know how to mediate between biological and psychological accounts; we do not know how to translate the code. We have no clue how the biochemical processes involved in psychopathology (or drug treatment) translate into psychological information and influence how the brain encodes and processes information. Nor do we know the opposite: how psychological information is encoded in specific patterns of neurotransmission and other biochemical processes. We can talk at a gross level about fairly unitary psychological states, like affects, and correlate those with some biological knowledge. For more complex psychological phenomena, we are at present woefully short of such correlations.[108] No one possesses more than extremely gross correlations between biological language and descriptions of psychological functioning like love, hate, denial, longing, reasoning, and so forth. Even less do we possess correlations between biological and psychological accounts of the complexities that compose a personality or its interactions with trying situations. In short, for most (perhaps all) of the problems of patients, scientific correlations between the psychological phenomena and biological explanations are nonexistent.

Unless everyone else is simply wrong—unless there are really no relationships between thought, action, personality, events that seem to precipitate psychopathology, and the states about which biological psychiatrists do have some biological knowledge—the biological accounts to date are extremely incomplete. To throw over existing psychological (and other) explanations in favor of some mythical promise that biology will someday explain these things is logically unjustified—and foolish. To deny fundamental explanatory power to theoretical and research efforts in psychological fields, in the name of the presumed superiority of biological explanation, is without any rational basis.

The point here is not the cliché that biological factors and psychological factors work together. The point is that we have two very different traditions of discourse, and there is no rational basis for assuming that biology will be able to offer adequate explanations of mental phenomena, including psychopathology.

---

[108] Two books that give exciting accounts of the state of neuroscientific research, how such research gets done, and the distance between neuroscience and our psychological and everyday accounts of mind are Daniel Alkon's *Memory's Voice* (1992) and Steven Rose's *The Making of Memory* (1992).

For one tradition of discourse to claim priority *a priori* is illogical and shortsighted.

An adequate science of psychopathology may require the creation of whole new sciences and vocabularies, analogous, perhaps, to the efforts that have begun to be made in the cognitive neurosciences. In all probability, the human race will have to evolve new vocabularies and a variety of new sciences to understand itself as the existing sciences progress. The most sophisticated efforts of psychologists and biologists will have to go into the creation of such sciences. For biological psychiatry to denigrate psychological explanations of psychopathology, prematurely claiming to know that biological explanations are fundamental, has little to commend it—especially since biological psychiatrists wobble back and forth between fragmentary biological discourse and speculative psychological discourse, without any known scheme of translation or rich body of detailed correlations. One can scarcely imagine this contributing to the development of more adequate science.

The Values of Biological Psychiatry

Biological psychiatry has a fairly *laissez-faire* attitude to the kind of psychotherapy used as an adjunct to medication (except for a fairly fierce antipathy to psychoanalysis), so long as medication comes first. We cannot really identify its recommendations about life with one or another form of psychotherapy. Biological psychiatry only insists that biological factors be given fundamental explanatory force and that drugs be seen as necessary to treatment. This insistence on the priority of biology and medication serves the culture's two basic values: to relieve distress and to restore medical privilege over mental health care. It also leads the culture into a confusion of values and a breathtaking hubris. The confusion and hubris, in turn, load the issue of medication with heavy moral and cultural freight that perhaps it should not have to bear.

We do not really know that drugs correct or compensate for biological deficiencies, but we do know that they frequently relieve distress. One frequent justification for biological psychiatry's claim to priority is that drugs give the quickest, most cost-effective relief. Our society is not satisfied with that view, however; it sounds too much like avoiding one's problems through drugs. The biological psychiatrists' view that drugs correct or compensate for deficits provides a more respectable justification. They say that drugs prescribed by psychiatrists differ from others drugs because they help patients toward what is normal. They claim that psychiatric drugs do not help people avoid their problems but remedy or manage problems that cannot be addressed in any other way. With this rationale, biological psychiatrists seem to move drugs out of the category of providing expedient relief into the category of attending to disease. They believe that the moral opprobrium we heap on avoiding problems through drugs does not apply to "properly prescribed" psychiatric drugs.

Here is the Hobson's choice of biological psychiatrists. If they admit that they do not know if drugs are addressing biological disease, they face our society's strong moral opposition. If they rescue drugs from this censure by claiming that they address biological abnormality, they speak falsely and interfere with the fullest possible understanding of distress—including the development of new and more sophisticated sciences. In either case, they make drugs problems as much as blessings in the quest to relieve psychopathology.

Biological psychiatry is confused as to its values. Rather than addressing in a straightforward way the issues raised by drugs, it avoids the fact that it foments a moral revolution more than a metaphysical one. The issue is not whether minds are brains. The issue is how we will understand "normal" life once we recognize that we have (at least some) power to change the material processes that constitute our psychological, social, "human-most" lives.

Biological psychiatry suffers its Hobson's choice and avoids facing its moral revolution because biological understanding of human life threatens (more acutely than talk therapy) to unravel the ambiguity at the foundations of mental health care. Biological psychiatry tries to conform to both sides of an incoherent idea—the Enlightenment ideal at the base of mental health care. We saw in chapter two that mental health care got its start, in part, from the Enlightenment notion that psychopathology amounts to deficits relative to one's "true nature." This ideal was profoundly incoherent, though, combining the transcendent philosophical and religious ideals of Western culture with a move toward nature as the locus of reality and source of truth. "Nature," in the Enlightenment notions, occupied a nebulous realm somewhere beyond how the natural world actually works but below the theological empyrean of transcendent ideals. The Enlightenment ideal wobbled between "nature" as "how we are supposed to be" and "nature" as "how the natural world works." These two ideas of nature were conjoined through the supposition that reality embodies the mind of God—the world works according to the ideas that God used in creating it. The laws of nature were the principles by which God intended the world to function, and science was thought to explicate the underlying logic of the world and therefore its "true nature." Isaac Newton's famous exclamation, "I am thinking God's thoughts after him" is a perfect expression of this. The modern ideal of science was thus thought to be consistent with humanity's stewardship over nature.

Biological psychiatry embodies this legacy of Western cultural tradition, claiming to help us toward our "true natures." But the "human nature" over which psychiatrists exercise stewardship is an equivocal concept—subsuming both the laws of nature by which human life functions and the notion that beyond what we *happen* to be is humanity's true and proper nature. Our traditional moral notions have to do mostly with the latter. The aim to explicate human nature and its pathologies through science has to do entirely with the former. Biological psychiatry wobbles between the two. When psychiatrists say that drugs are correcting for deficits, they are saying that they restore us to what we are supposed to be. Yet what we know about drugs has to do only with how they work, not with whether they restore anyone's true nature. In our society, we are uncomfortable with the idea of simply manipulating human nature by science; we want to believe that science should be used in accord with some higher plan. Biological psychiatry threatens to make clear that we can manipulate our lives through the fruits of science, without conforming to what we are "supposed to be." That idea is too frightening, especially in the realm of our mental life, so psychiatrists use the rhetoric of "correcting deficits" to flee back into the idea of making things what they should be.

As science, biological psychiatry could frankly say, "Whether or not these drugs remedy deficits, they do alter physical states in the following ways," and they could provide scientific explications of just what happens with drugs. Current drugs may not remedy any deficits in essential human functions (or perhaps they do, though we do not know it yet), but they make life much better. For a society still shaped by Western theology and Enlightenment ambiguity, that is not acceptable. "Better" seems to be unacceptably hedonistic, unless it is tied to some sort of transcendent ideal. By claiming to redress abnormality, biological psychiatry tries to dodge the issue, staying within the idea that human nature is supposed to be a certain way and disease is some deficit relative to that ideal. This lets it claim the moral legitimacy that our society has been loath to give to drug use. Properly prescribed psychiatric drugs just help us to be as we should; they help us fulfill our true nature.

The talk therapies can remain within the incoherent Enlightenment compromise more easily than biological psychiatry because they resemble, at least in form, moral and spiritual growth—growth toward one's true nature, toward what one is supposed to be. People have to "work through" their problems, facing unpleasant facts about themselves, getting themselves in line with reality and "health." In biological psychiatry, nothing resembling moral effort is required; the agent of change is a chemical. To remain within the Enlightenment compromise, biological psychiatrists have to say, in effect, that the drug merely brings one back to one's nature—in effect, to the transcendent ideal embodied in the laws of human nature. The price biological psychiatry pays to be acceptable in our society is an ideology that it is faithful to the Enlightenment idea that science discovers and serves the purposes of nature.

If we drop the idea that reality embodies the coherent principles by which creation came into being, and if we drop the idea that the principles that operate in human nature amount to a transcendent ideal to which we ought to aspire, we are faced with the prospect that human nature may include all sorts of problematic features—and that we can, if we wish, modify our natures. Psychoactive drugs give concrete reality to this consequence of our society's historical and technological development. Perhaps many of the problems that patients bring for treatment are not deficits relative to an ideal of human nature, but drugs help with them anyway.

To try to avoid the frightening possibility that nature cannot tell us what drugs should be used for, psychiatry and related life sciences frequently invoke evolution as the ideological basis for human design. Evolution, not God, designed us, and we need to conform to what evolution has made of us. In this way, it is thought, nature can still tell us what to do, including what to use drugs for. But invoking evolution actually increases the ambiguity of drugs and human nature rather than resolving it. Evolution is a doctrine of chance and "good enough" fit, requiring only that chance and natural selection cobble us together well enough that we survive and reproduce. Consider that many human problems seem to be by-products of evolution—the musculoskeletal problems that result from walking upright, for instance. Others are immune to the forces of natural selection—the problems of aging, for instance, that do not impede our capacity to reproduce and bring our offspring to the age at which they can take care of themselves. Is there any reason why at least some of our psychological problems might not be similar—the result, perhaps, of grafting our extraordinary cognitive capacities onto more primitive perceptual, emotional, and behavioral systems?[109]

Conceivably, psychoactive drugs do not compensate for deficiencies relative to what is normal but relieve distress that is a

---

[109] A debate among theorists and scholars of evolution concerns whether evolution guarantees "optimality," that is, whether the forms that successful species take is optimal for themselves in their environments. I am inclined against the idea that optimality is specific enough to be of much use in practical assessments (as in mental health care), for reasons beyond the scope of this book. Readers may consult *The Latest on the Best: Essays on Evolution and Optimality* (1987), edited by John Dupre, for this debate.

fairly inevitable result of normalcy (or to which the question of normalcy is quite irrelevant). The fact that the first medically acceptable psychoactive drugs addressed the problems of mental health patients may be an historical accident: Because we had mental health institutions in place, and because they already possessed a rationale that made drugs legitimate, drugs that alter psychopathology were given a place in these social institutions. Psychoactive drugs that have no special efficacy for psychopathology fall outside the socially legitimate institutions we happen to have. The rationale we use for medically accepted psychoactive drugs may be a fiction, however. Consider this prediction from Richard Restak:

> . . . the most interesting application of the new psychoactive agents may involve chemical attempts to modify character, personality, and habit patterns. Ordinarily these are very resistant to change, but drugs are in development that will help stimulate motivation, increase energy levels, and repair feelings of chronic low self-esteem—in short, make people who are not suffering from a definable mental illness feel better about themselves and the quality of their lives. . . . [T]his may not be a proper use for mind- and brain-altering drugs; we are not always the ideal judges of how best to improve ourselves. But properly and sensibly used, these drugs can help us achieve the goal that many philosophical and psychological systems have suggested is our best strategy for enduring and prevailing in an uncertain world: modifying not the world but our responses to it.[110]

We do not have to wait for the full fruition of drugs "in development" to face this issue. Since we do not know that our current drugs are correcting deficiencies, we already face it. They help us toward something we want.

Does this mean that they "let us avoid facing our problems"? We do not really know. As we have seen throughout this book,

---

[110] Richard Restak, *Receptors* (1994).

the talk therapies have no more scientific claim to our allegiance than biological psychiatry. If we knew that certain problems are due to psychosocial difficulties, and if we knew that they can be "confronted" and "worked out," it would make sense to say (for those problems) that when we use drugs to relieve them, we are avoiding our problems rather than resolving them. We generally do not know this. The issue of when drugs rather than psychosocial regimens more directly address the cause of one's problems cannot be decided scientifically at present.

Who, then, can be the "best judges of how to improve ourselves"—the judges of when drugs rather than some other regimen is the best way toward what we want? Biological psychiatrists already have the answer: They are. In the ideology of biological psychiatry, all patients should first consult a psychiatrist, who will decide whether drugs or psychosocial therapy is appropriate. As Wender and Klein put it:

> We advocate developing new methods of organizing care for those afflicted with mental disorders. The properly trained psychiatrist, we believe, is the best person to *evaluate* whether the troubled patient is suffering realistic unhappiness, personality limitations, or a psychiatric illness with a major organic component. . . ."

A few paragraphs later, they say, ". . . both evaluation and prescription absolutely require the services of a properly trained psychiatrist," and they repeat their call for reorganizing mental health care to give psychiatrists this hegemony.[111] (They emphasize in several places that "properly trained" means trained in biological psychiatry. Only those who have joined their particular culture are even considered competent psychiatrists.) Apparently, their views have not changed since 1981; their 1993 book, *Understanding Depression*, contains similar advice.

As we have seen, though, biological psychiatrists have no methods for ascertaining when to use drugs, other than their cul-

---

111 Paul H. Wender and Donald F. Klein, *Mind, Mood, and Medicine* (1981).

ture's habitual ways of interpreting behavioral and psychological signs. Their distinctions between biologically based problems and other problems are the lore of their culture, not the results of scientific discovery. We would be extremely naive to accept their claim to priority in deciding these issues without remembering two things: the medical profession's long and unlovely history of finding "appropriate" patients everywhere for the latest "next great cure" and its unflagging efforts throughout the century to prevent other mental health professions from encroaching on its market and social position. The belief of biological psychiatrists that they should decide who needs what kind of treatment has less to do with science than with the capacity of physicians to convince themselves of the prepotent importance of their preferred explanations and their wish to regain and solidify the social authority of psychiatry over other forms of mental health care.

Talk therapists are often reluctant to refer patients to psychiatrists, because they know that the patient is likely to receive some measure of indoctrination into the culture of biological psychiatry, which will undermine both the legitimacy and the effectiveness of their own form of therapy. This is not paranoia on the part of nonmedical therapists; Wender and Klein say (specifically in reference to treatment for depression):

> When psychotherapists refer patients for what they term "supportive" medication, a further problem arises because of the conflict over which of the therapists should be in charge of the treatment. We believe that the administrator of medication should have precedence . . . The patient who has been receiving psychotherapy usually has to go through a process of "unlearning" about the causes of his depression. The psychotherapist may have been emphasizing factors that are less relevant or even inaccurate.[112]

Medication, then, carries all the freight of the history and the current antagonism and rivalry among the mental health professions.

---

[112] Paul H. Wender and Donald F. Klein, *Understanding Depression* (1993).

We know, by this point, to be cautious about believing that a way of thinking that gives comfort, an appearance of reasonableness, and economic and social power to a particular culture of healing is true simply because the members of that culture assure us of their scientific integrity and benevolent intent. We also know that the biological psychiatrist's claims go far beyond anything known to be true. We see, as well, that the values of biological psychiatry are a reflection of Western culture's larger outlines and the professional self-image and ambitions of psychiatry. The upshot would seem to be that medication for psychopathology is a matter for society, not the mental health professions alone, to decide. The issues are pragmatic and moral as much as scientific, and none of the mental health professions are in a position to give advice uncolored by their professional interests.

Medication, Life, and Psychopathology

Psychoactive medications do not have to address biological abnormalities to be of use in mental health care. Where they do address biological illnesses, these need not be chronic or constitutional. We can easily conceive of persons whose inner turmoil, arising from psychological or social pressures or conflicts, is so debilitating that biochemical intervention is necessary if they are ever to find the resources to address their problems. We can easily conceive of psychosocial disorders that result in biological abnormalities, and we can conceive of medication that can ameliorate those abnormalities—even as the deeper psychosocial causes are being addressed by psychologically oriented therapy. Conceivably, some of the physiological processes that psychoactive drugs address could even be the consequences of the disruptions in biology that Freud predicted would be found to result from sexual and aggressive neuroses. We need not believe there has been a biological revolution in psychiatry or buy into the culture of biological psychiatry to value psychoactive medications— and to think carefully and responsibly about when to use them. When biological psychiatry loads onto medication its overweening ideology, it impedes our ability to do this.

Fortunately, many psychiatrists who do not accept the premises of biological psychiatry have incorporated medication into their treatment programs, and many of them willingly serve as medical consultants to nonpsychiatric therapists whose patients need drugs. For as long as the medical profession maintains its legal monopoly over the right to prescribe drugs (a monopoly they are not likely willingly to give up, since it is the only treatment—other than hospitalization—they can prescribe that other mental health professionals cannot), such consultants will be crucial to the work of all therapists. For as long as there is room within psychiatry for such practitioners, the imperial inclinations of biological psychiatrists and the defensiveness of nonmedical psychotherapists will be blunted. Still, society and patients—and mental health professionals in training—are presented with too much propaganda, colored too deeply by the vested interests of the competing professions, on the issue of medication.

As a society, we need to learn to think responsibly about psychoactive medications both in the treatment of psychopathology *and in other contexts*—for psychoactive medications may be useful even when no psychopathology is present. We can conceive of persons whose circumstances in life are sufficiently demanding and filled with conflict that psychoactive medications would be crucial to their meeting their obligations successfully, even if they suffer neither biological nor psychological abnormalities. Unless we have some adolescent illusion that life cannot be so filled with conflict that healthy, responsible persons must endure significant pain, we must acknowledge this possibility. We need to be able to think more clearly about when and how the use of psychoactive drugs may be morally justified for such people.

Similarly, we can legitimately hope that neurobiology will give us a more sophisticated understanding of the varieties of biological normality. Though this issue scares us—it is too easily taken hostage by racist, sexist, and other oppressive interests—we do need to understand better the various biological strains (as in strains of fruit flies or viruses) of humanity. Psychologists and others have begun to realize what mothers (and anyone else paying attention) have always known, that persons come with innate temperaments and proclivities. Some temperaments or proclivities may need biochemical help to meet the demands of life—or perhaps we would be wiser to take such discoveries as clues to how life in our society should be reorganized. To take a noninflammatory example, some people's circadian rhythms work on a twenty-five-hour cycle. What are the implications of this for people living in a society that works on a twenty-four-hour clock? Why not allow such people biochemical help in adjusting to life? Or would we prefer to reorganize society on flextime? Good neurobiology may help us think more wisely about many social issues and many issues of what individualism really means—unless it is commandeered by biological psychiatry for its own purposes.

The ideology of biological psychiatry has probably been necessary to establish the legitimacy of drugs, given Western culture's belief that life, following the principles by which God created nature, can be relatively coherent and free of unmanageable psychic pain. That belief led to the notion that using drugs rather than getting one's life in order represents some failure to live an appropriate life. Biological psychiatry has been shaped by the need to justify drugs against such notions. We can, if we wish, perpetuate such illusions and confusions (along with the ideology of biological psychiatry) to justify drug use. Or we can detach the issue of medication from such ideas and learn to think clearly and responsibly about when and why to alter life biochemically.

Chapter Seven

ANCILLARY MINDS:
From Authority to Resource

❋

HUMAN TROUBLES DO NOT YIELD EASILY TO
"CANNIBALS AND MISSIONARIES" TREATMENT.
BUT USUALLY THEY CANNOT BE PUT ASIDE UNTIL
THEY DO, THE WAY PROBLEMS IN SCIENCE CAN
BE, IN EXPECTATION THAT ONE DAY WE WILL
DO BETTER WITH THEM. THEY ARE USUALLY
ON OUR BACKS; WE CAN NEITHER SOLVE THEM
NOR WILL THEY GO AWAY. THEY ARE SIMPLY
PREDICAMENTS.

—*Jerome Bruner*
In Search of Mind

✻ SOME PERSONS ARE DERANGED, so clearly suffering the loss of basic faculties that we consider them insane. The mental health professions began by assuming custody of their care. Urbanization, industrialization, immigration, and other forces of modernization created new disruptions and problems that (along with almost anything else individuals wanted help with) were given over to the mental health professions for amelioration. The Enlightenment ideal, Protestant theology, and the emerging sciences of the nineteenth century provided a rationale for expanding the attentions of mental health professionals to care for the troubled sane: Human nature is rational, free, and progressive; certain problems reflect deficits relative to this ideal; each individual can move toward this perfection, with the help of science.

In effect our society created institutions called mental health professions and gave them custody over a heterogeneous assortment of difficulties. Because of the scientific tenor of the times, the charge to these professions was to deal with those problems scientifically.

The social mission of mental health care is not the only thing that has shaped it. Professions necessarily serve the needs of their own members, as well as their clients. Expanding one's market, securing one's image as uniquely qualified to address the needs of that market, acquiring respect in society, assuring oneself of one's competence, assuaging one's anxieties about one's tasks, and finding in one's work sufficient meaning to keep at it through its difficulties—these altogether human needs apply to mental health professions, as to any other. For the mental health professions, the humanitarian and scientific imperatives they serve set conditions on how they would go about meeting these needs for themselves. As the market expanded, new problems that came within their purview had to be interpreted as failures of essential human traits, which should be restored through the caring application of scientific knowledge. Legitimacy, respect, competence, security, and meaning all depended on cultivating an image of scientific knowledge in service to humanitarian ends.

We have shown that none of the major cultures of healing can claim scientific validity for most of what they teach patients. In each case, some plausible set of ideas or practices gives a culture a place in mental health care. As it secures its place, institutionalizing its beliefs and practices in training institutions and in the market, the original rationale fragments, dissolves, and gives way. New efforts arise within the basic cultural assumptions. The existence of the institutions, more than the power of the new ideas, keeps the culture going. Cultures of healing, like bureaucracies and social customs, are self-perpetuating.

Creating institutions to deal with problems seems obviously legitimate. The *hope* for a science of psychopathology—and for therapies based on such science—seems equally legitimate. Where we have gotten ourselves in trouble is pretending that we have science that we do not have. We have conflated two very different tasks: helping individuals with demonstrable problems, and developing a science of psychopathology and deriving therapies from it. This has led to mistaken assessments of what goes on in the helping process and how much we have accomplished scientifically.

We have probably also conflated many types of suffering under the metaphor of mental illness. The insane clearly suffer radical deficits relative to ordinary human capacities. We do not need science to tell us that; insanity was a folk term, a matter of commonplace observation, long before the mental health professions came into being. As care for additional problems has come under the aegis of the mental health professions, those problems have been interpreted as if they, too, were such deficits. Some of the problems of the troubled sane probably do reflect impairment in basic human functions, but many probably do not. We do not know very well which are which.

For all of that, the evidence seems fairly conclusive that mental health care helps. We do not possess a clear understanding of what that means, for we possess no widely agreed-upon concept of health or ways to measure improvement.

How Helpers Help

We face a complicated, confused situation. If we are to have a more accurate image of mental health care—and thus more wisely crafted attitudes toward it—we need to try to sort it out.

Perhaps we should start with what seems the most credible account of how the diverse cultures of healing manage to deliver relief. In *Persuasion and Healing*, perhaps the most enduring and influential work on the subject of how psychotherapy works, Jerome Frank says, "In our present state of ignorance the most reasonable assumption . . . is that all enduring forms of psychotherapy must do some good or they would disappear. While different therapies may have different effects on different problems, it is likely that the similarity of improvement rates across the board reflects features that are common to them all." In his view, the common features center on restoring hope, which itself involves (among other things) providing a system of beliefs that makes sense of the symptoms and treatment and implies a set of activities that the patient and therapist believe will redress the problems. The relationship between patient and therapist seems to Frank (as to many others) to be central. Frank says, "Indeed, to the extent that persons seeking psychotherapy are demoralized, they may respond to anyone with a modicum of human warmth, common sense, some sensitivity and a desire to help." As he points out, "No one type of training or background seems to foster therapeutic ethos more effectively than any other. Among those who have had professional training, moreover, psychiatrists, psychologists, and social workers seem to do equally well."[113]

What makes each culture of healing effective probably involves a number of elements. One may be its plausible, articulate

---

[113] Jerome D. Frank and Julia B. Frank, *Persuasion and Healing*, 3d ed. (1991). The earlier editions that established this view were the work of Jerome D. Frank alone.

rationale, which allows patients to conceptualize and address their problems. Psychoanalysis, behaviorism, and cognitive therapy certainly fulfill this requirement—or did, when they first arose. Even medication may work partly because the patient has been given an explanation of how and why it will relieve his problems. (This is probably true even in "double blind" studies. Test subjects generally know what kind of test they have become part of—a depression or anxiety medication test, for instance. Something we all know but that receives little overt recognition is the fact that test subjects and their physicians generally figure out quickly whether they are on the medication or the placebo. Psychoactive medications have side effects, and patients—and the physicians examining them—know whether patients are having them or not.) Another element involved in effectiveness is the basic human comfort we all take in an attentive, warm, supportive person who obviously wants to help. A third is the confidence we have in the abilities of an authoritative helper—an issue we address later in the chapter.

Perhaps the crucial issue is whether a particular therapist and patient "match." The patient needs to find in the therapist someone who manifestly understands him. He must find the therapist credible and worthy of respect, by his own lights. The rationale and plan of action that the treatment presents and embodies must be congruent with the patient's life and its problems, and with his talents, habits, and proclivities. Similarly, the therapist probably has to find in the patient someone worth helping, by her lights. The patient's temperament, habits of mind, values, and commitments probably have to be reasonably congruent with elements of herself that the therapist has worked out reasonably well. Therapists differ in the range of patients they have the flexibility, knowledge, and intelligence to understand, and "congruence" can be at a fairly general level, but it seems a safe bet that the therapist must be able to understand the particulars of the patient's reality. That will partly be a function of the therapist's own sense of reality.

Patients and therapists tend to sort themselves out so that they match. A therapist tends to develop a distinctive "voice," a repertoire of ways of analyzing, listening, addressing patients, and offering advice (directly or indirectly). Even biological psychiatrists do this. They develop their own respective ideas about what kinds of problems and characteristics are signs of each kind of biological process. They tend to become most familiar with certain drugs and to rely on them. We know that a particular patient may find little relief from one kind of therapy—even the kind that is "supposed" to help with his particular problems—while another works very well for him. We know that particular patients may find a modicum of help from one (or two or half a dozen) therapists, then find someone with whom the therapy succeeds spectacularly. We also know that a therapist's practice (or the practice of a particular group or clinic) develops through word of mouth, so that (presumably) persons who have found themselves well matched send their friends—who are presumably persons roughly similar to themselves. We can reasonably conjecture that therapists tend to find the patients to whom their voices speak. That makes for effective practices for individual therapists—and effective cultures, insofar as those repertoire influence how like-minded therapists practice.

That is all well and good, but notice: The rationale embodied in a culture of healing or a particular treatment does not have to be scientific to be effective. On reflection, this seems obvious: Even the most scientific cultures vastly exceed scientific knowledge. More important, a substantial number of cultures do not even purport to base themselves on science, but they manage to keep themselves in business and seem to help people.[114] What seems to matter is that the rationale be plausible, that it make sense of both the problems and the treatment, and that it give the patient a new set of thoughts and actions to address his problems. We might want to say that it has to be true, but we do not have much evidence for that and much reason to believe it is mistaken. Plenty of patients have been helped by therapies whose basic ideas have turned out to be wrong. Indeed, I

---

[114] The recent best sellers by Thomas Moore, *Care of the Soul* and *Soul Mates*, are good examples of a culture that is anything but scientific.

imagine that every therapist can identify a substantial number of patients she has helped on the basis of ideas she later realized were mistaken.[115] Truth, for good or ill, is probably not a therapeutic imperative.

At first blush, this is a profoundly disturbing conclusion. Perhaps, though, it disturbs only because of the intellectual pretensions we have built into the professions of healing. Perhaps our idea of expertise was always mistaken. An argument could be made that elitist notions of what constitutes adequate beliefs have infected mental health care. Perhaps belief need not be guided by anything so grand as truth. Perhaps an adequate belief is whatever works, in the judgment of whomever it works for. Perhaps reality is little concerned with the refined tastes of intellectuals and has much patience for figments of the imagination.

Consider the fact that basic human issues are handled in radically different ways in different societies—even in ways that are based on falsehoods. Though we know that most beliefs about the respective characteristics of men and women that justify traditional gender roles are false, a fair number of men and women managed to live fairly meaningful, well-formed lives under their guidance. We no longer countenance many of those practices or beliefs—just as we abhor many sexist practices in many cultures today. That does not change the fact that, as factually mistaken and morally troubling as traditional views were, they worked very well for a great many people, by their lights. We do not have to believe the ideologies and mores of those societies were accurate or right to admit that they worked, so far as many of their adherents were concerned. Conceivably, the

---

[115] Such an experience started me down the road that has led to this book. After finishing my training in psychoanalytic psychotherapy, I read Daniel Stern's *The Interpersonal World of the Infant* (1985), which claims to show (on the basis of serious research) that most psychoanalytic ideas about early development are wrong. I decided to try an experiment: to listen to and interpret my patients *as if* Stern were right and see what happened. I discovered that their symptoms and stories made just as much sense and they continued getting better in about the same way.

cultures of healing may handle psychopathologies on equally mistaken and morally questionable bases, but still work to the satisfaction of many.

This conclusion—that truth is not necessary to help patients feel better—coincides with one dimension of our argument: It calls for giving the mental health professionals *less* autonomy. If the ways helpers define patient's problems and treatment need not be true to be effective, we have all the more reason to insist on social and moral evaluation of the actions entailed. We may have to accommodate changes entailed by genuine discoveries, but we do not have to accept uncritically the impact of therapists' fictions. This conclusion also helps to make sense of the disparity between the scientific image of the cultures of healing and their actual scientific poverty. If truth is not necessary for making people feel better, scientific poverty is no great deficiency. Yet because our image of mental health care has taught us that effectiveness is a function of scientific truth, the cultures of healing have been able to convince themselves that they are fulfilling their mission. They think that people's getting better because of their work supports the truth of their ideas.

We could, if we wished, simply let the matter rest there: Anyone gets to teach and believe anything they want in mental health care, and the only functional criterion of choice is what works—for the persons for whom it works. Certainly this is not the worst possible conclusion, since a great deal of life is like this. To rest here, however, seems rather extreme and unwise. This conclusion is quite at odds with what we have expected our professions of healing to be, and we should adopt it only if there is no way to get from mental health care something more nearly like what we have wanted—namely, knowledge-based practices that let *all* of us (not just patients—customers—of particular practitioners) know how to think about and comport ourselves toward psychopathology. The sufferings of patients are real, and our society's wish to think about (and deal with) such suffering in informed ways is a mark of humanity in our cultural life.

Curiously enough, the way out of this bleak situation is precisely to give greater attention to the social and moral dimensions of mental health care.

The Social Mission of Mental Health Care

We can come to a less disillusioning conclusion by considering two things, both having to do with what we want, as a society, from the mental health professions: first, devotion to truthfulness and second, clear demarcation between mental health and illness, on the one hand, and notions of what constitutes desirable life and undesirable distress, on the other.

In demanding these two things of the mental health professions, we are imposing an issue of social policy upon the therapy process. If mental health care were strictly entrepreneurial, its professionals could say and do whatever individuals were willing to pay them to say and do. For better or worse, the mental health professions made of themselves something other than entrepreneurs when they looked to government for regulation, protection, and funding for training and research institutions, clinics, and hospitals. Mental health care is a social institution, and like all institutions it has made an implicit contract with the society that supports it.

The first quality we can ask of the mental health professions, then, is greater truthfulness. Even though truth is probably not an overriding imperative of therapy, part of the social contract between the mental health professions and society has been that these professions will provide us with accurate knowledge concerning distress and its amelioration. Cultures of healing may claim to have a way of thinking that demonstrably helps people overcome depression, anxiety, and so forth. As a society, we can demand to know whether it is true. If cultures of healing want society to accommodate itself to their ideas and recommendations, we can reasonably ask that they hold themselves to reasonable standards of truth. As a matter of social policy, we can make truth a condition of our support of these professions.

Second, we can specify just what mental health care is supposed to help us *with* and what it is supposed to help us *toward*. The basic concept of mental health care is that some distress results from failures in essential functions of being a person. Mental health care aims to restore (or compensate for) the deficit. We might want to say to the mental health professions, "It is not your job generally to relieve distress. Some distress has causes other than mental illness, and you have not been given license to address these. Your job is to identify essential human functions and their failures and to figure out how to correct them." We can say, "We did not agree to your role in providing a general palliative for the sufferings of individuals. We agreed to your existence because you offered to fulfill a certain task." We can demand that the mental health professions do both more and less than relieve distress. They could identify genuine mental disorders and treat those, and they could stop pretending that everything that offers relief from distress reflects some set of truths about mental illness and health.

What do we do, though, about the fact that the mental health professions do not possess knowledge sufficient to provide bases for practice, and that the cultures of healing have developed to fill in these gaps? What do we do about the fact that we lack sufficient knowledge about what is and is not mental illness to make any hard and fast rules about what mental health professionals can and cannot address? Society and the mental health professions have negotiated a social contract that cannot be fulfilled under present circumstances.

One thing we have to do, in amending our social contract, is to relax the demand for scientific validity. We can hold out a comprehensive science as a goal to which the mental health professions should aspire, but we must accept that in reality they are far from that goal. The way for the mental health professions to become truthful, at present, is to acknowledge exactly where they do and do not have scientific validation for their notions of health, illness, and cure. At least as important, they can clearly identify their beliefs and values and stop claiming they are more than that. The mental health professions should trade on honest communication of the substance of their beliefs, not on a mythical image of scientific authority. They need to become more culturally self-aware (of their beliefs and practices as functions of their cultures) and communicate with society on that basis.

We can also expect the mental health professions to make an assiduous effort to define health and illness accurately, and to distinguish between pathological distress and distress from other sources—however troubling it may be. But for most problems of most patients, we should not expect any clear knowledge of what is ill and what is healthy—nor should mental health professionals claim to know these things. Perhaps most important, patients should not invoke the authority of therapy to demand changes from others around them, nor should mental health professionals write books or give interviews telling people that mental health requires this or that change in how we live. We generally have a very different obligation to persons we are making ill than to persons with whom we are in conflict. The authority of mental health care should not be used to impose upon society or one's intimates an illusory obligation of "eliminating conditions that support pathology or impede health" where the problems of patients are not known to be matters of mental illness. We can easily conceive that for some persons, circumstance and social expectations clash with native (and altogether healthy) proclivities. Such distress needs to be addressed, but the patient should not be seen as ill—and working out such problems should not carry the connotation of "necessary for restoration of health" for those with whom he is in conflict. Similarly, we can easily conceive that a person's internal conflicts, cognitive confusions, and deficiencies of internal organization may cause turmoil so painful that they need help to resolve them. Yet conflicts, turmoil, and disorganization all can, more or less by definition, be resolved in a variety of directions—no one of which has much claim to be the "healthy" way to do it. We generally are not obliged to support the particularities of someone's solution to a personal quandary, even if we are obliged to allow that person to find *some* way out of her turmoil.

I am not recommending that we establish some government body to evaluate the truth of the claims of mental health professionals or release reports on their values and cultural characteristics. We can evaluate the mental health professions ourselves. We do not, after all, license historians, art critics, social commentators, advice columnists, and the like. We do not even license ministers and teachers (except those who want to teach in public schools, which probably ensures that public schools do not hire a great many able teachers), though presumably our souls and our

minds are fairly important. Nor do we need government evaluators to tell us who to listen to in mental health care. A social
mission for a profession does not entail government control.[116]
Rather, it entails a mutual responsibility between society and
those who execute tasks on its behalf. The responsibility of persons outside the mental health professions is to think carefully
about the claims made by those within them. The responsibilities
of those within the professions include making themselves open
to such scrutiny, not setting themselves apart and claiming special
knowledge that they do not, in fact, possess.

The point is that we cannot leave mental health care to "the
experts." Therapy can make people feel better without aspiring
to truth or to wisdom about the effects of its recommendations
on our social life. If we want the experts to do more than pronounce their opinions, we have to demand that they provide us
with good reasons for their opinions—and we need to participate
in shaping their opinions. If we want them to be socially responsible for the effects of their influence, we have to enter into
conversation with them about those effects. Certainly a person in
distress cannot take time to sit back and read up on all the varieties of mental health care available, passing judgment on each in
relation to her problems. We can, though, as a society subject the
claims of mental health care experts to rigorous scrutiny and
come to possess—about mental health professionals as about cars,
business establishments, and religious organizations—a general
body of knowledge and opinion.

---

[116] The issue of licensure is a complicated one, and many of the issues involved are beyond the
scope of this book. The biggest problem with licensure, I think, is that it creates the illusion that
there exists some body of objective knowledge that gives some people special competence. The
corollary illusion is that persons who have not done what is necessary to become licensed are
in some significant way lacking in competence. There is really no evidence for any of this.
Licensure serves mainly to give certain cultures government protection, I think. It is the professionals, not the public, that derives the greatest benefit from licensure. Robyn M. Dawes has
argued against most licensure, in *House of Cards* (1994). His arguments make sense but, lacking
in historical and sociological perspective, he fails to deal with the social policy ramifications of
what he recommends. Because the matter involves issues beyond the scope of this book, I do
not take any set position on the issue here.

■ ■ ■

Science, Other Disciplines, and Society

If we want our mental health professions to aim at truth, we have to consider what to do about the fact that in mental health care, as in life generally, we need beliefs on matters that the sciences that study mental illness and health have yet to illuminate. There are two sides to this: what we want mental health professionals themselves to do about it and what people in general should do as they bring the ideas of the mental health professions under scrutiny.

To start with, we need to look to a wider range of sciences for guidance on mental health issues. This, of course, presupposes that science is important. A fair number of people might think, to the contrary, that we should completely drop the value that we place on science. If science cannot give us what we need at present, should science continue to be given a principal place in what we expect of the mental health professions? Certainly the image of science as truth has lost some of its luster in recent decades. Anti-science therapists are not hard to find—though there is something quite paradoxical, and perhaps dishonest, about being anti-science while occupying positions of social power that depend on our society's belief that therapy is scientific. (This includes holding licenses, commanding authority, and collecting insurance payments that depend on the assumption of scientific legitimacy.) The use of science to develop weapons of war and the corruption of our natural environment through the fruits of science have been two major incentives for chastening our earlier worship of science. We have also undergone consciousness raising about ways that the sciences have been infected with many kinds of cultural bias—in the sorts of problems they have addressed and the hypotheses they have been willing to entertain, for instance. A variety of exposés and scholarly studies have shown how the politics of established science (as well as the egos and jealousies of scientists) influence what kind of research gets funded and published. Though it seems to me that the tide is shifting from disillusionment with science toward a less naive appreciation of its importance, sentiment against science is still significant. It seems to me profoundly unwise and illogical, nonetheless, to denigrate the central place of the sciences in dealing with the problems of life, including the excruciating problems that patients bring to therapists.

Modern science is fundamentally a social endeavor: an attempt to replace the idiosyncrasies of individual researchers with collaborative efforts of multiple researchers, who may not know each other personally, which are verifiable no matter which person happens to be doing the research. In the effort of modern science to surmount subjectivity and considerations of authority or status, there lies a deep belief that truth is fundamentally democratic. Thus, the institutions of peer review and the demand for replicability of findings are essential features of modern science. What counts is that the community of researchers adhere to common standards of investigation and that findings that conform to those standards are heard and considered. This august ideal operates in contravention of ordinary human loyalties, jealousies, self-seeking, and willfulness.

Like the system of checks and balances in American government, the methods of science have been (and continue to be) formulated with a recognition of the corruption to which human enterprises are prey. That science itself is prey to bias and willfulness should be no more surprising than the fact that American government suffers corruption. That science is not impeccable in reaching its ideals is no more reason to reject it than problems in democracy are good reason to revert to dictatorships. When we become disillusioned at the limitations of science itself, we need to remember that those limitations stem from precisely the all-too-human characteristics that science aims to fight against. Getting rid of science does not decrease those characteristics; it simply lets them function unencumbered by scientific discipline. Insofar as the quality of our lives depends upon the quality of our knowledge, that seems to me a dangerous thing.[117]

---

[117] I thought it best to forgo a disquisition on the esoteric debates in philosophy of science. My own view, after two decades of keeping up with such debates, is that C.S. Peirce came about as close as anyone to getting it right. I do not know of any better single essay, readable by most anyone, than his "The Fixation of Belief" (1877). This widely anthologized essay may be found in *Philosophical Writings of Peirce*, edited by Justus Buchler (1955), among other places.

In my estimation, current training programs and professional requirements demand far too little scientific knowledge of therapists. Only psychologists and psychiatrists have to learn science at all, and their requirements are fairly narrowly limited. I cannot imagine undertaking to estimate what is healthy and what is sick, for instance, without significant knowledge of anthropology and the evolutionary disciplines. Nor can I imagine discerning which suffering is a matter of something wrong within the individual without substantial knowledge of social psychology and sociology. Consider, for instance, the fact that for over a century mental health professionals have been diagnosing and prescribing healthy versus unhealthy sexual and mating patterns; they have even used their ideas on such matters as crucial categories in research. As data and data-based theory have begun to emerge from sciences outside clinical psychology and psychiatry— anthropology, sociology, and evolutionary disciplines—they do not square very well with much that mental health professionals even today see as "normal" or as signs of mental disorder.[118] Consider, furthermore, the solipsistic constriction of attention, in the mental health sciences, to the individual. Even the most scientific of clinical psychologists or psychiatrists is trained to understand the person's problems in terms of her individual traits, and science within the clinical disciplines is done in such terms. Yet other sciences have shown that distress can be explicated in terms of a person's social milieu. Clinicians do not, simply by virtue of their training in the sciences of clinical care, have expertise in understanding how social dynamics cause distress. Thus, individuals are taught to interpret their distress in terms of their personal characteristics, even when a non-clinical

---

[118] See, for instance, Helen Fisher, *The Anatomy of Love* (1993), and David M. Buss, *The Evolution of Desire* (1992). Special notice should be taken that what is natural is not necessarily morally desirable, but what is morally undesirable is not a mark of mental illness. When the sciences show that some unsavory characteristic is part of our natural equipment, we may still want to proscribe it. We should not, though, take its occurrence as anything other than an expression of something natural to humans. Mental illness, it would seem, involves failures of essential human traits. Thus, traits that are part of the ordinary genetic make-up of our species should not be seen as signs of psychopathology, even when they are traits we work hard to minimize in society.

■ ■ ■

scientist could easily offer at least as strong an explanation of the problem without seeing the individual as a salient variable.[119]

We also need to look beyond the sciences to the humanistic disciplines, for these provide both important information and important methods of disciplining belief. We endanger our ability to have sound belief by confining ourselves within what is thought—or even genuinely known—within the sciences at present. Actually, this is not dangerous so much as impossible: So much of what we need ideas about has yet to yield to scientific inquiry that we cannot avoid holding all sorts of beliefs that are beyond the current reach of scientific validity. What is dangerous is failing to recognize that we are going beyond science. For when we delude ourselves that our ideas are scientifically valid, they escape discipline by other forms of scrutiny. The genuine danger of valuing science is that it can lead us to devalue other ways of disciplining our thinking and perpetuate our delusion that we know more than we do.

The sciences are not necessarily the best source of true ideas. The sciences are not the best way to come up with true ideas so much as they are *in principle* the best way to avoid falsehood. A true idea is true, whether or not we have ascertained that (scientifically or otherwise), and true ideas can come from anywhere. Most ideas have to be thought of before they can be tested, so even scientists come up with all sorts of true ideas prior to tests. The problem is that we have to figure out which of our ideas are true and which are false, and science seems the best way to make this assessment. That does not mean it is the only way, or even that *at present* the sciences are the best way in all areas. We do

---

[119] The therapy encounter itself constitutes a social setting with its own social dynamics. As we have seen, the patient is enculturated to see herself in terms of the therapist's culture. I believe that much of what happens in the therapy room should be understood in terms of the social dynamics of the encounter, not in the terms that therapists use to understand it. Becoming a patient induces an immense variety of strange experiences, which the patient is taught to interpret in consonance with the culture of the therapist. Perhaps in many cases what is going on has less to do with anything true of the patient and more to do with a therapist (like an evangelist at a revival) both inducing an experience and providing a way to interpret it.

not yet have the methods or basic science to approach many areas or questions of life, but we do have many other forms of sophisticated intellectual discipline to approach many of those issues. We expect far too little broader humane knowledge of mental health professionals. Social and historical provinciality, for instance, would seem to be serious impediments to understanding many basic issues of what is normal and what is sick. We do not expect mental health care professionals to know enough of history or other cultures to be able to distinguish fashions of our time from essential human traits, conflicts of our place from disturbance in normal life. Intelligent philosophic interrogation of ethical, religious, and social interests of persons would seem a fairly important element of understanding issues of health and illness. We do not find the institutions of mental health care encouraging great sophistication about these issues.

Before the effort to understand life became the work of a motley assortment of narrowly focused, fractious, competing academic professions, there were intellectuals who thought they needed to understand the best that had been thought and said—across the board. Insofar as providing mental health care depends upon the quality of the therapist's beliefs, therapists need to be such old-style intellectuals. That, it seems to me, is the best way both to marshal the resources of many sciences and to discipline our beliefs on matters of importance that have yet to yield to scientific inquiry—and the best way to escape the blinders of current science and recognize the limitations of our current knowledge. In the best of all possible worlds, our mental health professions would probably not be divided along the lines they are now. All mental health professionals would study roughly the same body of information, even though they would come at it from different perspectives and derive from it different views.

The need for a more general intellectualism in mental health care seems profound; this is one of two major reasons why the substantive beliefs of the mental health care professions need to be opened to social and cultural criticism. Obviously, no one person can encompass everything that needs to be known—"the best that has been thought or said" now exceeds the grasp of individuals. What we can reasonably hope, though, is that our beliefs about mental health and illness might become the products of a conversation among many disciplines (and among interdisciplinary and nonacademic thinkers). As we renegotiate the social contract between society and the mental health disciplines, we can insist that the latter end their insular pretense of delivering singular truths and make such a conversation integral to their training and professional discourse. Ideally, mental health care should not be the province of any of the current disciplines that claim to deliver truths about it. Mental health care needs to be much more interdisciplinary and informed by a much broader range of influences than it currently is.

Mental health care should be open to this wider influence not only for intellectual but for moral reasons. Its influence on how people live should, like any recommendation for living, be subject to evaluation by those whose lives it touches. Individuals can, of course, hire whomever they want to give them whatever guidance they want in working out their lives, whatever the moral acuity of those helpers may be. As a social institution, mental health care has to be shaped by concerns beyond the pleasure of those who hire therapists—or the therapists who hire themselves out. When mental health care professionals claim to have discovered impediments to mental health, they need to be taken seriously—as are nutritionists who discover deleterious consequences of our eating habits or bacteriologists who discover deficits in public hygiene. Since so little of what mental health professionals say amounts to conclusive science, though, evaluating such claims calls for more circumspect thinking by a wider range of thinkers. What historians or philosophers think about mosquitos and malaria, for instance, is fairly irrelevant—the facts are the facts. Whether social customs, such as suppressing anger toward (or deferring one's interests in favor of) one's parents or spouse cause psychological deficits is usually a far less scientifically clear issue. As a society, we have a legitimate interest in whether and how such things are taught to patients under the authority of mental health care.

What I am suggesting for the mental health professions, though, goes as well for all of society, insofar as it plays a role in determining the status, beliefs, and practices of mental health care professions. We need a more general intellectualism in society at large—including greater scientific and humanistic learning. We need this intellectualism to be deployed in questions of mental health care. We will not, of course, suddenly (or perhaps ever) become a society of intellectuals. We need a larger number of the bright and able among us, though, to concern themselves with more than the knowledge base of their particular professions. In mental health care, as in politics and social change, we need a substantial body of persons to concern themselves with the welfare of our society. One need not be a politician to be a policy analyst, political activist, or participant in discussions that shape politics. Even so, one need not be a member of a mental health profession to participate in its study and shape.

The institutional arrangements—training and accreditation regulations and the like—could take any of a number of forms. Some existing discipline could transform itself into a more interdisciplinary arena, or new interdisciplinary training programs and credentials could be created. The institutional particulars are not important for the purposes of this book; if such reform were to transpire, we can be sure it would be determined by multifarious sociological and political compromises and enterprises, and there is no point trying to predict what they would produce. The important thing is to realize that the intellectual content of mental health care must come from a much more extensive range of thought than it currently does.

Is there anything, though, about which mental health professionals can claim special expertise? Is there room for any professional privilege for mental health care providers? Perhaps we should assiduously pry apart the intellectual, moral, and pragmatic aspects of the mental health professions and see them as three distinct concerns that intersect in mental health care. Intellectual and moral issues require a broader conversation among many kinds of scientists, other intellectuals, and society at large. Clinicians can claim special expertise only over the pragmatics of helping.

The Clinician as Ancillary Mind

If mental health care were to work as I suggest, the clinician delivering care could be seen as delivering the benefits of the broad conversation that shapes mental health care to distressed individuals. We could think of the clinician (including the physician who helps one decide whether to take medication) as an ancillary mind. This, I think, allows us to understand the legitimacy of clinical care.

Every person—whether his problems are severe and unrelenting, nagging and chronic, acute and transient, or mild and temporary—faces the task of using his mind to try to find solutions. That is a fundamentally legitimate task of humans. The clinician is a resource for persons who have to perform that task within a context of debilitating distress. The legitimacy of clinical care lies in this: The clinician helps the distressed person perform the clearly legitimate task of puzzling out changes intelligently. The clinician is necessary to this task because of the distress and debility under which the patient labors and the substantial level of knowledge needed to deal with her problems. If the patient knew what the therapist knows and could look at her problems without immediate threat to her welfare (and if she could order medications other than alcohol, nicotine, caffeine, sucrose, and the like), she would not need a therapist. Everything the therapist can offer, she could do for herself. But no one can consider her own problems without urgent concern for the ways they affect her own life, and no one but a therapist gets to spend her life trying to learn things relevant to therapy.

Thus, the therapist provides an "expert" outside resource in service to very ordinary human activities of puzzling out one's life and its needs. These ordinary activities take place in extraordinary circumstances; people generally do not seek out professional help unless their problems are severe and debilitating. Nonetheless, the therapist is simply a resource for ordinary activities undertaken in extraordinary circumstances.

Clinicians depend on others to develop special expertise in science, morals, or social concerns, but as ancillary minds they must be able to bring to the patient's aid sophisticated knowledge of such issues. Otherwise, they help patients become foolish, morally inept, or socially obtuse. The unique expertise of the clinician lies in knowing how to be present to persons in pathological (or other severe) distress, to deploy what he has learned from scientists and others in order to understand the patient, and to communicate to the patient the ideas and actions that will address his problems. Each clinician is, as it were, a point at which the conversation constituting our beliefs about mental health crystallizes into a particular perspective. Each treatment of each patient is a dialogue between the clinician, as emissary of the conversation constituting a therapeutic culture, and a specific individual in distress. This dialogue delivers the teachings of the current conversation, as the particular clinician has crystallized it *and* as the characteristics of that patient shape that specific dialogue. In an ideal world, such highly particular dialogues feed back into the larger conversation, through the ways in which they shape the clinician and the ways in which the patient later participates in our social discourse on mental health.

Knowing how to be present to persons in pain, how to distill a workable perspective into something understandable to the patient, how to support and instigate therapeutic change are not minor skills. Bertrand Russell (and many others since) distinguished between "knowing that" and "knowing how." For "knowing that"—what some philosophers call "declarative" knowledge—clinicians have no claim to a privileged knowledge base about mental health and illness. This declarative knowledge (or opinion) needs to be the product of the wider conversation I am recommending. For "knowing how"—sometimes called "procedural knowledge"—clinical training and experience are crucial. This is (and always will be) the distinctive knowledge of mental health professionals. Being an ancillary mind for persons in pathological distress, like riding a bicycle, is an acquired capacity.

Thus, we can understand mental health care as fully legitimate, precisely insofar as it is an institution created by our society to bring the resources of the sciences and other ways of knowing to bear on the completely ordinary human task of puzzling out solutions to one's difficulties, in the peculiar circumstances of debility posed by psychological distress. Bringing these resources to bear in these circumstances calls for the clinical skills—the procedural knowledge—of clinicians.

The Authority and Power of the Mental Health Professions

If the mental health professions do not deserve the authority that they have claimed—the authority of scientific validity—we have to consider what kind of authority they can rightly claim. More important, we need to consider what authority they can be granted. One of the necessary conditions of effective treatment, it seems, is the patient's confidence in the clinician, and part of that confidence comes from the authority that society places with the professions. Further, the authority we place with the professions partially determines their power, over patients and in society. Because the mental health professions shape how people understand themselves, their inherent power is substantial—the power to shape how people (or society) think about how they are and need to be goes to the heart of determining the quality of life. We augment or qualify this power by the authority we place with the mental health professions.

Any limitation we place on the power of the mental health professions is especially important because of this: The mind of a patient is, by definition, impaired, so (insofar as a patient accepts the basic premise of mental health care) the patient can trust his own judgment only to a limited degree. When a person consults a financial advisor, an architect, or an internist, he recognizes that the advisor has greater technical knowledge than he. He does not have to accept, as a premise of the consultation, that his capacity to think clearly is impaired. In mental health care, the patient's admiration or skepticism may be a function of the very impairment for which he seeks help. To the extent that the therapist, in effect, gets to define where the patient's ways of thinking are impaired, she gets to judge where the patient needs to be brought into agreement with her. To the extent that clinical care enjoys great authority, we expect patients to defer to the judgment of the therapist. If we decrease the authority of the therapist too much, we may give the patient too much latitude to evaluate treatment using the impaired capacity that treatment is needed to correct. If we increase the therapist's authority, we encourage the unjustified presumption that the therapist should be acceded to.

As the mental health professions now stand, decreasing their authority radically seems to me rationally necessary. Because the cultures of healing have mistaken their cultural creations for natural facts, they have not generally evaluated those cultural creations in the appropriate manner. In general, acceding to the role of patient is analogous to women or African-Americans acceding to their culturally created roles. While the intentions of the mental health care professions may be less self-serving than the intentions of men and whites, the necessity of most of what patients are told is (for all we now know) probably about the same as the necessity of traditional gender and race roles.

Recognizing this may (and should) decrease the confidence of society and patients in the mental health profession. The confidence of individual patients in their helpers, for now, should be a function of the particular relationships between them, not a function of a general faith in the profession. At present, the only functional criteria for a patient to evaluate a therapist (or a therapist to evaluate herself) are the evident breadth of a particular therapist's learning, care in forming opinions, and intellectual honesty (with herself and the patient); her evident sensitivity to the patient's problems, personality, and circumstances; and her devotion to the welfare of the individual.

Such issues will always be important in determining a patient's faith in an individual therapist, but if the mental health professions reformed themselves along the lines I am suggesting—opening themselves to the social and interdisciplinary conversation I call for—we could eventually have significant faith in the professions *per se*. We would not be able to assume they pronounce the truth, but we could be confident that they do the best that can be done. That, for good or ill, is all we can rightly ask. Even within such reformed mental health professions, authority would be tempered by the professions' need to rely on all those outside the professions who contribute to the conversation constituting the context of care. Unless and until the sciences of psychopathology and mental health give us comprehensive, conclusive, univocal understanding, the authority of the mental health care professions cannot be autonomous.

Diversity of Cultures

The problem with cultures of healing is not that they are cultures. The problem is both that they do not know they are cultures and that they claim to be more than cultures. Implementing what I recommend would not change the fact that much of what would be believed in mental health care would be cultural creations rather than facts about nature. We should therefore not expect only one culture of healing to come into existence. For as long as we are creating culture, we should (unless we appoint a Therapy Czar) expect diversity.[120]

As in political culture, diversity of parties, as it were, is not necessarily a harmful thing. In the reformed world of mental health care I am suggesting, each culture would be a way of precipitating from the conversation constituting that world a coherent, critically careful way of making sense of mental illness and health. Because they would all both result from and be open to widespread scrutiny (and determination by multiple sciences and disciplines), we would know fairly clearly how to regard each. Diversity does not entail provinciality (though our current cultures are highly provincial); each culture would be comprehensive in its considerations but make of them something distinctive. Indeed, there is no reason to desire a single culture of healing; having only one would not be intrinsically sounder, and diversity within a comprehensive conversation should promote development of better viewpoints.

The real problem of diversity would be an excessive number of microcultures, more than public discourse could evaluate. At present, the claim of the cultures to scientific authority impedes

---

[120] Even if the day comes when the basic science about human nature and its pathologies has been completed, there will probably be (in a different sense than we have been concerned with here) different clinical cultures. Human nature is probably so highly general that different cultures will be needed to deliver care in different times and places. The difference between those cultures and current cultures is that they will all be informed by the same general scientific principles.

sound social and cultural criticism, but so does the fact that cultures spring up willy-nilly. So long as that continues, many cultures will influence people without the benefit of wider evaluation and without patients really understanding what they are signing on for.

The magnitude of the current problem is immense, especially because of widespread eclecticism among clinicians. A great many studies have shown that a substantial number of clinicians (some surveys put the number at over fifty percent) identify themselves as eclectic. We can understand why: Each culture of healing is too confining, and as clinicians confront the problems of patients they have to grope around for whatever works. Especially as they gain more experience, clinicians look beyond the confines into which their training enculturated them. While eclectics tend to keep some basic orientation from their original training (an eclectic former psychoanalyst tends to be a very different animal from an eclectic former behaviorist), eclecticism essentially means that the therapist makes up her own version of therapy. A homebrewed regimen, made up while one also conducts a practice, will not be thought through as carefully as one that is shared across a community of professionals. The treatment also will not be subject to the scrutiny of a wider community. We can, as social and cultural critics (or as scientific thinkers), evaluate the general attributes of each major culture of healing. To the extent that therapists maintain fidelity to the culture that spawned them, such an evaluation will apply to their work. It is a safe bet that most eclectic therapists never have their peculiar syntheses subjected to the scrutiny of a wide community of critics.[121]

---

[121] Eclecticism also tends to be an incoherent hodgepodge. Though eclectics frequently say (and seem to have the self-image) that they "take what is best from each school," they rarely say how they picked this best. Since we do not possess any general method of evaluating cultures, it is a safe bet that this claim is false. Eclectics also sometimes say (and seem to have the self-image) that they "do what is best for a particular patient." We do not possess any valid criteria for delineating which patients are best for which forms of treatment, so it is a safe bet that *this* claim is false. Since eclectics rarely give a defensible account of the criteria by which they cobbled together their (in reality) seat-of-the-pants repertoire, and since we know that the cultures of healing hold radically disparate notions of illness, health, and treatment, it seems a safe bet that eclecticism is rarely a considered and coherent whole.

Unfortunately, there is no obvious remedy for either eclecticism or proliferating microcultures at present. Perhaps if we had a diversity of cultures that were comprehensive, not provincial, in their considerations, this would be less of a problem. We cannot really predict that. All we can do is recognize that diversity within a more general conversation is a good thing, whereas the indiscriminate babble of too many voices is not.

Where This Leaves Us

If the argument of this book is accurate, why should anyone now consult a mental health care professional at all? If the cultures of healing are all so many optional ways of looking at life, each of them a biased mélange of scientific fragments, guesses, and wishful thinking, why bother? Why submit oneself to someone else's version of life? The simple answer is this: When a person is in pain and cannot find a way out on his own, he needs help. For good or ill, the mental health professions are our society's principal answer to this sort of pain. They do seem to work. Even though we cannot specify exactly what this means, we know that most people who engage in a course of treatment suffer less afterwards than before.

That a person in chronic or debilitating pain usually needs help from outside herself seems a reasonable assumption: If one's own ways of thinking, feeling, and acting, or one's own physiology, constitute a part of the problem—if one is, in fact, a significant variable in one's own distress—it would seem reasonable to assume that relying solely on one's own devices may perpetuate the problem. One's own devices, after all, are at least part of the source of the problem. The question we face is why mental health professions should be seen as the help of choice for what we have come to call psychopathology. Why join one of these cultures, rather than some other culture—some religion, some alternative way of living, some particular regimen offered by any of the various gurus or reformists?

It would be hard to prove that professional mental health care works *better* than other conceivable ways of coping with or ameliorating debilitating distress.[122] The fact is, though, that except for those from quirky families that "believe in" mental health care, sending everyone to therapy, most people who come under the care of a mental health professional have already tried most everything else they could think of to relieve their pain. Career moves, romantic changes, further education, self-help regimens, exercise routines, new habits, twelve-step programs, religious activities, charitable volunteer work, chewing friends' ears off, stoic diligence, and all sorts of other things precede most people's entry into care. Some of these desperate souls find relief through professional mental health care. It would seem to follow that, at least for some people, therapy works better than those alternative ways of coping.

Our concern in this book, though, has not been the relief care can offer so much as the influence it exerts. A patient can be reasonably confident of finding some measure of relief if she finds a therapist with whom she feels rapport—who makes sense to her and seems to understand her, and whom she can trust and respect. Can a patient be confident that the therapist's ways of understanding her problems are sound? Can the patient be confident in the therapist's notions of illness and health—what needs changing and what does not—and what one is well advised to do? Can a patient be reasonably confident that the influence a therapist exerts will be optimal?

I think it very unwise to take an affirmative answer for granted. Will a person be advised to be "more rational," when perhaps he needs to become more imaginative? Will she be taught to pay more attention to sources of pleasure and pain in her environment, when she needs a deeper sense of her personal history and

---

[122] In general, even the best studies of therapy effectiveness do not test for this. In the best studies, persons who receive care are compared to some sort of control group. However, within the control group, *alternative* ways of improving one's life are not uniform. At best, all of the controls receive some dummy treatment, some sort of placebo. It would probably be impossible to design a control in which all members of the control group undergo conversion to a religion that suits them, find the right mates, get a better work life, or whatever. It is, then, conceivable that one or more of these other ways of improving one's lot might work as well as therapy, for some substantial body of persons, but research to date would not have been able to capture this fact.

personal projects that will make her less bound by immediacy? Will he be brought to exquisite sensitivity to the presence of the past, when he needs to make the present and future more determinative of his sense of worth? Will she be taught that she has a chronically misshapen neurobiology, when she needs to learn assertiveness and hope? Will he be taught to value and respect his feelings, when he needs to control and shape them? Will the opposite of each of these scenarios, instead, take place? I think, as things stand now, each of these is an everyday occurrence. This is not because clinicians are incompetent, but because they see the world through the filters of their own enculturation.

Whether one finds a therapist whose influence is just what one needs is partly a matter of chance and circumstance. The culture of healing a particular therapist or researcher will join also depends on chance and circumstance. What teachers one happens to run across in college, what (because of the peculiarities of one's history) seems attractive when one is applying to graduate school, where one is accepted for training, what seminars or workshops ones happens across at moments one is open to new influences— all these matters of chance and circumstance affect the views a clinician comes to hold. A book one happens across in a book store, that one has never seen reviewed in the journals of one's own culture, may change one's ways of thinking and practicing. Even what gets published, in professional journals or in books, depends significantly on chance: Which journal referee a paper gets sent to (and whether she happens to be in a foul or expansive mood when reviewing it) or whether the editor reviewing a book proposal happens, at that time, to need a book like the one proposed on her list of titles (at least as much because of current fashions in the market as anything else) or has a personal interest in a book like that at that particular time.

The fact that choices of culture (and the formative events within cultures) are at least partly matters of chance and circumstance is, for most people, likely to be rather disturbing. In America, we are especially squeamish about chance, fate, and similar notions. We relish the myth that each of us can be master of our fate, that our public institutions and private beliefs can be shaped by free and deliberate rational choice. We do not like to face the enormous role that the chance influence of others—not just mental health care professionals—plays in shaping our lives. In mental health care, though, chance is really far too clear to hide—the incoherent babble of therapeutic voices makes it so. The fact that persons thinking of seeking help usually feel weak and confused exacerbates their fear of being influenced in the "wrong" direction, for they already feel mastery over their fate to be slipping away. This conflict is all the more poignant because it is partly our illusory faith that we can master our fate, and that mental health care can help us do it, that makes the United States far and away the most therapized country on Earth.

The reality of chance, it seems to me, is inescapable. We have to face the fact that chance exists; the therapist one happens to see will exert an influence, and the influence exerted will not be effective because it is "right." The influence of an effective treatment carries great weight precisely because it makes one feel so much better—even though a substantially different treatment, with a different influence, could also have brought relief. The shape of each clinician's or researcher's career, including spectacular success or even fame (or failure and oblivion), has much to do with chance.

The reality of chance, though, is not a reason to avoid mental health care, as patient, practitioner, or researcher. Chance is pervasive. To avoid mental health care because of it makes as much sense as avoiding dating, choosing a mate, associating with friends, taking a new job, moving to a new city, or buying a new book. That is, it makes no sense at all. To forgo chance influence is to avoid life.

What does make sense is to evaluate one's culture of healing as carefully and assiduously as one evaluates other major influences on one's life. Vesting uncritical faith in care makes as much sense as arranged marriages or going to a particular college solely because of the status it confers. One can do one's life that way. Why, though, would anyone think that was a good idea? Chance and circumstance are inevitable, but within that context we can think carefully and critically and choose wisely—or not. We should think about mental health care as deeply and with as much critical attention as we think about other major determinants of the quality of our lives.

We should not be disheartened that the mental health professions are not so scientific as we would like to think. Cultures of healing, like larger human cultures, work out ways of looking at and acting within life, discharging pressing needs, and letting those who partake of them handle the problems that beset them. Cultures of healing may differ in how they teach their members and the pilgrims who wander through them to think and live— but what human concern is free of such variation? In cultures of healing, we may do better or worse in formulating beliefs and practices, but that is simply how life is. Most of us, most of the time, in most cultures, manage to get on with life well enough— well enough that it beats the alternative. Most practices of most cultures sustain life without the help of special sciences. We should applaud, cherish, and assiduously defend every effort to achieve better knowledge about the problems that beset us. In mental health care, as in life generally, we do the best we can— and the evidence is clear that mental health care does good things. The important thing is to learn how to think as we need to think, to formulate the best ideas, and make the best decisions we can—and to be honest with ourselves about what we know and the choices we make.

IMPLICATIONS FOR CHOOSING
OR CHANGING A THERAPIST

✺

THOUGH THIS BOOK has been about the status of mental health care as a social matter, the issues we have addressed would not arise at all were treatment not a profoundly personal matter. Choosing a therapist—or choosing to leave or change therapists—rightly seems to most people a weighty matter. The therapist will shape how a patient views some significant portion of her life. The influence of therapy on a patient's life can be wide-ranging and fundamental. This book has several messages for individuals who are choosing a therapist or reevaluating their therapy.

In general, the views of mental health professionals are functions of their cultures, not matters of scientific knowledge. This does not mean that such views are not worth listening to—very little of life, after all, is based on scientifically valid ideas. However, it does mean that one should not assume that one's therapist is delivering objective truths.

Since mental health care has labored under a mistaken self-image (that it is scientifically based) and practitioners have been enculturated into particular ideas and practices, one cannot count on a prospective therapist to know the difference between the beliefs and values of his culture and sound knowledge of what is ill, what is healthy, and what procedures are helpful in getting from one to the other.

The recommendations of mental health professionals may be understood as moral and social recommendations—recommendations on how it would be good to be. Unfortunately, the mistaken image of mental health care has allowed the professions to avoid justifying their recommendations in moral and social terms. Thus, they frequently justify as "healthy" what would be more accurately described as "how we think it would be good to be."

There exists no general consensus in the mental health community on most matters of concern to patients. The multitude of schools of care offer a variety of views on almost every issue. Thus, the views the particular therapist to whom one entrusts one's well-being are quite optional; one could just as easily go to some other equally well-trained, reputable therapist who would offer quite a different view of one's problems and possibilities.

Yet the fact is that substantial research indicates that persons who undergo treatment usually benefit from it. Why this should be the case is not clear, but it seems likely that the effectiveness of treatment has to do with the relationship between the patient and therapist, the utility of the therapist's views in helping the patient think about her particular problems, and the value to the patient of having an outside observer "on her side."

The conclusion of this book is that the legitimacy of treatment rests with the mental health professional's role as an "ancillary mind." We all must use our minds to ferret out changes in our lives that resolve our problems. Hiring someone to serve as an assistant in this process is certainly legitimate. None of us can know as much as it is possible to know about resolving our own problems, and none of us can look at our own problems with disinterest. A therapist is someone who brings to the process of changing a person's life resources and perspective that he cannot possess alone.

We can use these central messages to arrive at some guidelines for choosing a therapist and evaluating a particular course of therapy.

First, you—the prospective patient—need to be as clear as possible about what you want help with, what you are happy about in your life, and what your central values and commitments are. You should seek a therapist whose views are consistent with these. If the therapist is to be *your* ancillary mind, she must be able to enter into what you want done in a way that is as consistent as possible with who you are. If you do not take the time and effort to think about these matters, finding the right therapist will be purely and completely a matter of chance.

This is not as difficult as it may seem. Most of us know a great deal about ourselves, even when we are in acute distress. We know, for instance, whether we are generally admiring or critical of our society's dominant ways of life, whether we are religious, whether we believe romantic commitments are important, whether our friends are as important to us as our work, whether we are generally conservative or liberal, whether we value rationality more than emotion, and the like. We know something of the choices we have made in our lives and the values that have guided them.

You should not be reticent to ask a prospective therapist about his views and values. A significant body of research shows that in a successful treatment, the patient's views and values shift in the direction of those of the therapist. It is well within one's rights to ask what one is buying into, and submitting oneself to the care of someone who will not or cannot discuss these matters in a nondefensive, nonauthoritarian way is probably not wise. Furthermore, going into treatment with someone whose views or values are distinctly different from your own is probably not a good idea. For instance, if intellectual pursuits are fundamental moral matters for you, a therapist who devalues these in favor of emotionality may be a bad match. If you are deeply committed to artistic, aesthetic, or other non-ratiocinative ways of apprehending life, you probably should not be in treatment with someone who sees these as frills or trivia or mere entertainments. Nor is it a good idea to go into treatment with someone who has strong views about something that is a source of confusion for you. A person who is in a serious quandary about his religious commitments or the place of religion in his history, for instance, probably should not be in treatment with someone who believes religion is by nature neurotic—or essential to good health, for that matter. He should probably be in treatment with someone who understands the issues and recognizes what conditions would make for a valid resolution in either direction.

A therapist should be able and willing to identify to patients what her values and assumptions are, and she should consider this a professional obligation. A therapist who is unwilling to discuss such matters with a prospective patient (or with a current patient who is questioning the treatment) is arrogating to herself the right to sell the patient a bill of goods.

Ideally, the therapist should know the difference between his own therapeutic values and what is known about mental health. A therapist who mistakes his values for how people are supposed to be is not dangerous if those values match yours, but the likelihood of getting wise advice from such a person is small if they do not.

A therapist certainly has a right to a private life, and many things about the therapist are none of the patient's business. Marital or parental status, sexual orientation, family relations, hobbies, and matters of personal history are certainly not matters about which every prospective patient has a right to ask. Yet a patient has a right to ask about the therapist's general attitudes toward such matters. If a therapist is generally skeptical of marriage or believes that an existing marriage should be preserved, the patient has a right to know this. If the therapist has a view of sexual orientation at odds with the patient's own, the patient has a right to know this. If the therapist believes that people should try to remain part of the communities from which they originated, or believes that such affiliations are usually best gotten past, the patient has a right to know this. A patient does well to think through her central values and obligations and ask where the therapist stands on them. A therapist should be responsive to such requests, while honoring his own right to privacy.

Second, you should not approach a prospective therapist as an authority figure, nor should you enter therapy with a therapist who seems to want to be seen this way. We have seen in this book that what therapists say is usually optional, and therapists say substantially different things. You should not assume that what a prospective therapist says is necessarily true. You should not graciously defer to the putative expertise of your helper. Both patient and therapist need to recognize that the therapist is a helper in the patient's life, and they should have attitudes appropriate to the helping relationship—not attitudes appropriate to the relationship between authority and subject.

While a patient may happen across just the right therapy from someone who is a true believer in her therapeutic ideology, such a therapist will lacking something in intellectual honesty, breadth of knowledge, or ability to live with the truth. No therapist who faces honestly the state of the art can really believe that her views are right. They may be the most reasonable she is capable of, they may work better than others for the sorts of patients she enjoys working with, they may serve her better as a therapist. But she cannot reasonably hold that those views are right and all or most others are wrong. As a patient, what you can reasonably trust is your therapist's intellectual honesty and good judgment. Thus, it is probably wise to avoid therapists who do not recognize the fact that their views are optional.

At the same time, no therapist can work at all without some coherent point of view. Thus, a patient should expect a therapist to have thoughtful, coherent views to which he is not inalterably wedded. The therapist should be open to surprise and to changing views. He should be conversant with other views, even if he does not use them. That is a minimal condition for holding views rationally—unless one knows and can see the merits of alternative views, one can scarcely claim to have arrived at one's own views through a rational process. A patient need not be a genius to discern whether a therapist studies and thinks broadly and deeply, holds considered views, and recognizes the provisional nature of those views.

The therapist should also be able to tell a patient how she was trained and how she has departed from that training—and why. Training colors one's work long after one believes oneself to have departed from it, for it provides the basic categories of care that shape one's journey as a therapist.

The therapist might also be expected to explain how his views reflect his temperament and proclivities. This would seem an essential part of recognizing that one's views are not entirely objective. While a therapist may justifiably decline to discuss such personal matters with a new patient, an ability to do so is probably a good indicator.

Therapists who show a straightforward ability to discuss their basic assumptions and values and how their work was shaped by their training and further study, and who show a willingness to consider a wide variety of views and sources of evidence, are probably fairly reliable people to put one's trust in.

Reasonably self-aware therapists know that they are not good for all patients who walk through the door. They know what matters to them and what they are adept at helping people toward. If you meet such a therapist and her values seem reasonably consistent with your own, and if you find that this therapist understands, respects, and says things that seem illuminating to you, the treatment is probably worth a try.

When considering therapy, most patients have a variety of questions about whether to seek long-term or short-term treatment, whether medication is called for or avoidable, what kinds of credentials the therapist should have, and how much the treatment is going to cost. If your therapist is to serve as your ancillary mind, she must be able to think with you, and accommodate your thinking, on these matters.

Research indicates fairly clearly that the specific kind of professional degree a therapist holds is not an important variable. Psychiatrists, psychologists, social workers, and trained lay therapists all get good results—and all these professions have their ineffective or unhelpful therapists. For many patients, relatively short-term work yields good results, but for some patients long-term work is highly beneficial.[123] Medication is probably essential for the treatment of schizophrenia and manic-depression, and a short course of medication (six months or so) is probably a good idea for debilitating depression that lasts more than a few weeks. Medication is probably a good idea if your therapy helps you achieve positive changes in how you live and think but does not relieve your emotional distress. Given these facts, it is not the best idea to see a practitioner who is inflexible or strongly biased

---

[123] Substantial transitions in one's life generally take a few years to accomplish, and they are made more difficult by previously unresolved conflicts or poorly handled development, as Daniel Levinson and his colleagues discovered in their ground-breaking work on the adult life cycle. (See *Seasons of a Man's Life* [1978].) If we think of the therapist as an ancillary mind, it would make sense that in many cases assistance is needed throughout a major transition. This is a different notion than the psychoanalytic insistence on unraveling infantile conflicts. The current emphasis on short-term work, and the disrepute into which psychoanalysis has put long-term work, militate against persons getting the help they need through a substantial transition.

on these issues. Working with someone who assumes that all good therapy is long-term, or that long-term treatment is generally uncalled for, is not wise. Nor is it optimal to see someone who wants to put all patients on medication or who believes medication is generally a bad idea.

A patient is also unwise to sign on for treatment that is more expensive than you can afford. It is probably irrational to see someone who is more expensive than you can afford simply because she is one sort of professional (psychiatrist, psychologist, etc.) rather than another. It is also irrational to sign on with someone who does not take your financial limitations seriously. Where there are significant financial constraints, a therapist should agree to work in a short-term format, if she cannot reduce her fee sufficiently to make a more open-ended format viable. A therapist who cannot do this is not a good choice for the financially limited. An ancillary mind that cannot think responsibly about your financial condition and act accordingly is a dangerous auxiliary in your effort to solve your problems.

Persons in therapy frequently have questions about the therapy they are getting; indeed, a person for whom such questions do not arise is probably not thinking. No therapist can be perfect for a patient all the time, and the thinking patient will therefore have points of disagreement to consider.

Perhaps the most acute problem in evaluating your discomfort in treatment is whether that discomfort reflects your problems rather than a problem with the treatment. A second problem is whether this discomfort reflects some difference between you and the therapist that can be worked through or worked around, or whether it is an issue over which you should leave treatment. Many patients never get to the second question; they get stuck on the first and assume that their discomfort reflects some neurotic problem.

While these questions have to be answered on a case-by-case basis, a patient can use much of what we have already said to think about them. If the difference is over some basic value or some long-standing commitment, you should be very cautious about concluding that the therapist is right. Sometimes she will be; we all have basic values and commitments that need revision. However, you should consider the moral, social, and personal reasons for continuing or changing your commitment, not just the allegedly psychological reasons. If a therapist cannot talk in these terms but insists on invoking "health" as the deciding issue, she is not talking in a self-aware, probative manner, for most recommendations of most therapists are as much moral and social as psychological. Similarly, if the therapist cannot consider the intellectual merits of a point of disagreement, but mainly tries to show why the points you are raising are distractions from (or resistance to) the treatment, she is failing to take seriously the optional nature of her views and the legitimacy of your thinking. If, for instance, you come across a book or article that seems to shed light on your problems, but your therapist cannot or will not discuss this with you as an intellectual issue—if she insists that your concerns only reflect your problems—then she is probably violating her role as *your* ancillary mind and revealing closed-mindedness. A therapist's inability to think in moral or social terms or to think beyond the confines of her culture may coincide with some real problem you have—your concerns may, in fact, reflect your problems. However, if these matters cannot be discussed in moral, social, and intellectual terms, there is no way to tell where the problem lies. It is irrational under such conditions to acquiesce in the view that your discomfort reflects your problem.

You should not undergo a treatment that does not make sense to you, nor should you suspend your considered opinion in deference to the alleged expertise of the therapist. You should not undergo a treatment that gives a secondary (or lower) place to the moral and social structure of your life. If a therapist cannot relate to you as an intelligent, socially involved person with values that deserve serious consideration, then he is the wrong therapist for you.

Perhaps more important, a therapist may be very honest, careful, thoughtful, and respectful of you, yet see the world in a way that is at odds with things that are important to you. One can be in therapy with a very good, admirable, honest person who is not the right therapist. Deciding whether to continue a treatment is not necessarily to evaluate the therapist's competence, ethics, or quality as a person. You may think very highly of your therapist and rightly so. That does not mean he is right for you. This cuts both ways. The therapist may recognize a difference in values, and he may believe it is wise to end the treatment because of this difference. Patients should not take such an occurrence as a "judgment," for therapists are not authorities. Therapists are persons who, like all persons, must work from their own perspectives. You should take such an occurrence as a reflection of the therapist's honest regard for your best interests and honest recognition of an obstacle to your working together. Ideally, when there is a genuine conflict of values or central beliefs, the patient and therapist should be able to discuss the matter with mutual regard and part ways amicably.

Finally, no one should hesitate to try more than one therapist or more than one type of therapy. There are more variables in the therapy process than anyone understands, and you may find success with another therapist or another form of therapy. To stay in a therapy that does not seem to be working well is irrational. To conclude from one unsatisfying experience that therapy is not worth trying is equally irrational. Nor should you refuse to give something that has not worked especially well in the past another try. What works or does not work for you at a particular time may have a very different outcome later.

Life is not easy, and getting whatever help with it that you can is often a good idea. If you are wise in choosing a therapist, and if you are wise in deciding when to disagree with your therapist, therapy can be of immense help with life's difficulties. You must, though, be thoughtful and responsible, and it is not wise simply to submit oneself to some form of treatment. Pretending that therapy cannot lead you down personally, morally, or socially destructive paths—not necessarily because of therapeutic incompetence but because of a mismatch between patient and therapist—makes no sense. A treatment at odds with what is most important to you, a treatment that is based on views that are too narrow, a treatment that undermines your own judgment and commitments—such a therapeutic encounter can be a debilitating mistake. This is not a reason to avoid seeking help, though, but a reason to be thoughtful. You can try therapy and discontinue any treatment that seems unwise. So long as you recognize that the therapist is an assistant in your own efforts, not an authority, and so long as you do not suspend your judgment or violate your values, therapy will in all probability augment your life.

REFERENCES

Abramson, Lyn K., Martin E. P. Seligman, and John D. Teasdale. "Learned Helplessness in Humans: Critique and Reformulation. *Journal of Abnormal Psychology* 87 (1978).

Adelson, Joseph. "The Social Sciences and the Humanities." In *Challenges to the Humanities*, edited by Chester E. Finn, Jr., Diane Ravitch, and P. Holley Roberts. New York: Holmes and Meier, 1985.

Alkon, Daniel. *Memory's Voice: Deciphering the Mind-Brain Code*. New York: Harper Collins Publishers, 1992.

Andreasen, Nancy C. *The Broken Brain: The Biological Revolution in Psychiatry*. New York: Harper & Row, 1984.

Aronson, Eliot. *The Social Animal*. 6th ed. New York: W. H. Freeman and Company, 1992.

Bandura, Albert. *Principles of Behavior Modification*. New York: Holt, Rinehart, & Winston, 1969.

Bandura, Albert. *Social Foundations of Thought and Action: A Social Cognitive Theory*. Englewood Cliffs, N.J.: Prentice-Hall, 1986.

Barondes, Samuel. *Molecules and Mental Illness*. New York: Scientific American Library, 1993.

Beck, Aaron T., and Gary Emery. *Anxiety Disorders and Phobias: A Cognitive Perspective*. New York: Basic Books, 1985.

Beck, Aaron T., and Marjorie Weishaar. "Cognitive Therapy." In *Comprehensive Handbook of Cognitive Therapy*, edited by Arthur Freeman, Karen M. Simon, Larry E. Beutler, and Hal Arkowitz. New York: Plenum Press, 1989.

Beck, Aaron T. *Cognitive Therapy and the Emotional Disorders*. New York: International Universities Press, 1976.

Beck, Aaron T., A. John Rush, Brian F. Shaw, and Gary Emery. *Cognitive Therapy of Depression*. New York: The Guilford Press, 1979.

Bellack, Alan S., Michel Hersen, and Alan E. Kazdin, eds. *International Handbook of Behavior Modification and Therapy*. 2d ed. New York: Plenum Press, 1990.

Bellack, Leopold. "Teaching Psychoanalysis as Science." In *Psychoanalysis at 100*, edited by Gerd Fenchel. Washington, D.C.: University Press of America, 1993.

Bergmann, Martin S., and Frank R. Hartman, eds. *The Evolution of Psychoanalytic Technique.* New York: Basic Books, 1976.

Beutler, Larry E., and Paul D. Guest, "The Role of Cognitive Change in Psychotherapy." In *Comprehensive Handbook of Cognitive Therapy,* edited by Arthur Freeman, Karen M. Simon, Larry E. Beutler, and Hal Arkowitz. New York: Plenum Press, 1989.

Bruner, Jerome S. *Acts of Meaning.* Cambridge, Mass.: Harvard University Press, 1990.

Bruner, Jerome S. *Beyond the Information Given.* New York: W. W. Norton, 1973.

Bruner, Jerome S. *In Search of Mind: Essays in Autobiography.* New York: Harper and Row, 1983.

Buss, David M. *The Evolution of Desire: Strategies of Human Mating.* New York: Basic Books, 1994.

Calvin, William H. *The Cerebral Symphony: Seashore Reflections on the Structure of Consciousness.* New York: Bantam Books, 1990.

Cooper, Jack R., Robert H. Bloom, and Floyd E. Roth. *The Biochemical Basis of Neuropharmacology.* 6th ed. New York: Oxford University Press, 1991.

Corsini, Raymond J., and Danny Wedding. *Current Psychotherapies.* 4th ed. Itasca, Ill.: F. E. Peacock, Publishers, 1989.

Coyne, James C. "Thinking Postcognitively about Depression." In *Comprehensive Handbook of Cognitive Therapy,* edited by Arthur Freeman, Karen M. Simon, Larry E. Beutler, and Hal Arkowitz. New York: Plenum, 1989.

Crits-Christoph, Paul, and Jacques P. Barber, ed. *Handbook of Short-Term Dynamic Psychotherapy.* New York: Basic Books, 1991.

Dain, Norman. *Concepts of Insanity in the United States, 1789–1865.* New Brunswick, N.J.: Rutgers University Press, 1964.

Dawes, Robyn M. *House of Cards: Psychology and Psychotherapy Built on Myth.* New York: Free Press, 1994.

Degler, Carl N. *In Search of Human Nature: The Decline and Rise of Darwinism in American Social Thought.* New York: Oxford University Press, 1991.

Dennett, Daniel C. *Consciousness Explained.* Boston: Little, Brown and Company, 1991.

Drinka, George. *The Birth of Neurosis: Myth, Malady, and the Victorians.* New York: Simon and Schuster, 1984.

Dupre, John, ed. *The Latest on the Best: Essays on Evolution and Optimality.* Cambridge, Mass.: MIT Press, 1987.

Eagle, Morris N. *Recent Developments in Psychoanalysis: A Critical Evaluation.* Cambridge, Mass.: Harvard University Press, 1984.

Ehrenwald, Jay, ed. *The History of Psychotherapy.* Northvale, N.J.: Jason Aronson, 1991.

Ellman, Steven J. *Freud's Technique Papers: a Contemporary Perspective.* Northvale, N.J.: Jason Aronson, 1991.

Eysenck, Hans. "A Critique of Contemporary Classification and Diagnosis." In *Contemporary Directions in Psychopathology: Toward the DSM-IV,* edited by Theodore Millon and Gerald Klerman. New York: Guilford Press, 1986.

Eysenck, Hans. *The Decline and Fall of the Freudian Empire.* New York: Viking, 1985.

Eysenck, Hans. *The Effects of Psychotherapy.* New York: International Science Press, 1966.

Eysenck, Hans, and Glenn D. Wilson. *The Experimental Study of Freudian Theories.* London: Methuen, 1973.

Fancher, Raymond E. *Psychoanalytic Psychology: The Development of Freud's Thought.* New York: W. W. Norton, 1973.

Fieve, Ronald R. *Moodswing.* Rev. and exp. ed. New York: Bantam Books, 1989.

Fisher, Helen E. *The Anatomy of Love: The Natural History of Monogamy, Adultery, and Divorce.* New York: W. W. Norton, 1992.

Fisher, Seymour, and Roger P. Greenberg. *The Scientific Credibility of Freud's Theories and Therapy.* New York: Basic Books, 1977.

Flanagan, Owen. *The Science of the Mind.* 2d ed. Cambridge, Mass.: MIT Press, 1991.

Frank, Jerome D. *Persuasion and Healing.* 2d ed. Baltimore: The Johns Hopkins University Press, 1973.

Frank, Jerome D. and Julia B. Frank. *Persuasion and Healing.* 3d ed. Baltimore: The Johns Hopkins University Press, 1991.

Freeman, Arthur, Karen M. Simon, Larry E. Beutler, and Hal Arkowitz. *Comprehensive Handbook of Cognitive Therapy.* New York: Plenum Press, 1989.

Friedman, Lawrence J. *Menninger The Family and the Clinic.* New York: Alfred A. Knopf, 1990.

Gardner, Howard. *The Mind's New Science: A History of the Cognitive Revolution.* New York: Basic Books, 1985.

Garfield, S. L. "Problems in Diagnostic Classification." In *Contemporary Directions in Psychopathology: Toward the DSM-IV,* edited by Theodore Millon and Gerald Klerman. New York: The Guilford Press, 1986.

Garfield, S. L., and A.E. Bergin. *Handbook of Psychotherapy and Behavior Change.* 3d ed. New York: John Wiley and Sons, 1986.

Gay, Peter. *Freud: A Life for Our Times.* New York: W. W. Norton, 1988.

Gazzaniga, Michael. *Mind Matters.* Boston: Houghton Mifflin, 1988.

Gazzaniga, Michael. *Nature's Mind.* New York: Basic Books, 1992.

Goldfried, Marvin R., ed. *Converging Themes in Psychotherapy: Trends in Psychodynamic, Humanistic, and Behavioral Practice.* New York: Springer Publishing, 1982.

Goldfried, Marvin R., and Wendy Padawer. "Current Status and Future Directions in Psychotherapy." In *Converging Themes in Psychotherapy,* edited by Marvin R. Goldfried. New York: Springer Publishing, 1982.

Gosling, F. G., *Before Freud: Neurasthenia and the American Medical Community, 1870–1910.* Urbana and Chicago: University of Illinois Press, 1987.

Grob, Gerald. *From Asylum to Community: Mental Health Policy in Modern America.* Princeton, N.J.: Princeton University Press, 1991.

Grob, Gerald. *The Mad Among Us: A History of the Care of America's Mentally Ill.* New York: Free Press, 1994.

Grob, Gerald. *Mental Illness and American Society, 1875–1940.* Princeton, N.J.: Princeton University Press, 1983.

Grosskurth, Phyllis. *The Secret Ring: Freud's Inner Circle and the Politics of Psychoanalysis.* Reading, Mass.: Addison-Wesley, 1991.

Hale, Nathan, Jr. *Freud and the Americans: The Beginnings of Psychoanalysis in the United States, 1876–1917.* New York: Oxford University Press, 1971.

Hersen, Michel, and Cynthia G. Last. *Behavior Therapy Casebook.* New York: Springer Publishing, 1985.

Hobson, J. Allan. *The Dreaming Brain.* New York: Basic Books, 1988.

Hunt, Morton. *The Story of Psychology.* New York: Doubleday, 1993.

Izard, Carroll E., Jerome Kagan, and Robert B. Zajonc. *Emotions, Cognition, and Behavior.* Cambridge, England, and New York: Cambridge University Press, 1984.

Jacobson, Neil S. "Cognitive and Behavioral Therapists in Clinical Practice: An Introduction." In *Psychotherapists in Clinical Practice: Cognitive and Behavioral Perspectives,* edited by Neil S. Jacobson. New York: The Guilford Press, 1987.

Jacobson, Neil S., ed. *Psychotherapists in Clinical Practice: Cognitive and Behavioral Perspectives.* New York: The Guilford Press, 1987.

Johnson-Laird, Philip N. *Mental Models.* Cambridge, Mass.: Harvard University Press, 1983.

Kalish, Harry I. *From Behavior Science to Behavior Modification.* New York: McGraw-Hill, 1981.

Kazdin, Alan E. *Behavior Modification in Applied Settings.* 4th ed. Pacific Grove, Calif.: Brooks/Cole Publishing, 1989.

Kazdin, Alan E. *History of Behavior Modification.* Baltimore: University Park Press, 1978.

Klerman, Gerald. "Classification and DSM-III-R." In *The New Harvard Guide to Psychiatry,* edited by Armand Nicholi, Jr. Cambridge, Mass.: The Belknap Press of Harvard University Press, 1988.

Klerman, Gerald. "Historical Perspectives on Contemporary Schools of Psychopathology." In *Contemporary Directions in Psychopathology: Toward the DSM-IV,* edited by Theodore Millon and Gerald Klerman. New York: The Guilford Press, 1986.

Kline, Paul. *Fact and Fantasy in Freudian Theory.* London: Methuen, 1972.

Kline, Paul. *Psychology and Freudian Theory: An Introduction.* London: Methuen, 1984.

Kosslyn, Stephen E., and Oliver Koenig. *Wet Mind: The New Cognitive Science.* New York: The Free Press, 1992.

Kramer, Peter D. *Listening to Prozac.* New York: Viking, 1993.

Kuhn, D., J. Langer, L. Kohlberg, and N.S. Haan. "The Development of Formal Operations in Logical and Moral Judgment." *Genetic Psychology Monographs* 95 (1977).

Levinson, Daniel J., with Charlotte N. Darrow, Edward B. Klein, Maria H. Levinson, and Braxton McKee. *The Seasons of a Man's Life.* New York: Knopf, 1978.

Lickey, Marvin E., and Barbara Gordon. *Medicine and Mental Illness: The Use of Drugs in Psychiatry.* New York: W. H. Freeman and Company, 1991.

Luborsky, Lester, and Thomas McClellan, et al. "Therapist Success and Its Determinants." *Archives of General Psychiatry,* 1985.

Malcolm, Janet. *Psychoanalysis.* New York: Knopf, 1981.

McGovern, Constance M. *Masters of Madness: The Social Origins of the American Psychiatric Profession.* Hanover, N.H.: University Press of New Hampshire, for the University of Vermont, 1985.

Millon, Theodore. "On the Past and Future of DSM-III: Personal Recollections." In *Contemporary Directions in Psychopathology,* edited by Theodore Millon and Gerald Clerman. New York: The Guilford Press, 1986.

Millon, Theodore, and Gerald Klerman, eds. *Contemporary Directions in Psychopathology: Toward the DSM-IV.* New York: The Guilford Press, 1986.

Moore, Thomas. *Care of the Soul.* New York: Harper Collins Publishers, 1993.

Moore, Thomas. *Soul Mates.* New York: Harper Collins Publishers, 1994.

Neisser, Ulric. *Cognition and Reality: Principles and Implications of Cognitive Psychology.* New York: W. H. Freeman and Company, 1975.

Neisser, Ulric. *Memory Observed: Remembering in Natural Contexts.* New York: W. H. Freeman and Company, 1982.

Nicholi, Armand M., Jr., ed. *The New Harvard Guide to Psychiatry.* Cambridge, Mass.: The Belknap Press of the Harvard University Press, 1988.

Nisbett, R. E., and L. Ross. *Human Inference: Strategies and Shortcomings of Social Judgment.* Englewood Cliffs, N.J.: Prentice Hall, 1980.

Nozick, Robert. *The Nature of Rationality.* Princeton, N.J.: Princeton University Press, 1993.

O'Leary, K. Daniel, and G. Terence Wilson. *Behavior Therapy: Application and Outcome.* 2d ed. Englewood Cliffs, N.J.: Prentice Hall, 1975.

Peirce, C. S. "The Fixation of Belief." In *The Philosophical Writings of Peirce,* edited by Justus Buchler. New York: Dover, 1955.

Perry, Helen Swick. *Psychiatrist of America: The Life of Harry Stack Sullivan.* Cambridge, Mass.: The Belknap Press of Harvard University Press, 1982.

Peterson, Christopher, Steven F. Maier, and Martin E. P. Seligman. *Learned Helplessness.* New York: Oxford University Press, 1993.

Plomin, Robert, J. C. DeFries, and G. E. McClellan. *Behavioral Genetics: A Primer.* 2d ed. New York: W. H. Freeman and Company, 1990.

Posner, Michael I., ed. *Foundations of Cognitive Science.* Cambridge, Mass.: The MIT Press, 1989.

Quinn, Susan. *A Mind of Her Own: The Life of Karen Horney.* Reading, Mass.: Addison-Wesley. 1988.

Rachman, S. J. *Fear and Courage.* 2d ed. New York: W. H. Freeman and Company, 1990.

Reisman, John M. *A History of Clinical Psychology.* 2d ed. New York: Hemisphere Publishing, 1991.

Restak, Richard. *Receptors.* New York: Bantam Books, 1994.

Rogow, Arnold A. *The Psychiatrists.* New York: G. P. Putnam's Sons, 1970.

Rose, Steven. *The Making of Memory: From Molecules to Mind.* New York: Doubleday, 1992.

Sapolsky, Robert M. *Why Zebras Don't Get Ulcers.* New York: W. H. Freeman and Company, 1994.

Schafer, Roy. *The Analytic Attitude.* New York: Basic Books, 1983.

Schafer, Roy. *Retelling a Life.* New York: Basic Books, 1991.

Schweder, Richard. *Thinking through Cultures.* Cambridge, Mass.: Harvard University Press, 1991.

Scott, Charles. *Boundaries in Mind: A Study of Immediate Awareness Based on Psychotherapy.* American Academy of Religion Studies in Religion, no. 27. New York: The Crossroads Publishing Company and The Scholar's Press, 1982.

Seligman, Martin E. P. *Helplessness: On Development, Depression and Death.* New York: W. H. Freeman and Company, 1992.

Seligman, Martin E. P. *Learned Optimism.* New York: Alfred A. Knopf, 1991.

Shepherd, Gordon M. *Neurobiology.* 2d ed. Oxford: Oxford University Press, 1988.

Skinner, B. F. *Beyond Freedom and Dignity.* New York: Alfred A. Knopf, 1971.

Skinner, B. F. *About Behaviorism.* New York: Random House, 1974.

Smith, M. L., G. V. Glass, and T. I. Miller. *The Benefits of Psychotherapy.* Baltimore: The Johns Hopkins University Press, 1980.

Snyder, Solomon H. *Drugs and the Brain.* New York: Scientific American Library, 1986.

Spence, Donald P. *The Freudian Metaphor: Toward Paradigm Change in Psychoanalysis.* New York: W. W. Norton, 1987.

Spence, Donald P. *Narrative Truth and Historical Truth: Meaning and Interpretation in Psychoanalysis.* New York: W. W. Norton, 1982.

Starr, Paul. *The Social Transformation of American Medicine.* New York: Basic Books, 1982.

Stern, Daniel. *The Interpersonal World of the Infant.* New York: Basic Books, 1985.

Strupp, Hans, and Grady I. Blackwood, Jr. "Recent Methods of Psychotherapy." In *Comprehensive Textbook of Psychiatry*, 4th ed., edited by Harold I. Kaplan and Benjamin J. Sadock. Baltimore: Williams & Wilkins, 1985.

Tavris, Carol. *The Mismeasure of Woman*. New York: Simon and Schuster, 1992.

Taylor, S. E. *Positive Illusions: Creative Self-Deception and the Healthy Mind*. New York: Basic Books, 1989.

Unger, Roberto Mangabeira. *Passion: An Essay on Personality*. New York: The Free Press, 1984.

Valenstein, Elliot S. *Great and Desperate Cures: The Rise and Decline of Psychosurgery and Other Radical Cures for Mental Illness*. New York: Basic Books, 1986.

Wender, Paul H., and Donald F. Klein. *Mind, Mood, and Medicine: A Guide to the New Biopsychiatry*. New York: Farrar, Strauss, and Giroux, 1981.

Wender, Paul H., and Donald F. Klein. *Understanding Depression*. New York: Oxford University Press, 1993.

Wertsch, James V. *Voices in the Mind: A Sociocultural Approach to Mediated Action*. Cambridge, Mass.: Harvard University Press, 1991.

Wills, Christopher. *The Runaway Brain: The Evolution of Human Uniqueness*. New York: Basic Books, 1993.

Wilson, G. Terence. "Behavior Therapy." In *Current Psychotherapies*, edited by Raymond J. Corsini and Danny Wedding. Itasca, Ill.: F. E. Peacock, Publishers, 1989.

Wolpe, J. *The Practice of Behavior Therapy*. New York: Pergamon Press, 1969.

Wolpe, J. *Psychotherapy by Reciprocal Inhibition*. Stanford, Calif.: Stanford University Press, 1958.

Wolpert, Lewis. *The Unnatural Nature of Science: Why Science Does Not Make (Common) Sense*. Cambridge, Mass.: Harvard University Press, 1993.

INDEX

�֍

Printed in the United States
by Baker & Taylor Publisher Services